Teaching Ideas
and
Classroom Activities
for Health Care

Teaching Ideas
and
Classroom Activities
for Health Care

Lee Haroun, Ed.D

Susan Royce, MS (Education)

THOMSON

DELMAR LEARNING

Australia   Canada   Mexico   Singapore   Spain   United Kingdom   United States

THOMSON

DELMAR LEARNING

Teaching Ideas and Classroom Activities for Health Care

by Lee Haroun and Susan Royce

Vice President of Health Care:
William Brottmiller

Editorial Director:
Cathy L. Esperti

Acquisitions Editor:
Marah Bellegarde

Developmental Editor:
Jennifer Conklin

Marketing Director:
Jennifer McAvey

Channel Manager:
Lisa Osgood

Marketing Coordinator:
Kip Summerlin

Production Manager:
Barb Bullock

Production Coordinator:
Catherine Ciardullo

Art/Design Coordinator:
Jay Purcell

Project Editor:
Bryan Viggiani

COPYRIGHT © 2004 by Delmar Learning, a division of Thomson Learning, Inc. Thomson Learning™ is a trademark used herein under license.

Printed in the United States of America
1 2 3 4 5 XXX 07 06 05 04 03

For more information, contact Delmar Learning, 5 Maxwell Drive, Clifton Park, NY 12065
Or find us on the World Wide Web at http://www.delmarlearning.com

ALL RIGHTS RESERVED. No part of this work covered by the copyright hereon may be reproduced or used in any form or by any means—graphic, electronic, or mechanical, including photocopying, recording, taping, Web distribution or information storage and retrieval systems—without the written permission of the publisher.

For permission to use material from this text or product, contact us by
Tel (800) 730-2214
Fax (800) 730-2215
www.thomsonrights.com

Library of Congress Cataloging-in-Publication Data

Haroun, Lee.
  Teaching ideas and classroom activities for health care / Lee Haroun, Susan K. Royce.
    p.   cm.
  Includes index.
  ISBN 0-7668-4490-0
  1. Medicine—Study and teaching—Activity programs.   2. Medical care,—Study and teaching—Activity programs.
I. Royce, Susan K. II. Title.
R834.H336 2004
610'.71'1—dc21

                        2003047386

International Divisions List

Asia (Including India):
Thomson Learning
60 Albert Street, #15-01
Albert Complex
Singapore 189969
Tel 65 336-6411
Fax 65 336-7411

Australia/New Zealand:
Nelson
102 Dodds Street
South Melbourne
Victoria 3205
Australia
Tel 61 (0)3 9685-4111
Fax 61 (0)3 9685-4199

Latin America:
Thomson Learning
Seneca 53
Colonia Polanco
11560 Mexico, D.F. Mexico
Tel (525) 281-2906
Fax (525) 281-2656

Canada:
Nelson
1120 Birchmount Road
Toronto, Ontario
Canada M1K 5G4
Tel (416) 752-9100
Fax (416) 752-8102

UK/Europe/Middle East/Africa:
Thomson Learning
Berkshire House
1680-173 High Holborn
London WC1V 7AA
United Kingdom
Tel 44 (0)20 497-1422
Fax 44 (0)20 497-1426

Spain (includes Portugal):
Paraninfo
Calle Magallanes 25
28015 Madrid
España
Tel 34 (0)91 446-3350
Fax 34 (0)91 445-6218

Notice to the Reader

Publisher does not warrant or guarantee any of the products described herein or perform any independent analysis in connection with any of the product information contained herein. Publisher does not assume, and expressly disclaims, any obligation to obtain and include information other than that provided to it by the manufacturer.

The reader is expressly warned to consider and adopt all safety precautions that might be indicated by the activities described herein and to avoid all potential hazards. By following the instructions contained herein, the reader willingly assumes all risks in connection with such instructions.

The publisher makes no representations or warranties of any kind, including but not limited to, the warranties of fitness for particular purpose or merchantability, nor are any such representations implied with respect to the material set forth herein, and the publisher takes no responsibility with respect to such material. The publisher shall not be liable for any special, consequential, or exemplary damages resulting, in whole or part, from the reader's use of, or reliance upon, this material.

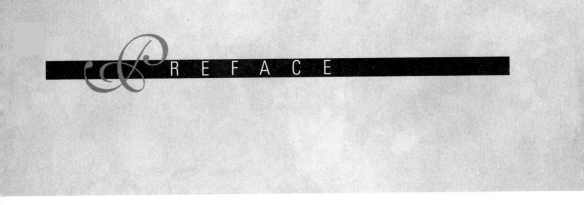

WHO IS THIS BOOK FOR?

Teaching Ideas and Classroom Activities for Health Care is intended for busy instructors who are looking for innovative classroom activities to help them teach and reinforce the basic concepts needed by students in nursing and allied health care occupations. This book is designed to support and enhance the material presented in textbooks. The activities were developed to serve a number of educational purposes:

- Respond to the trend in education for increased hands-on learning.
- Help future health care workers think and apply what they learn in the classroom.
- Engage students in using a variety of learning styles.
- Make learning more enjoyable.
- Provide materials for teaching topics not always addressed in subject-matter textbooks.

Most of the activities herein address the general skills needed in a variety of health care occupations.

WHAT DOES THIS BOOK CONTAIN?

Teaching Ideas and Classroom Activities for Health Care contains more than 200 activities presented in a wide variety of forms:

Case studies	Role-play scenarios
Games	Small group discussions
Hands-on projects	Team contests
Individual assignments	Worksheets
Internet activities	Whole class projects
Puzzles	

Most activities stand on their own. No unit or chapter depends on the completion of any other. Instructors may pick and choose activities in almost any order to support the subjects they are teaching.

The activities range from the lighthearted (Activity 1-6, Body-Part Hokey Pokey) to the serious (Activity 18-8, What Do You Think?, which is a discussion of legal and ethical issues). Not all activities will be suitable for all groups. Instructors should consider both individual student preferences and class dynamics when selecting activities their students will enjoy and that will help them learn.

Some activities can be used to introduce new topics (Activity 11-8, Brainstorming), while others are summary in nature and best used to review material the students have already studied (Activity 3-2, Vital Facts).

A minimum of the instructor's time is required to select, prepare for, and conduct activities to increase students' knowledge and skill level. Support materials are listed for every activity. For example, games include the questions; group discussions include the case studies, class presentations include the transparency masters, and many activities include instructor sheets with answer keys and other helpful information.

HOW IS THIS BOOK ORGANIZED?

The activities are organized into chapters by topics that represent the knowledge areas and skills needed by health care students. Each activity is presented in a complete, instructor-friendly format that includes:

- Student learning objectives
- List of materials needed
- Step-by-step instructions on how to prepare for and conduct the activity
- Suggested answers to all questions used in games, quizzes, and worksheets
- Instructor sheets
- Student handouts
- Transparency masters
- Discussion questions

Note: The authors did not include the time needed for each activity because factors such as the size of the class, ages of the students, instructor's purpose for using the activity, and time available will dictate the actual time needed to complete an activity. In some cases, students can begin work on a project in class and then complete it at home. In others, you may ask students to prepare in advance before the activity is conducted in the classroom.

HOW CAN YOU BEST USE THIS BOOK?

- Do your best to match the activities to the personality of the class. Not all students will respond to all types of activities. For example, many students of all ages have great fun playing games like Body-Part Hokey Pokey. Others find them inappropriate.
- Be sure students understand the purpose of the activity and what they are supposed to be learning.
- Conduct follow-up discussions. These are often the most important part of the activity because they give students opportunities to draw conclusions and make the connection between the content of the activity and its application to their future occupation.

This book can serve as a collection of recipes to be followed or as a stimulus for your own ideas. We hope you enjoy using it and welcome your comments, suggestions, and ideas for additional activities.

Lee Haroun has a master of arts degree in education from Portland State University (Oregon), a master of business administration degree from National University in San Diego, and a doctoral degree in education from the University of San Diego. The focus of her dissertation was to study the needs of new postsecondary health care instructors as they transition from the field to the classroom.

Lee has more than 30 of years experience in teaching and educational administration. She has developed health care curriculum for a variety of postsecondary programs, including occupational therapy assistant, health administration, insurance coder, and patient care technician. She has a special interest in working with students to help them reach their maximum potential in school, career, and life. She is the author of *Career Development for Health Professionals* (W. B. Saunders Company); co-author of *Introduction to Health Care* with Joyce Mitchell (Delmar Learning); and co-author of *Occupational Therapy Fieldwork Survival Guide: Strategies for Success* with Bonnie Napier-Tibere (F. A. Davis Company).

Susan R. Royce has a bachelor's degree in psychology from the University of California at San Diego and a master of science degree in education from National University. Her master's thesis explored the role of service dogs in the emotional and social development of children in the classroom.

Susan has more than 16 years of experience in health care, including education, management, and curriculum writing and consultation. She has worked in ophthalmology and orthopedics as an office manager and front and back office assistant. With her health care background, Susan has consulted throughout the United States on the topics of insurance reimbursement and compliance for ophthalmologists.

Susan has taught and written curriculum for courses in medical terminology, anatomy, medical reception, medical billing, medical insurance billing, accounting, management, computer applications, career readiness, and English. As an administrator, Susan served as a program director and was responsible for five allied health programs with more than 700 students (including 350 medical assistant students). She held the position of director of education for a college with more than 1,000 students, most of whom were enrolled in health care programs. Susan currently works as the director of education for a postsecondary school that teaches allied health and computer networking programs.

Dedication

To David, whose unfaltering optimism in the face of all odds has taught me that anything is possible.

—Lee Haroun

To my husband, Steve, and daughter, Laura, for all the support they continue to give me no matter how much I take on to do. And to all those wonderful educators who helped me by sharing ideas, especially Suzette, Sandra, and Lisa.

—Susan Royce

ACKNOWLEDGMENTS

The authors wish to acknowledge the help and support of Jennifer Conklin and Sherry Gomoll at Delmar Learning. A special thank you to all the reviewers who offered many wonderful suggestions:

Larry Hudson, Ph.D.
Associate Professor
University of Central Florida
Orlando, Florida

Detna K. Kacher
Health Occupations Instructor
Friendswood High School
Friendswood, Texas

Rita Michelson, R.N.
Instructor
Aaron Manor
Chester, Connecticut

Peggy Ulrich, R.N.
Medical Academy Instructor
Titusville High School
Titusville, Florida

CONTENTS

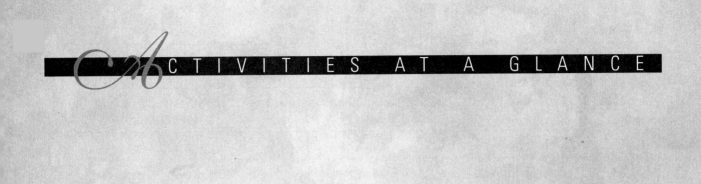

Chapter 1   Medical Terminology

Activity	Title	Topic	Type
1-1	We Know More Than We Think	Recognizing already-known medical terms	Whole class or groups, (create words) (written & discussion)
1-2	What's on TV	Medical terms	Individual, observation (TV program)
1-3	Create New Words	Working with word elements to make new terms	Groups, oral (create words)
1-4	It's a Matter of Combining	Word elements	Groups, written (create medical terms)
1-5	Body-Part Simon Says	Medical terms	Whole class, physical (game)
1-6	Body-Part Hokey Pokey	Medical terms	Whole class, physical (dance)
1-7	Word Flash!	Terms or word elements	Whole class, oral (flash cards)
1-8	Picture This!	Terms or word elements	Groups, written (drawings)
1-9	Haven't I Seen You Somewhere?	Medical terms	Groups, research (create word lists)
1-10	Catch That Word	Terms or word elements	Whole class, physical (game)
1-11	Word (Un)Scramble	Word elements	Whole class, physical (flash cards)
1-12	That's My Word!	Terms or word elements	Pairs, physical (flash cards)

Chapter 2   Anatomy and Physiology

Activity	Title	Topic	Type
2-1	How Bionic Can We Become?	Transplant/replacement organs	Individual, research (report or project)

Activity	Title	Topic	Type
2-2	Where Are Our Taste Buds?	Taste (tongue)	Groups, hands-on (experiment)
2-3	Smell and Taste	Smell and taste	Whole class, hands-on (experiment)
2-4	Endocrine System Skits	Endocrine system	Groups, physical (skit)
2-5	Using a Pinhole	Vision	Groups, hands-on (experiment)
2-6	The Eye: Testing for the Blind Spot	Eye	Individual, hands-on (experiment)
2-7	Blood Circulation	Cardiovascular system	Groups, hands-on (art project)
2-8	Mini-Dissection	Major organs	Groups, hands-on (experiment)
2-9	What Am I?	Anatomy	Whole class, physical (game)
2-10	What Am I? 10 Questions Version	Anatomy	Whole class, oral (game)
2-11	Human Body Scavenger Hunt	Anatomy	Pairs, written (worksheet)
2-12	That's Amazing!	Anatomy and physiology	Whole class, oral (game)
2-13	Body Pathways	Anatomy and physiology	Whole class, physical (game)
2-14	Name That Disease	Physiology	Whole class, oral (contest)
2-15	Anatomy Bingo	Anatomy	Whole class, oral (game)
2-16	Anatomy Challenge	Anatomy	Whole class, oral (game)

Chapter 3   Vital Signs, Wellness, and Prevention

Activity	Title	Topic	Type of Activity
3-1	Monitoring Vital Signs	How physical activity affects vital signs	Pairs, hands-on (experiment)
3-2	Vital Facts	Vital signs as indicators of health status	Whole class, oral (contest)
3-3	Wellness Crossword Puzzle	Wellness vocabulary	Individual, small group, or whole class, written (puzzle)
3-4	Wellness Word Search	Wellness vocabulary	Individual, small group, or whole class, written (puzzle)

Activity	Title	Topic	Type
3-5	Wellness Posters	Lifestyle habits that promote wellness	Groups, research & hands-on (art project)
3-6	Wellness Projects	Lifestyle habits that promote wellness	Individual, research & hands-on (projects)
3-7	Personal Wellness Plan	Developing lifestyle habits that promote wellness	Individual, written (worksheet)
3-8	How Healthy Are My Eating Habits?	Good nutrition, eating habits	Individual, written (worksheet)
3-9	Healthy Bites	Good nutrition, healthy snacks	Individual & whole class, hands-on (eating)
3-10	The Benefits of Exercise	Physical exercise	Groups, oral & written (create lists)
3-11	The Effects of Exercise	Physical exercise	Groups, physical (experiment)
3-12	Relax!	Muscle relaxation exercise	Whole class, physical (experiment)
3-13	Meditation	Health benefits of meditation	Whole class, physical (experiment)
3-14	Race for Prevention	Strategies for prevention of disease	Whole class, physical (contest)

Chapter 4   Standard Precautions and Emergency Procedures

Activity	Title	Topic	Type of Activity
4-1	Crossword Puzzle	Standard precautions and emergency vocabulary	Individual, group, or whole class, written (puzzle)
4-2	Break That Chain!	Chain of infection and prevention of spread of infection	Individual, written (worksheet)
4-3	Collect Those Cards!	Transmission and control of infection	Groups, physical (game)
4-4	Safety Fashion Show	Personal protective equipment	Groups, physical (presentation)
4-5	Rationale, Please	Rationale for specific emergency and first aid procedures	Whole class, oral (contest)
4-6	Emergency Match	Appropriate first aid procedures for specific conditions	Whole class, physical & oral (presentation)
4-7	Building a First Aid Kit	Items needed in a basic first aid kit	Whole class & individual, hands-on (project)

Activity	Title	Topic	Type
4-8	How Well Do I Follow Directions?	Following written instructions	Individual, listening (worksheet)
4-9	Following Verbal Directions	Listening and following directions	Individual, listening & written (drawing)

Chapter 5   Math Review

Activity	Title	Topic	Type
5-1	Sharing Fears	Math fears	Groups, oral (discussion)
5-2	Fear Not!	Math fears	Whole class, physical (contest)
5-3	Overcoming Math Anxiety	How to overcome math anxiety	Groups, oral (discussion)
5-4	When Will I Use Math?	Using basic math skills	Whole class, oral (discussion)
5-5	Forming Fractions	Understanding fractions	Individual, hands-on (problem solving)
5-6	Playing with Factions	How fractions relate to a whole	Individual, hands-on (problem solving)
5-7	Comparing Fractions	Fraction equivalencies	Individual, hands-on (problem solving)
5-8	Multiplication Models for Fractions	Multiplication of fractions	Individual, hands-on (problem solving)
5-9	Acting It Out—Dividing Fractions	Division of fractions	Groups, physical (presentation)
5-10	Visualizing Decimals	Decimal place values	Individual, written (problem-solving)
5-11	What a Difference a Decimal Point Makes!	Decimal point placement	Groups, hands-on (project)
5-12	Ordering Decimals	Decimal numerical values	Groups, physical (presentation)
5-13	Decimal Number Line	Decimal numerical values	Whole class, physical (presentation)
5-14	Percentage Grids	Relationship between percentages, decimals, and fractions	Individuals & pairs, written (project)
5-15	Learning the Metric System	Comparing metric and English systems	Groups, whole class, hands-on (experiment & discussion)
5-16	Conversion Sayings	Comparing metric and English systems	Individual, whole class, written (worksheet & discussion)

Activity	Title	Topic	Type
5-17	Fun with Numbers	Number patterns and characteristics	Individual, whole class, written (worksheet & discussion)
5-18	Math Baseball	Problem solving	Whole class, physical (contest)

Chapter 6   Diversity

Activity	Title	Topic	Type of Activity
6-1	How Do I See the World?	Recognizing and understanding different viewpoints	Individuals, written (worksheets)
6-2	What Is Special about My Culture?	Cultural differences	Whole class, oral (discussion)
6-3	Cultural Values	Values of various cultures	Whole class, oral (discussion)
6-4	Reflections	Physical appearance is only part of who we are	Groups, oral (discussion)
6-5	Who Am I?	Preconceptions based on physical appearance	Individuals, written & oral (experiment)
6-6	Who Is This Person?	Preconceptions based on physical appearance	Whole class, oral (experiment)
6-7	Stereotypes	Common stereotypes	Individuals, written (worksheet)
6-8	What Do We Have in Common?	Commonalities among individuals	Pairs, oral (interviews)
6-9	This Is Me	Exploring one's background	Individuals, hands-on (art project)
6-10	Peer Coaching	Helping others	Groups, oral (teaching & learning)
6-11	Who Are the People Around Me?	Exploring diversity	Individuals, hands-on (experiment)
6-12	Animal Farm	Respecting differences	Individuals, physical & oral (discussion)
6-13	Celebrating Culture	Practices of various ethnic groups	Whole class, hands-on (projects)
6-14	Door Decorating	Practices of various ethnic groups	Whole class, hands-on (projects)
6-15	Let's Eat!	Potluck meal	Whole class, hands-on (eating)

xviii ● ACTIVITIES AT A GLANCE

Chapter 7 Empathy

Activity	Title	Topic	Type of Activity
7-1	Understanding Physical Limitations	Relating to the experiences of patients	Whole class, hands-on (experiments)
7-2	Understanding the Experience of Illness	Relating to the experiences of patients	Individual, research & written (experiential)
7-3	Be Me	Understanding the needs of patients	Groups, oral (discussion of scenarios)
7-4	What Would It Be Like?	Understanding the experience of living with health problems	Groups, oral (discussion of scenarios)
7-5	Walk a Mile in My Shoes	Understanding the experience of receiving a negative health report	Whole class, listening (experiential)
7-6	Empathy Role Play	Empathetic responses	Groups, oral (role-play)
7-7	Verbal Barriers to Empathy	Inappropriate verbal responses	Groups, oral (role-play)
7-8	My Empathy Score	Exploring personal level of empathy	Individual, written (questionnaire)
7-9	How Does It Feel?	Understanding the experience of being excluded	Groups, oral (experiment)
7-10	We All Share Similar Feelings	Ridicule and its effects	Whole class, oral (discussion)
7-11	What Are the Rules?	Social and group rules and customs	Whole class, oral (experiential)
7-12	Active Listening Practice I	Listening comprehension (aural)	Individual, listening & written (worksheet)
7-13	Active Listening Practice II	Listening comprehension (verbal)	Pairs, listening & oral (experiential)

Chapter 8 Working as a Team Member

Activity	Title	Topic	Type
8-1	Strengths Target	Discovering individual strengths	Individual & group, written & oral (experiential)
8-2	What Are My Strengths?	Discovering individual strengths	Groups, written (experiential)
8-3	Blind Walk	Trusting others as part of a team	Pairs, physical (experiment)
8-4	Blindfold Tag	Trusting others as part of a team	Pairs, physical (experiment)

Activity	Title	Topic	Type
8-5	Wheelchair Race	Trusting others as part of a team	Groups, physical (experiment)
8-6	Balloon Game	Working toward a common goal	Groups, physical (cooperative effort)
8-7	Making the Job Easier	Teamwork makes jobs easier	Groups, physical (cooperative effort)
8-8	Braiding	Importance of leadership; teamwork gets the job done	Groups, physical (cooperative effort)
8-9	Values for Successful Teams	Team consensus	Groups, oral & written (discussion)
8-10	Getting Consensus	Team consensus	Groups, oral & written (create list)
8-11	Consequences	Importance of keeping commitments	Groups, oral (discussion)
8-12	Teamwork in Today's Health Care Workplace	Importance of teamwork in health care delivery	Groups, oral (discussion)
8-13	Drawing on One Another	Advantages of teamwork	Individuals, pairs, & groups, written (experiment)
8-14	Together It Works: Group Teaching Project	Working toward a common goal	Groups, written (project)

Chapter 9   Dealing with Conflict

Activity	Title	Topic	Type of Activity
9-1	What Color Is Conflict?	Personal feelings about conflict	Individuals or groups, oral (discussion)
9-2	I Represent Conflict	Personal reactions to conflict	Whole class, physical (experiment)
9-3	Putting Up a Fight	Personal values	Whole class, oral (discussion)
9-4	Concentrate on the Positive	Positive feedback	Pairs, oral (sharing)
9-5	Constructive Conflict	How conflict can be constructive in the workplace	Groups, oral (generate ideas)
9-6	Conflict Posters	Constructive conflict	Groups, hands-on (art project)
9-7	I-Messages	Communicating feelings without blaming	Pairs, oral (role-play)
9-8	Try to See It My Way	Considering the viewpoints of others	Pairs, oral (role-play)
9-9	Conflict Role-Play	Using communication skills	Small-groups, oral (skits)

Chapter 10   Critical Thinking

Activity	Title	Topic	Type
10-1	It's an Illusion!	How perceptions influence what we see	Whole class, observation (experiment)
10-2	Interactive Stroop Effect Experiment—or—You Often Get What You Expect!	Experience influences what we see	Whole class, observation (experiment)
10-3	Describe an Object I	We view the world in a general way	Individual, drawing (experiment)
10-4	Describe an Object II	We each see things based on our own perceptions	Individual, drawing (experiment)
10-5	What Happened Here?	Perceptions affect beliefs	Individuals, observation (experiment)
10-6	Thinking Outside the Box	Assumptions limit what we see	Individual, observation (puzzles)
10-7	Whose Shoes?	Stereotypes can lead to incorrect conclusions	Groups, oral (experiment)
10-8	The Power of Stereotypes	Stereotypes influence our perceptions	Whole class, oral (discussion)
10-9	Things Aren't Always As They Seem	Assumptions can lead to unfair or incorrect conclusions	Groups, oral (discussion of scenarios)
10-10	Facts versus Opinions	Recognize the difference between facts and opinions	Whole class, oral (discussion of statements)
10-11	It's Logical!	Using logic to determine if a statement is true, false, or indeterminable	Whole class, oral (discussion of conclusions)
10-12	What's Wrong with This Logic?	Recognizing statements with false premises	Whole class, oral (discussion of statements)
10-13	There's Always More Than One Side	Controversial issues have more than one side	Whole class, oral (debate)
10-14	What's the Problem?	Many things motivate our behaviors	Whole class, oral (discussion of scenarios)

Chapter 11   Problem Solving and Decision Making

Activity	Title	Topic	Type of Activity
11-1	Hitting the Jackpot	Making group decisions	Groups, oral (decision making)
11-2	Creative Collaboration	Working as a group to apply creativity to a project	Group, hands-on (project)

Activity	Title	Topic	Type
11-3	Thinking outside the Box	Solving problems using creativity	Individuals, hands-on (puzzles)
11-4	More Fun with Toothpicks	Developing problem-solving strategies and predicting consequences	Pairs, hands-on (game)
11-5	Line Them Up	Nonverbal communication in group problem-solving tasks	Whole class, physical (problem solving)
11-6	How Tall Are You?	Verbal communication in group problem-solving tasks	Whole class, physical (problem solving)
11-7	What Kind of Problem Solver Are You?	Personal problem-solving styles	Individual, written (self-assessment)
11-8	Brainstorming	Using brainstorming for problem-solving tasks	Groups, oral (brainstorming)
11-9	What's the Problem?	Identification and clarification of problems	Individual & whole class, written & oral (worksheet & discussion)
11-10	The Five-Step Problem-Solving Process	Using the five-step process for problem solving	Whole class, oral (problem solving)
11-11	I've Got a Problem!	Using the five-step problem-solving process	Groups, oral (problem solving)
11-12	Decisions, Decisions!	Using a decision matrix	Whole class & individual, written (decision making)

Chapter 12   Communication with Patients, Co-workers, and Supervisors

Activity	Title	Topic	Type of Activity
12-1	Nonverbal Signals	Common nonverbal gestures	Whole class, physical (contest)
12-2	What Is It?	Nonverbal communication	Whole class, physical (determining meaning)
12-3	Silence!	Nonverbal communication in a group	Groups, hands-on (project)
12-4	Reading Body Language	Messages communicated by body language	Groups, physical (determining meaning)
12-5	Clothing Clues	Messages sent by clothing and appearance	Individuals, physical (presentation)
12-6	Listening Between the Lines	Listening and applying reasoning and logic	Individuals, listening & written (worksheet)
12-7	Words of Wisdom	Influence of culture on interpretation (proverbs)	Individual, written (worksheet)

Activity	Title	Topic	Type
12-8	Collage	Self-identity	Individual, hands-on (art project
12-9	Checking for Understanding	Using oral feedback techniques	Groups, oral (role-play)
12-10	Assertive Messages	Assertive communication	Pairs, oral (role-play scenarios)
12-11	Gossip Begone	Dealing with gossip in the workplace	Pairs, oral (role-play scenarios)
12-12	Patients with Special Needs	Communication techniques for patients with various limitations	Groups, oral (role-play)
12-13	Which Word Do I Use?	Commonly confused words	Individual, written (worksheet)

Chapter 13   Telephone Technique

Activity	Title	Topic	Type of Activity
13-1	What's Helpful, What's Not	Importance of good telephone technique	Groups, oral & written (generate list of ideas)
13-2	Great Telephone Technique	Characteristics of good telephone manners	Whole class discussion, oral (generate list of characteristics)
13-3	Telephone Technique Questions	Facts about good telephone technique	Whole class, physical (game)
13-4	Handling Routine Calls	Handling typical calls appropriately	Pairs, oral (role-play scenarios)
13-5	Special Telephone Techniques	Transferring calls, putting callers on hold, handling emergency calls	Groups, oral (role-play scenarios)
13-6	Handling Challenging Calls	Handling calls from patients with problems	Pairs, oral (role-play scenarios)
13-7	Telephone Scavenger Hunt	Gathering information by telephone	Individual, research (make phone calls)
13-8	Vocal Clues	Not judging people by the sound of their voices	Whole class, listening & written (worksheet)

Chapter 14   Patient Education

Activity	Title	Topic	Type of Activity
14-1	What's Available on the Internet?	Locating resources for patient education	Individual or pairs, research & written (worksheet)

Activity	Title	Topic	Type
14-2	What's Available Locally?	Finding local sources of information for patient education	Individual or groups, research (telephone calls, visits)
14-3	What's My Learning Style?	Identifying individual learning styles	Individual, written (self-assessment)
14-4	Take Advantage of Learning Styles	Learning styles and instruction	Groups, oral (brainstorm ideas)
14-5	Giving Instructions	Giving clear instructions	Pairs, oral (giving instructions)
14-6	You're the Teacher	Preparing and presenting a lesson	Groups or individual, oral (presentation)
14-7	Create a Pamphlet	Preparing written information and instructions	Individual or groups, written (project)
14-8	Games That Teach	Developing creative teaching ideas	Groups, hands-on (project)
14-9	Learning about Heart Disease	Using questionnaires in patient education	Individual, written (create a questionnaire)
14-10	Am I Doing It Right?	Teaching by demonstration	Whole class and groups, oral (skits)
14-11	Word Scramble	Developing teaching aids	Individual, written (create a puzzle)

Chapter 15   Documentation

Activity	Title	Topic	Type of Activity
15-1	Docu-Match	Medical records vocabulary and concepts	Whole class, physical (match pairs, presentation)
15-2	Good Documentation	Characteristics of good documentation	Whole class, oral (generate a list of characteristics)
15-3	Subjective versus Objective Information	Correctly charting subjective and objective information	Groups, written (worksheet)
15-4	What If?	Correct medical charting procedures	Groups or individual, oral or written (answer questions)
15-5	How Do I Chart It?	Correct way to state information on medical chart	Individual, written (worksheet)
15-6	How Do I Report This?	Health conditions that must be reported to local authorities	Individual, research (create list)

Activity	Title	Topic	Type
15-7	Drug-Related Abbreviations	Common abbreviations used with pharmaceuticals	Individual, written (worksheet)
15-8	Prescriptions, Please	Format for prescriptions	Individual, physical & written (prescriptions)

Chapter 16 Attitude and Personal Motivation

Activity	Title	Topic	Type
16-1	Philosophies of Life	Different life philosophies through quotes	Whole class, oral (discussion or reports)
16-2	Self-Talk	Self-talk can affect what we do	Individuals, written (worksheet)
16-3	Give It a Positive Spin	Looking for the positive in all we do	Groups or pairs, physical (game)
16-4	What Are My Strengths?	What others see in us that is good	Whole class, written (compliments)
16-5	Success/Failure	To distinguish between success and failure	Groups, oral (generate ideas)
16-6	Dream Board	Developing strategies for self-motivation	Individuals, hands-on (art project)
16-7	Appreciation	Focusing on what is right about our lives	Groups, oral (discussion)
16-8	Happiness and Health	How happiness is related to general well-being	Whole class or groups, oral or hands-on
16-9	Happy Skits	Positive ways to increase happiness	Groups, oral (skit)
16-10	Affirmations	Achieving goals through affirmations	Individual, oral (experiential)

Chapter 17 Time Management and Goal Setting

Activity	Title	Topic	Type
17-1	RUMBA	Writing effective personal goals	Individual, written (worksheet)
17-2	Simple Goal Setting	Setting short- and long-term goals	Individual, written (worksheet)
17-3	Share Your Good News!	Setting and clarifying 5-year goals	Individual, written (letter/report)
17-4	Action Plans	Creating action plans to help achieve goals	Individual, written (worksheet)
17-5	Hitch Your Goals to the Stars	Sharing goals with others	Individual, hands-on (art project)

Activity	Title	Topic	Type
17-6	The Universe Got in My Way	Dealing with problems that interfere with goals	Individual, written (personal report)
17-7	Reaching My Goals	Developing a plan to reach goals	Individual, written (personal plan)
17-8	Sharing Helpful Hints	Strategies for personal organization and time management	Whole class, oral (sharing ideas)
17-9	How Do I Spend My Time?	Analyzing time management	Individual, written (worksheet)
17-10	Managing Your Precious Time	Analyzing time management	Individual, written (self-assessment)
17-11	Procrastination	Breaking the procrastination habit	Whole class, oral (generate ideas)

Chapter 18   Work Habits, Ethics, and Confidentiality

Activity	Title	Topic	Type
18-1	If I Were the Boss	The impact of employee behavior in the workplace	Groups, oral (discuss scenarios)
18-2	If I Were the Patient	The impact of employee behavior on the patient	Groups, oral (discuss scenarios)
18-3	Outstanding Employees	Behaviors exhibited by outstanding employees	Whole class, oral (generate list of characteristics)
18-4	It's the Law	Facts about federal employment laws	Groups, research & oral (presentation)
18-5	Sexual Harassment Questionnaire	The nature of sexual harassment	Individual, written (questionnaire)
18-6	Rumors	Information becomes distorted as it passes from one person to another	Whole class, oral (experiment)
18-7	Ethical Principles	Guiding principles for health care ethics	Groups, oral (discussion)
18-8	What Do You Think?	Ethical and legal issues can be complex	Whole class, oral (discussion of cases)
18-9	It's Confidential	Protecting patient confidentiality	Groups, oral (generate ideas)
18-10	Where Do I Stand?	Understanding personal ethics	Whole class, written & oral (discussion of cases)
18-11	Show Your Ethics	Dealing with ethical situations presented in the office	Groups, oral (skit)

CHAPTER 1

Medical Terminology

INTRODUCTION

Learning the language of medicine is an important component of the health care student's education. Yet many students find medical terminology difficult to master because doing so requires learning many new words that look and sound quite different from English. Helping students discover how much they already know about medical terms and offering a variety of activities makes mastering this new language less overwhelming.

ACTIVITY 1-1
WE KNOW MORE THAN WE THINK

What Students Will Learn

- We use medical terminology every day without even realizing it. The general population usually understands words such as "tonsillitis" and "appendectomy."
- Students will become confident about their ability to learn medical terminology.

What You Will Need

- A whiteboard, chalkboard, or overhead projector.

What To Do

1. This activity is especially effective at the beginning of a terminology course before students learn too many elements. They will need to understand the concept that different meanings are conveyed by the various parts of words.
2. The activity can be conducted with the entire class, or you can divide the class into groups. If you use small groups, you can make the activity a contest.
3. Ask students to think of every medical term they can and call them out. Write them on the board, or transparency for viewing with overhead projector.
4. After you provide examples of identifying the components of a word, have students divide each term into its elements and define each element. If someone suggests "appendectomy" and knows it means "removal of" the appendix, ask which part of the word means "removal." Give other words using "-ectomy" to demonstrate the concept of using suffixes to modify and/or add meaning.
5. If the activity is done in groups, have them take turns sharing their lists with the whole class. The group that comes up with the most correctly defined words wins.
6. Combine, copy, and distribute the lists to all students.

Follow-up Discussion

1. How did you determine the meanings of the various word parts?
2. What clues were there within the words themselves?
3. How do you think you might use this strategy when learning medical terminology?

ACTIVITY 1-2
WHAT'S ON TV?

What Students Will Learn

- Medical terminology is used in medical and health care settings to ensure understanding and clear communication among health care professionals. (This activity works best when students have some knowledge of medical terms.)

What You Will Need

- Ask students to watch a medical TV show before class, or show a tape of a program or movie that has medical terms in it.

What To Do

1. Students watch a medical show or movie and write down each medical term they hear. Terms must be spelled correctly and defined.
2. Discuss the definitions and any lessons about word elements that can be drawn from the examples they supplied.
3. Make copies of the lists to share with all students.

Follow-up Discussion

1. In what types of situations was medical language used?
2. Did the health care workers use another level of language when they spoke with patients?
3. Why do health care workers use different levels of language on the job?

ACTIVITY 1-3
CREATE NEW WORDS

What Students Will Learn

- The concept of combining word elements to create new words that convey specific meanings.

What You Will Need

- Students: creative imaginations.
- Students: A good medical dictionary and a medical terminology text.

What To Do

1. Ask students to use their new knowledge of medical terminology elements to create humorous words. For example, find a medical term for "foot in mouth." Students can really have fun while they practice using medical word elements.
2. This is an especially effective activity for students to do in small groups.
3. Consider awarding small prizes for the most or funniest words created.

Follow-up Discussion

1. How can knowledge of medical terminology help you outside of your new career?

ACTIVITY 1-4
IT'S A MATTER OF COMBINING

What Students Will Learn

- Adding prefixes and suffixes to root words and combining forms to create medical terms.
- The meanings of a variety of root words, common combining forms, prefixes, and suffixes. (These will already have been presented and studied.)

What You Will Need

- A copy of Student Handouts 1-1, Common Suffixes, and 1-2, Common Prefixes, for each student.
- A list of combining forms that are parallel in meaning for assigning to student groups, such as the following:
    1. cardi/o
    2. derm/o
    3. enter/o
    4. gastr/o
    5. hepat/o
    6. nephr/o
    7. my/o
    8. neur/o
    9. oste/o
    10. pneum/o
- Students: Each group of students needs a medical dictionary or terminology text that includes an alphabetical list of combining forms and elements.

Student Handout **1-1**

Student Handout **1-2**

What To Do

1. Divide students into groups of three or four.
2. Give each group the handouts of prefixes and suffixes to review for 5 minutes.
3. After the 5 minutes, give each group a different combining form.
4. Instruct the groups to make up as many correct medical terms as possible by adding suffixes or suffixes and prefixes to the combining form using the lists of suffixes and prefixes.
5. Once they have finished compiling their lists, the students can use the dictionary to ensure that these are actual words and that they are spelled correctly.
6. The team with the most correct words at the end of a given period of time is the winner.
7. More challenging version: Give each group the lists of prefixes and suffixes to review for 5 minutes.
8. After 5 minutes, give each group a different combining form.
9. Groups work for a designated period of time to make up as many correct medical terms as possible by adding suffixes or suffixes and prefixes. They are not to look at the handout lists but use as many as they can remember. They may not use the dictionary.

10. The teams must know the meanings of the terms they create. The winning group is the one with the most correct words.

Follow-up Discussion

1. Did you find that hearing words made up by other students helped you to think of new words?
2. Is your medical vocabulary larger than it was when you began this class?

ACTIVITY 1-5
BODY-PART SIMON SAYS

What Students Will Learn
- Medical terms for body parts.

What You Will Need
- A list of terms for various body parts that students can move or shake in response to commands from "Simon," such as:

carpals	radius
cranium	scapula
deltoid	tarsals
fibula	tibia
humerus	triceps
patella	ulna

What To Do

1. This activity is a variation of the old children's game, Simon Says. Students stand in an area large enough for them to move their arms and legs.
2. The instructor or a student is "Simon" and asks students to move various body parts as he or she calls them out, using the appropriate medical term.
3. If the term is preceded by "Simon says," students move that particular part. If the term is not preceded by "Simon says," they should not move it.
4. Students who move the incorrect part or move without the "Simon says" statement sit down.
5. The game can be played until only one student remains standing or for a designated period of time.

Follow-up Discussion

1. Do you find physical movement helpful in learning the terms?
2. How can you use movement to learn other important information?

ACTIVITY 1-6
BODY-PART HOKEY POKEY

What Students Will Learn
- Medical terms for various body parts.

What You Will Need
- The words to Hokey Pokey:

You put your _____ in,
You put your _____ out,
You put your _____ in,
And you shake it all about.
You do the hokey pokey,
And you turn yourself around.
That's what it's all about.
(Clap three times.)

What To Do

1. Have students stand in a circle. They must leave enough space between themselves to move their arms and legs.
2. The instructor or a student calls out body parts that students are to move in and out of the circle and "shake all about." Students sing or chant the words, filling in the body-part term that has been called out.

Follow-up Discussion

1. Do you find physical movement helpful in learning the terms?
2. How can you use movement to learn other important information?

ACTIVITY 1-7
WORD FLASH!

What Students Will Learn

- The meanings of a given set of words or word elements.
- The learning strategy of using repetition over time to master new material, such as medical terminology.
- That one-time review and cramming are not effective for long-term retention.

What You Will Need

- Lightweight cardstock to make flash cards large enough for the entire class to see; 4 × 8 inches is a good size.
- Marking pens in various dark colors.
- A list of words or elements you want students to learn or a list of those that have been particularly difficult for your students.

What To Do

1. Prepare flash cards using marking pens. On one side, write the medical term; on the other, write the definition or layman's term. (You may omit the definition and simply call it out when prompting students for the medical term.)
2. Review the terms for a few minutes each class session. Students can respond to prompts as a group, row, or individually.
3. Keep the pace moving along and create two stacks of cards: (1) the words or elements that everyone seems to know and (2) those that still need review.
4. Continue reviewing each class session until all words are in pile number one.

Follow-up Discussion

1. How quickly were you able to learn the words by frequently repeating them?

ACTIVITY 1-8
PICTURE THIS!

What Students Will Learn
- The meanings of a given set of words or word elements.
- Using visual clues as associations to remember difficult words.

What You Will Need
- A list of words or word elements you want students to learn. Divide the list into groups of up to 10 words.

What To Do
1. Divide the class into groups of three to five students.
2. Distribute the lists to the groups and have students devise visual associations as reminders of each word, for example:
   - cranium: a large skull being lifted by a crane
   - hem/o: a big man (he-man) fainting at the sight of blood
   - gastr/o: the stomach in the form of a gas can with a pouring spout
   - ot/o: big ears sitting at a desk in the classroom. "My ears are working over-time (OT) in this class listening to these new words!"
3. After creating the clues, each group shares its list with the rest of the class. Lists can be copied for distribution to all class members.
4. If students can draw quick sketches on the board or act out their clues, the exercise will be even more effective for providing a visual picture of the terms.

Follow-up Discussion
1. How helpful did you find visualization for learning terminology?

ACTIVITY 1-9
HAVEN'T I SEEN YOU SOMEWHERE?

What Students Will Learn
- That many words, both medical and nonmedical, have common roots that give clues to their meaning.
- The learning strategy of using spelling clues or familiar parts of words as associations to remember new words.

What You Will Need
- Students need access to lists of medical terms such as in their textbooks or medical dictionaries. Or you can prepare lists of words you want students to learn that have similarities to commonplace words, for example:
  - supra-, contains the word "up"
  - sub-, a *sub*marine goes under the water
  - tri-, *tri*ple
  - –plasty, surgical repair (*plast*ic surgery)

What To Do
1. Divide the class into groups of three to five students. Each group needs to have at least one textbook or medical dictionary.

2. Assign a different section of the book or dictionary to each group. Instruct each group to search for and list words that are related to commonplace words.
3. If you have prepared a list of words or elements to use in the activity, divide it so that each group has a separate list.
4. When groups have completed their findings, have them share with the class.
5. Copy the lists to distribute to all students.

Follow-up Discussion

1. Why do you think many words have common elements?
2. How can you apply this knowledge to make it easier to learn medical terminology?

ACTIVITY 1-10
CATCH THAT WORD

What Students Will Learn

- The meanings (in review) of a given set of words or word elements.

What You Will Need

- A list of words that students have already studied.
- A ball made of soft material such as foam rubber.

What To Do

1. Distribute a copy of the list to each student and give them a few minutes to review.
2. Have the students stand up. Toss the ball to a student and call out either a medical term or definition from the list.
3. The student must respond with either the appropriate definition or term. If it is correct, he or she may choose a word or definition from the list, then toss the ball to another student who must supply the appropriate answer.
4. If any student cannot supply the answer, he or she returns the ball to the person who asked the question and then sits down. The last person standing is the winner.
5. An alternate version is to have students remain standing, even if they miss, and simply play the game for a designated period of time.

Follow-up Discussion

1. Did you find a competitive game motivated you to learn the terminology?

ACTIVITY 1-11
WORD (UN)SCRAMBLE

What Students Will Learn

- The concept of adding prefixes and suffixes to root words and combining forms to create medical terms.

What You Will Need

- Using a list of medical terms the students have already studied, create cards for each element of each word. For example, "echocardiogram" would have three cards:

echo	cardio	gram

You need one card for each student.

What To Do

1. Give each student one card. It is important that all cards comprising each term be distributed.
2. Have students walk around the room and try to form complete medical terms by correctly combining their cards with those held by other students.
3. When a word is completed, students write it on the board and then sit down.
4. When everyone is finished, ask each group of students to stand up, hold up their cards, and give the correct pronunciation and definition of the completed term.

Follow-up Discussion

1. Why is it better to learn word elements and how to put them together rather than simply memorizing whole medical words?
2. What are some other methods you could use to learn the word elements?

ACTIVITY 1-12
THAT'S MY WORD!

What Students Will Learn

- The meanings (in review) of a given set of medical terms.

What You Will Need

- A list of words that students have already studied.
- 3 × 5 cards in two colors.

What To Do

1. Mark a pair of cards for each term on the list: the medical terms on one color and the definitions on the other. (Or, students can prepare the cards as a pre-activity assignment.)
2. Version # 1: Distribute one card to each student. Be sure to hand out all the cards so that all terms will have a matching definition.
3. Students walk around the class to find their match. Once they pair up, they write the term on the board and sit down.
4. Version # 2: Students with definition cards stand up and read the definition. The student who has the matching word stands up and says, "That's My Word!"

Follow-up Discussion

1. Can you think of other physical activities that can help you to learn medical terminology?

REFERENCES

Mitchell, J. & Haroun, L. (2002). *Introduction to health care.* Clifton Park, NY: Delmar Learning.

Common Suffixes

Suffix	Meaning
-ac, -al, -ar, -ary, -eal, -iac, -ic, -ical, -ose, -ous, -tic	pertaining to
-algia	pain
-centesis	surgical puncture to remove fluid
-cide	to kill, destroy
-cyte	cell
-ectomy	removal of
-emia	blood condition
-gram	record, image
-graph	an instrument used to record, image
-graphy	process of recording, imaging
-ia	condition, especially an abnormal state
-ism	condition
-itis	inflammation of
-lithiasis	presence of or formation of stones
-logy	study of
-megaly	enlargement
-oid	resembling
-oma	tumor
-otomy, -tomy	surgical incision
-pathy	disease
-plasty	surgical repair
-plegia	paralysis
-pnea	breathing, respiration
-rrhea	drainage, flow
-scope	examination, instrument
-scopy	examination using a scope
-stasis	stoppage
-stomy	surgically create an artificial mouth or stoma (opening)

Source: Adapted from Mitchell, J. & Haroun, L. (2002). *Introduction to health care.* Clifton Park, NY: Delmar Learning.

Common Prefixes

Prefix	Meaning
a-/an-	without, not
anti-	against
auto-	self
bi-	two, double
brady-	slow
dys-	bad, difficult, painful
epi-	above (location)
eu-	good, normal
hemi-	half
hyper-	higher than normal, excessive
hypo-	less than, under
inter-	between
intra-	within
multi-	many
non-	not
peri-	around
poly-	many, much
post-	after, behind
pre-	before, in front
pseudo-	false
quadri-	four
semi-	half
sub-	under, below
supra-	above, over
tachy-	fast, rapid
tri-	three

Source: Adapted from Mitchell, J. & Haroun, L. (2002). *Introduction to health care.* Clifton Park, NY: Delmar Learning.

CHAPTER 2

Anatomy and Physiology

INTRODUCTION

The study of the fundamentals of anatomy and physiology involves learning many new terms that students often find difficult and somewhat tedious. This chapter provides a variety of ways for students to learn and review new terms and increase their understanding of how our bodies function.

ACTIVITY 2-1
HOW BIONIC CAN WE BECOME?

What Students Will Learn
- To identify organs that are available for transplant or replacement.
- To identify nonhuman items that can be transplanted (such as heart valves and replacement knees and hips).

What You Will Need
- Access to a good library and/or the Internet for research.

What To Do
1. Students are to do some research and do one of the following:
   - Write a paper.
   - Create a poster.
   - Put on a skit.
   - Give an oral report.
2. Explain to the students that the purpose of this activity is to teach others what body parts can now be replaced by organ or joint transplant or replacement. An example of a creative project is for students to draw a large outline of a body and mark on it the locations of body parts that can be replaced such as the heart, lungs, kidney, knee joint, hand joints, hip joint, skin, and cornea.
3. Specify that the information given should include whether the replacement part is from another human or an animal (such as a pig valve), or is artificial.
4. Schedule time for students to share their projects with the class.

Follow-up Discussion
1. What are some of the new body parts that will be available for transplant or replacement in the next few years?

ACTIVITY 2-2
WHERE ARE OUR TASTE BUDS?

What Students Will Learn:

- Where the four types of taste buds (bitter, sour, salty, and sweet) are located on the tongue.*

What You Will Need

- Food to represent each of the four different types of taste buds: bitter, sour, salty, and sweet. Food ideas include a small cup of black coffee, a small cup of lemon juice or vinegar, saline solution, honey or sugar dissolved in water.
- Four short (about four inches) pieces of straw for each student.
- Transparencies 2-1, Location of Taste Buds, and 2-2, Diagram of a Taste Bud.

What To Do

1. This activity may be done with the entire class or with groups of four or five students.
2. Choose one student to sit in the front of the group.
3. Using a piece of straw as a dropper, drop one of the liquids on different areas of the tongue.
4. Have students map each area of the tongue to show what type of taste buds it has.
5. When students have completed the activity, have them check their taste bud maps against Transparency 2-1, Location of Taste Buds. Then show Transparency 2-2, Diagram of a Taste Bud, to show what a taste bud looks like.

Follow-up Discussion

1. Where are the taste buds for salty?
2. Where are the taste buds for sweet?
3. When you place something salty on a sweet taste bud, how does it taste?

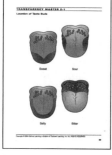

Transparency Master **2-1**

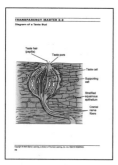

Transparency Master **2-2**

ACTIVITY 2-3
SMELL AND TASTE

What Students Will Learn

- The relationship between the senses of smell and taste.†

What You Will Need

- A blindfold.
- Grated apple.
- Grated carrot.
- Grated potato.
- Three bowls.
- Spoon.

---

* *Source:* A. Smith (Ed.). (1996). Adapted from *The Usborne big book of experiments*. Oklahoma: EDC Publishing.

† *Source:* A. Smith (Ed.). (1996). Adapted from *The Usborne big book of experiments*. Oklahoma: EDC Publishing.

What To Do

1. Put grated apple, carrot, and potato in different bowls.
2. Blindfold a student and ask him to hold his nose.
3. Spoon a little of each food, one at a time, into the student's mouth.
4. Ask the student to identify the food by taste alone (without being able to see or smell the food).
5. Students will have difficulty identifying what they are eating because the tongue can only taste sweet, sour, bitter, or salty. Without the senses of sight and smell, it is difficult to know exactly what one is eating.

Follow-up Discussion

1. Why is it difficult to tell what each food is when you cannot see or smell it?
2. Where in the brain are the senses of smell and taste located?

ACTIVITY 2-4
ENDOCRINE SYSTEM SKITS

What Students Will Learn

- The glands of the endocrine system and their functions.

What You Will Need

- A resource with detailed information about the endocrine system. Access to the Internet would be helpful.

What To Do

1. Divide the class into groups of about six students.
2. Assign each group an endocrine gland (adrenal, pancreas, pituitary, testes, ovaries, thymus, pineal, parathyroid, or thyroid).
3. Have students put together a skit that explains what their gland does and what happens when it malfunctions or is diseased. For example, students assigned the pancreas can demonstrate the release of insulin and what happens when insulin is not released or is not absorbed properly by the body when it is released.

Follow-up Discussion

1. What are some of the diseases caused by a malfunctioning endocrine system? (hyperthyroidism, diabetes, e.g.)
2. What is some of the newest research in the area of diabetes?

ACTIVITY 2-5
USING A PINHOLE

What Students Will Learn

- How light rays on the retina affect vision.

What You Will Need

- 3 × 5 cards.
- Hat pin or other device for punching a small hole.

- An eye chart.
- Students who are nearsighted to act as patients.
- Saline solution and contact lens cases (you can ask students to bring their own if you do not have access to any).
- Transparency 2-3, Light Rays and Vision

What To Do

1. Divide students into groups of two or three, being sure that each group includes a student who is nearsighted (wears glasses or contact lenses).
2. Give each group a card and have them punch a small pinhole in each card.
3. Have each group test the vision of its nearsighted group member while wearing her glasses or contact lenses. Chart the result.
4. Next have the patients remove their glasses or contact lenses. (Be sure students removing contact lenses wash hands first and have a clean and safe place to store the lenses.)
5. Have the groups check uncorrected vision and chart the results.
6. Now, have the patients read the eye chart without correction, but while looking through the pinhole. Record vision.
7. Point out that vision through the pinhole should be close to the corrected vision of the patient. When a person has difficulty seeing, she often squints, producing an effect similar to looking through a pinhole. Vision through a pinhole will not be any better than the best corrected vision, but it will generally show how well a person can see if she has adequate corrective lenses. Students with no diseases of the eye, but with corrective lenses that need a prescription change, may have better vision with the pinhole than while wearing their current corrective lenses.

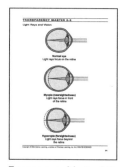

Transparency Master **2-3**

Follow-up Discussion

1. Why does a pinhole work?

Instructor's Note: When a person is nearsighted (has difficulty with distance vision), light rays are focused in front of the retina rather than on it. Using a pinhole narrows the group of light rays entering the eye and focuses them on the retina so the person can have clear vision. Pinholes only correct for refractive errors such as myopia and presbyopia, not other diseases of the eye. Use Transparency 2-3, Light Rays and Vision, to demonstrate how light rays focus on the retina in both normal and defective vision.

ACTIVITY 2-6
THE EYE: TESTING FOR THE BLIND SPOT

What Students Will Learn

- Facts about the structure and function of the eye.

What You Will Need

- One unlined 3 × 5 card for each class member.
- Transparency 2-4, Structures of the Eye.

What To Do

1. On the 3 × 5 cards, place a large dark dot one inch to the left of center and a large cross one inch to the right of center. Or distribute blank cards and have students draw the dot and cross. See the accompanying illustration.
2. Have students close their right eye and look at the cross with their left eye.
3. Instruct them to move the card toward their faces until the dot disappears. (This shows where the blind spot is in the left eye.)

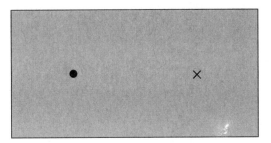

Follow-up Discussion

1. Why do we have a blind spot?
2. What medical conditions can affect the size of the blind spot? (glaucoma)

Instructor's Note: The blind spot is at the intersection of the optic nerve and the retina. Use Transparency 2-4, Structures of the Eye, to show its location. Also explain that the dot disappears because our brains fill in the space with white from the card. It is for this reason that we do not notice our blind spot, even when we are looking with only one eye.

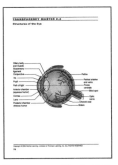

Transparency Master **2-4**

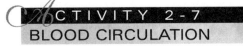

ACTIVITY 2-7
BLOOD CIRCULATION

What Students Will Learn

- How blood flows through the heart and body.

What You Will Need

- Butcher paper (enough to draw one body for every two students in class).
- Magic marker or other drawing implement.
- Large space where students can lie on paper to be traced.
- Colored pencils or pens, including red and blue.
- Reference showing the heart and circulatory system.

What To Do

1. Divide students into groups of two (the groups can be larger, if you wish).
2. Give each group a set of colored pencils and a piece of butcher paper large enough to trace a person on.
3. Have one student lie on the paper and the other student trace his entire body. (If students trace two bodies and cut them out, they can stuff paper inside and staple the two together to make a "person." This is not necessary for learning, but it is fun.)
4. Have students draw the heart, showing the chambers; the lungs; and the major arteries and vessels.

5. Using red (oxygenated blood) and blue pencils (oxygen-poor blood), students can show the flow of blood through the heart and lungs and throughout the body. For more interest, have students draw hair on their "person" and decorate him or her any way they like. These can then be displayed around the room.

Follow-up Discussion

1. What is the normal heart rate?
2. What is normal respiration?
3. Do you draw arterial or venous blood when you do venipucture?

ACTIVITY 2-8
MINI-DISSECTION

What Students Will Learn

- The anatomical structure of various body parts.*

What You Will Need

Instructor's Note: A local butcher shop or specialty meat market may be able to supply some, if not all, of the animal parts.

- A variety of beef, chicken, or turkey bones, such as leg and neck.
- Turkey leg with meat attached.
- Beef heart.
- Kidneys.
- Beef tongue.
- Beef or sheep brains.
- Cow eye.
- Cutting boards.
- Scalpels.
- Access to water, soap, paper towels for cleanup.
- A copy of Student Handout 2-1, Mini-Dissection Picture Guide, for each student.
- Disposable gloves for each student.

What To Do

1. Before the class session designated for this activity, set up stations with cutting boards, scalpels, and animal parts.
2. At the time of the activity, divide the class into pairs or groups of three or four students, depending on the size of the class and number of stations.
3. Distribute Student Handout 2-1, Mini-Dissection Picture Guide.
4. Explain to the students that the handout contains drawings of human anatomy, which may not be exactly the same as the animal parts they will be dissecting (especially true for the turkey leg).
5. Instruct students to dissect the animal parts at their stations. Ask them to look for the structures illustrated on the handout.

Source: Adapted from L. Keir, B. A. Wise, & C. Krebs (1993). *Medical assisting: Administrative and clinical competencies,* (3rd. ed.). *Teacher's resource kit.* Clifton Park, NY: Delmar Learning.

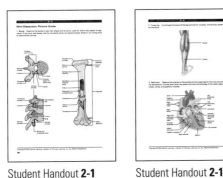
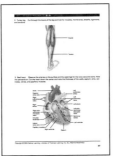
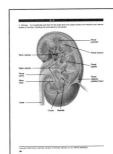
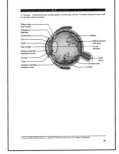

Student Handout **2-1**   Student Handout **2-1**   Student Handout **2-1**   Student Handout **2-1**
                                 (*Continued*)   (*Continued*)   (*Continued*)

Follow-up Discussion:

1. How were the parts you dissected similar to or different from what you saw in the human anatomy drawings?

2. Which parts were the most difficult to identify?

ACTIVITY 2-9
WHAT AM I?

What Students Will Learn

- The characteristics and functions of various body parts.

What You Will Need

- Cards or pieces of paper with the names of various body parts written on them to serve as labels. You or the students can make these, using words they have found to be difficult or that need to be reviewed.
- Tape or pins.

What To Do

1. Students tape or pin labels on each other's backs without revealing the label to the wearer.

2. Students then walk around the classroom and ask each other questions that can be answered with a "yes" or "no" in an attempt to guess what part they are. Examples: "Am I an organ?" "Am I part of the digestive system?"

3. An easier version is to have all words belong to one system or one category, such as organs, glands, bones, and so on.

Follow-up Discussion

1. What was hardest to guess: bones, organs, or glands?

ACTIVITY 2-10
WHAT AM I? 10 QUESTIONS VERSION

What Students Will Learn

- The functions of various body structures.

What You Will Need

- Enough 3 × 5 cards, each containing the name of an anatomical part that students need to review, for every student to have at least one.

What To Do

1. Distribute the cards to the students. They should not disclose to anyone else what is on their card.
2. Call them one at a time to the front of the class. The other students can ask up to 10 yes or no questions in an attempt to guess the anatomical structure the student represents.

Follow-up Discussion

1. Are 10 questions enough to be able to guess the body structures?

ACTIVITY 2-11
HUMAN BODY SCAVENGER HUNT

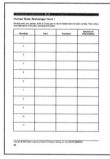

Student Handout **2-2**

What Students Will Learn

- The function and quantity of various body parts.

What You Will Need

- A copy of Student Handout 2-2, Human Body Scavenger Hunt I, or Student Handout 2-3, Human Body Scavenger Hunt II, for each student.
- Anatomy/physiology texts or reference books

What To Do

1. Explain that the activity is to match numbers with various parts of the body. (For example, 1 heart, 3 types of muscles.)
2. Answers can include categories, such as the number of types of tissue.
3. It is called a scavenger hunt because some of the answers will require some searching.
4. Have the class divide into pairs. Working together, they are to fill in Student Handout 2-2. Student Handout 2-3 is a more challenging version. The purpose of including the source is to make checking the answers, if necessary, easier.

Student Handout **2-3**

Follow-up Discussion

1. Review with students the functions of the different anatomical structures.

ACTIVITY 2-12
THAT'S AMAZING!

What Students Will Learn

- Interesting facts about the human body.*

---

*_Source:_ A. S. Scott & E. Fong (1998). _Body structures and functions,_ (9th ed.). Clifton Park, NY: Delmar Learning.

What You Will Need

- A list of facts about the human body, along with corresponding false facts. For example:
    1. Each day the lungs take in approximately 12,000 quarts of air. (Suggested false fact: 5,000 quarts.)
    2. The lungs produce about 1 quart of mucous every 24 hours. (Suggested false fact: 1 cup.)
    3. Cilia move at a rate of 1,500 beats per minute. (Suggested false fact: 200 beats per minute.)
    4. If all the air sacs in the lungs could be spread out, side by side, they would occupy the size of a tennis court. (Suggested false fact: the size of a football field.)
    5. The heart of the average person beats over 115,000 times each day. (Suggested false fact: 85,000 times.)
    6. The average person eats at least 35 tons (70,000 pounds) of food in a lifetime. (Suggested false fact: 10 tons or 20,000 pounds.)
    7. The average human head contains at least 100,000 hairs. (Suggested false fact: 500,000 hairs)
    8. Hair grows faster during the day than during the night. (Suggested false fact: hair grows at the same rate day and night.)
    9. Almost half the bones in the body are contained in the hands and feet. (Suggested false fact: the hands and feet contain about one-fourth of the total number of bones in the body.)
    10. The 3 smallest bones in the body are in the ears. (Suggested false fact: in the hands.)
    11. Nerve impulses can travel at speeds of up to 426 feet per second. (Suggested false fact: 50 feet per second.)
    12. At rest, the body consumes about ½ pint of oxygen per minute. (Suggested false fact: 1 quart.)
    13. If the small intestine were stretched out, it would measure about 23 feet. (Suggested false fact: 75 feet)
    14. The skin weighs twice as much as the brain. (Suggested false fact: the skin weighs about the same as the brain.)
    15. A full stomach can hold about 1½ quarts. (Suggested false fact: about 4 quarts.)
    16. Muscles make up about half the total weight of the body. (Suggested false fact: muscles make up about a quarter of the total weight of the body.)
    17. The human eye can see about 7 million shades of color. (Suggested false fact: 100,000 shades.)
    18. The heart of an average person beats more than 36 million times a year. (Suggested false fact: 50 million times.)
    19. If all the capillaries were lined up end to end, they would stretch more than 16,000 miles. (Suggested false fact: 10,000 miles.)
    20. The most common disease in the United States is tooth decay. (Suggested false fact: heart disease.)
    21. The human nose can detect about 10,000 different smells. (Suggested false fact: about 2,000 different smells.)
    22. Smell accounts for approximately 90% of what we think of as taste. (Suggested false fact: 50%.)
    23. There are about 9,000 taste buds on the tongue. (Suggested false fact: about 1,000.)

24. The brain is 2% of the average body's total weight but uses up to 20% of its fuel. (Suggested false fact: 2% and 10%.)

What To Do

1. Divide the class into two teams.
2. Using the list of facts, read aloud either a fact or false statement.
3. The teams may alternate turns to answer the question or press buzzers after the question is read aloud.
4. The team member whose turn it is states whether the fact is true or false.
5. The team to earn the most points, after all the questions are asked, is the winner.

Follow-up Discussion

1. What is the most surprising fact you learned?
2. Do you know other interesting facts about the body you can share with the class?

ACTIVITY 2-13
BODY PATHWAYS

What Students Will Learn

- The anatomy and physiology of various body systems.

What You Will Need

- Sets of cards or papers on which are written, large enough to be seen by the entire class, the components of various body systems. One word or word set should be written on each card. (So, for example, Set 1 should have 11 cards.)

  Set 1: Urinary System: Pathway of Urine—renal artery, glomerulus, Bowman's capsule, renal tubule, collecting tubule, renal pelvis, ureter, urinary bladder, urethra, urinary meatus.

  Set 2: Digestive System: Pathway of Food—oral cavity, pharynx, esophagus, cardiac sphincter, stomach, pyloric sphincter, duodenum, ileum, jejunum, ascending colon, transverse colon, descending colon, sigmoid colon, rectum.

  Set 3: Respiratory System: Pathway of Respiration—nasal cavity, pharynx, larynx, trachea, bronchus, bronchioles, alveoli.

  Set 4: Special Senses: Pathway of Hearing—auricle, external auditory canal, tympanic membrane, malleus, incus, stapes, cochlea, auditory nerve, temporal lobe of brain.

  Set 5: Special Senses: Pathway of Vision—pupil, cornea, lens, retina, optic nerve, occipital lobe of brain.

- Transparencies 2-5 through 2-9: Pathway of Urine, Pathway of Food, Pathway of Respiration, Pathway of Hearing, and Pathway of Vision.
- A whiteboard, chalkboard, or overhead projector.

What To Do

1. Distribute one of the cards to each student. Be sure to distribute all the cards in each set used.

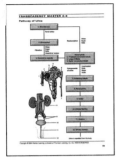
Transparency Master **2-5**

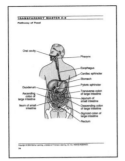
Transparency Master **2-6**

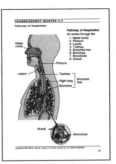
Transparency Master **2-7**

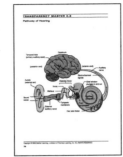
Transparency Master **2-8**

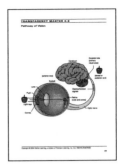
Transparency Master **2-9**

2. Display the categories of the sets distributed on the board or using an overhead projector.

3. The first part of the activity is for students to form groups by walking around the classroom and finding students who have cards that belong together in the same category, using the list on the board as a guide.

4. When all groups are formed, ask the students to move to the front of the classroom, one group at a time, and line up in the correct order to demonstrate the indicated pathway.

5. The students in the lineup should then briefly explain the function of the components on their cards. Show Transparency 2-5, Pathway of Urine, Transparency 2-6, Pathway of Food, Transparency 2-7, Pathway of Respiration, Transparency 2-8, Pathway of Hearing, and Transparency 2-9, Pathway of Vision, to illustrate the pathways.

Follow-up Discussion

1. What is the pathway of the urine?
2. How does air enter and leave the body?
3. What does the lens do in the eye?

ACTIVITY 2-14
NAME THAT DISEASE

What Students Will Learn

- Common diseases that affect various body systems.

What You Will Need

- Textbooks or reference books that contain information about common diseases.
- A copy of Student Handout 2-4, Diseases and Disorders, for each student.
- 40 4 × 6 (or 4 × 8) inch cards (more if you wish to add diseases and conditions to the list provided).

What To Do

1. Distribute one or more cards and a copy of Student Handout 2-4 to each student.

2. Have students count off, write their number on their card, and write the name of the disease from the numbered list on Student Handout 2-4 that corre-

Student Handout **2-4**

sponds to their number. The count-off can continue until students have more than one number in order to cover all the conditions listed on the handout.

3. Allow several minutes for students to list five clues about their disease(s) on the card(s). The clues may be signs, symptoms, the body system involved, common treatment, prevention techniques, and so on.

4. When students have completed their lists, collect the cards.

5. To play the game, divide the class into two or more teams. Students from each team alternately take turns playing.

6. The instructor draws a card and reads one sign or symptom at a time. The student has an opportunity to guess the disease after each is read.

7. The points awarded are the numbers of clues needed before the disease is correctly identified. Therefore, the team with the *lowest* score is the winner after all cards are drawn or time is up. If the disease is not identified after all clues have been read, the team receives six points.

Follow-up Discussion

1. How many symptoms do you usually need to hear to be able to name the disease?

2. Were there many disorders that had the same symptoms? If so, how do you think this influences the diagnosis of disorders?

ACTIVITY 2-15
ANATOMY BINGO

What Students Will Learn

- Review of various body structures and functions.

What You Will Need

- A Bingo card for each student. Copy from Student Handout 2-5.
- Two copies of Instructor Sheet 2-1, Anatomy Bingo Caller List. Cut up one copy to use the pieces for the call outs. Use the second copy to track what you have called.

What To Do

1. Play like traditional Bingo.
2. Students are to match the definitions called out with the words on their cards.
3. The first student to mark a row and define each word in the row correctly is the winner.

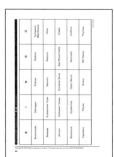

Student Handout **2-5**

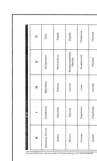

Student Handout **2-5**
(*Continued*)

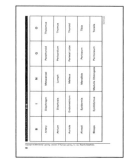

Student Handout **2-5**
(*Continued*)

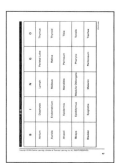

Student Handout **2-5**
(*Continued*)

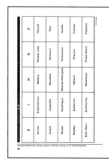

Student Handout **2-5**
(*Continued*)

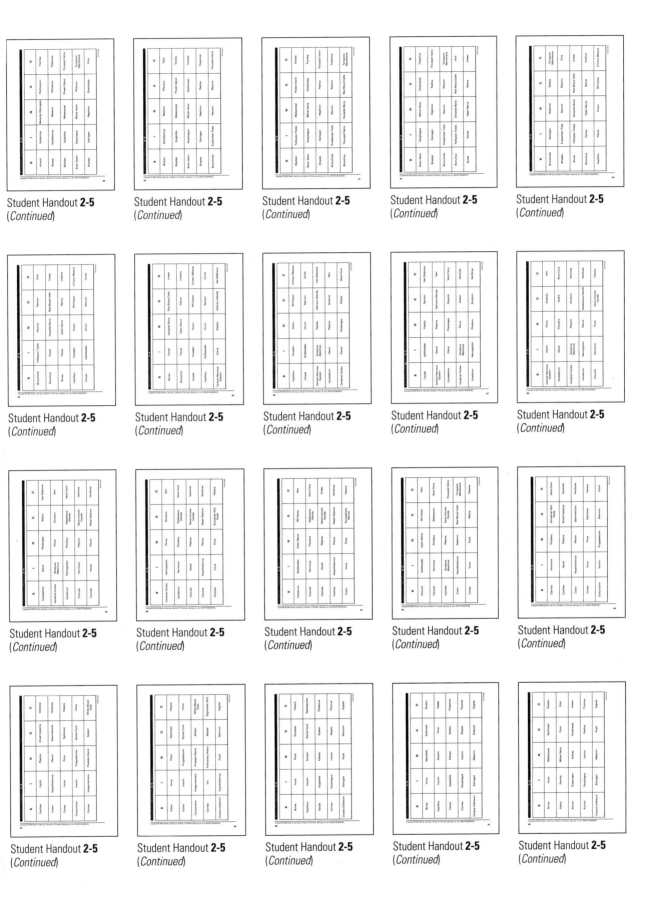

Student Handout **2-5**
(*Continued*)

Student Handout **2-5**
(*Continued*)

Student Handout **2-5**
(*Continued*)

Student Handout **2-5**
(*Continued*)

Student Handout **2-5**
(*Continued*)

Student Handout **2-5**
(*Continued*)

Student Handout **2-5**
(*Continued*)

Student Handout **2-5**
(*Continued*)

Student Handout **2-5**
(*Continued*)

Student Handout **2-5**
(*Continued*)

Student Handout **2-5**
(*Continued*)

Student Handout **2-5**
(*Continued*)

Student Handout **2-5**
(*Continued*)

Student Handout **2-5**
(*Continued*)

Student Handout **2-5**
(*Continued*)

Student Handout **2-5**
(*Continued*)

Student Handout **2-5**
(*Continued*)

Student Handout **2-5**
(*Continued*)

Student Handout **2-5**
(*Continued*)

Student Handout **2-5**
(*Continued*)

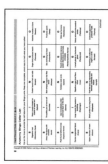

Instructor Sheet **2-1**

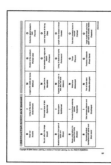

Instructor Sheet **2-1**
(*Continued*)

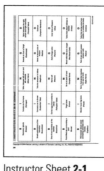

Instructor Sheet **2-1**
(*Continued*)

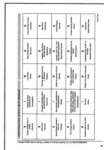

Instructor Sheet **2-1**
(*Continued*)

Instructor Sheet **2-1**
(*Continued*)

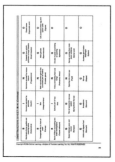

Instructor Sheet **2-1**
(*Continued*)

4. They may write on the cards or use markers.
5. Prizes are fun but optional.

Follow-up Discussion

1. Why is it important to learn the vocabulary related to the various body systems?
2. When might you use this vocabulary in your future occupation?
3. What are other games or activities you might use to learn anatomy?

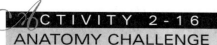

ANATOMY CHALLENGE

What Students Will Learn

● Review of various body structures and functions.

What You Will Need

● Body system category charts made with Transparencies 2-10, or 2-11, Anatomy Challenge Categories I and II. Or you can list the categories and points on the board or on a large chart.
● A list of answers (prompts) and questions (correct answers) for each category (Instructor Sheet 2-2).

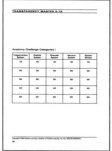

Transparency Master **2-10**

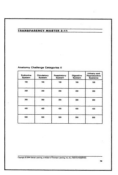

Transparency Master **2-11**

What To Do

1. Challenge is a game in which a panel of contestants choose categories and the point values. Referring to Instructor Sheet 2-2, the host gives a prompt from that category in the form of an answer. The contestant must supply the question that the prompt answers. For example:
   Host: Synapse
   Contestant: What is the space between nerve cells through which impulses are transmitted?
2. Four contestants play at a time. The first contestant to play can be chosen at random or by answering a question.
3. The first contestant chooses a category and value. If the question is answered correctly, the points are awarded and the contestant continues until missing a question.

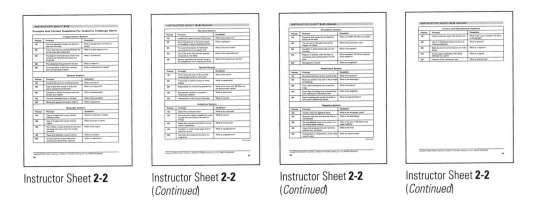

Instructor Sheet **2-2**

Instructor Sheet **2-2**
(*Continued*)

Instructor Sheet **2-2**
(*Continued*)

Instructor Sheet **2-2**
(*Continued*)

4. In the case of an incorrect answer, the value of the question is deducted from the contestant's score and the next contestant has an opportunity to select a category and value.

5. The game continues until all questions have been attempted. The winner is the contestant with the highest score.

Follow-up Discussion

1. Ask students to write one or two new challenge questions and answers to be used the next time the game is played.

REFERENCES

Colbert, B. J., Ankney, J., Wilson, J., & Havrilla, J. (1997). *An integrated approach to health sciences: Anatomy and physiology, math, physics, and chemistry.* Clifton Park, NY: Delmar Learning.

Keir, L., Wise, B. A., & Krebs, C. (1993). *Medical assisting: Administrative and clinical competencies* (3rd. ed.). *Teacher's resource kit.* Clifton Park, NY: Delmar Learning.

Muschla, G. R., & Muschla, J. A. (1996). *Hands-on math projects with real-life applications.* West Nyack, NY: The Center for Applied Research in Education.

Scott, A. S., & Fong, E. (1998). *Body structures and functions* (9th ed.). Clifton Park, NY: Delmar Learning.)

Smith, A. (Ed.). (1996). *The Usborne big book of experiments.* Oklahoma: EDC Publishing.

VanCleave, J. (1995). *The human body for every kid.* New York: Wiley.

Anatomy Bingo Caller List

Cut on the lines to provide the call letters for your Bingo game. Keep one complete, uncut copy to track what you have called.

B	**I**	**N**	**G**	**O**
Digestive tract (Alimentary Canal)	Major muscle located on outside of upper arm (Deltoid)	Protein found in hair and nails (Keratin)	Organ that produces insulin (Pancreas)	Attaches muscles to bone (Tendon)
Artery that leaves left ventricle (Aorta)	Threadlike part of nerve cell (Dendrite)	Bean-shaped organs that filter blood (Kidneys)	Sac enclosing the heart (Pericardium)	Produces sperm (Testes)
Fluid found behind cornea (Aqueous Humor)	Lies immediately under outermost layer of the skin (Dermis)	Contains vocal cords (Larynx)	Branch of autonomic nervous system that slows down body processes (Parasympathetic Nerves)	Male sex hormone (Testosterone)
Carries oxygenated blood (Artery)	Large muscle that assists in breathing (Diaphragm)	Digestive organ that filters blood (Liver)	4 small glands in the thyroid gland (Parathyroid)	Relays stimuli to the cerebral cortex (Thalamus)
Upper chamber of heart (Atrium)	Shaft portion of a long bone (Diaphysis)	Fluid that acts as intermediary between capillaries and tissues (Lymph)	Pertaining to walls of an organ or cavity (Parietal)	Endocrine gland that produces T-cells (Thymus)

(continues)

B	I	N	G	O
Outer ear (Auricle)	Lining of the uterus (Endometrium)	**N** Largest of 3 middle ear bones (Malleus)	**G** Division of the cerebrum (Parietal Lobe)	**O** Endocrine gland located in neck (Thyroid)
Tiny air cells in the lungs (Aveoli)	Outermost layer of skin (Epidermis)	**N** Lower jaw bone (Mandible)	**G** Area between the vagina and rectum (Perineum)	**O** Lower long bone of the leg (Tibia)
Muscle located in front part of upper arm (Biceps)	Stores sperm (Epididymus)	**N** Pigment that gives color to hair, skin, and eyes (Melanin)	**G** Lining of abdominal cavity (Peritoneum)	**O** Lymph tissue located in throat (Tonsils)
Stores urine before it is excreted from body (Bladder)	Prevents food from entering trachea (Epiglottis)	**N** Wrist bone (Metacarpal)	**G** Throat (Pharynx)	**O** Tube that connects larynx to bronchi (Trachea)
Connects cerebral hemisphere with spinal cord (Brain stem)	Tube between pharynx and stomach (Esophagus)	**N** Part of brain stem (Medulla oblongata)	**G** Produces melatonin (Pineal Gland)	**O** Large muscle that runs from upper neck to shoulder blades (Trapezius)

(Continues)

B	I	N	G	O
B Mammary glands (Breasts)	**I** Female sex hormone (Estrogen)	**N** Valve between left atrium and left ventricle (Mitral Valve)	**G** Muscle on front of thigh (Quadracep)	**O** Valve between the right atrium and right ventricle (Tricuspid Valve)
B Small subdivisions of the bronchus (Bronchiole)	**I** Connects ear to throat (Eustachian Tube)	**N** Tubular structure in kidney (Nephron)	**G** Bone on thumb side of forearm (Radius)	**O** Eardrum (Tympanic Membrane)
B One of two branches of the trachea (Bronchus)	**I** Carries eggs from ovaries to uterus (Fallopian Tubes)	**N** Nerve cell (Neuron)	**G** End of large colon (Rectum)	**O** Inner bone of forearm (Ulna)
B Fluid-filled sac surrounding a joint (Bursa)	**I** Thigh bone (Femur)	**N** Bone in back of head (Occipital Bone)	**G** Blood cells that carry oxygen (Red Blood Cells)	**O** Tubes that attach kidneys to bladder (Ureter)
B Microscopic blood vessel connecting arterioles with venules (Capillary)	**I** Slender lower-leg bone (Fibula)	**N** Nerve that carries impulses from eye to brain (Optic Nerve)	**G** Part of eye which contain receptor cells (Retina)	**O** Tube that carries urine from bladder to outside the body (Urethra)

(Continues)

B	I	N	G	O
B Opaque middle layer of eyeball (Choroid)	**I** Pigment of blood containing iron (Hemoglobin)	**N** The Auricle (Pinna)	**G** Sack holding testicles (Scrotum)	**O** Lower chamber of heart (Ventricle)
B Collar bone (Clavicle)	**I** Chemical messenger with a specialized function (Hormone)	**N** Pea-sized gland at the base of the brain (Pituitary)	**G** Located in the dermis. Secretes sebum (Sebaceous Glands)	**O** Back Bone (Vertebrae)
B Spiral-shaped passage in inner ear (Cochlea)	**I** Bone between mandible and Laryngopharynx (Hyoid)	**N** Straw-colored part of blood (Plasma)	**G** Located in inner ear – they help maintain equilibrium (Semi-circular canals)	**O** Internal Organs (Viscera)
B Part of large intestine (Colon)	**I** Located below thalamus. Regulates body temp., autonomic nervous, and other systems (Hypothalamus)	**N** Multilayered membrane surrounding lungs (Pleura)	**G** Cartilage separating the two nostrils (Nasal Septum)	**O** Female external genitalia (Vulva)
B Receptor cells of the retina (Cones)	**I** The anvil (Incus)	**N** Bridge at the base of the brain (Pons)	**G** Establishes basic rhythm of the heart (Sinoatrial Node (SA))	**O** Leukocytes (White blood cells)

(Continues)

B	I	N	G	O
B Bone of wrist (Carpal)	**I** Loose skin covering end of penis (Foreskin)	**N** Female gonad (Ovary)	**G** An antigen substance in blood (RH Factor)	**O** Outer opening of urethra (Urinary Meatus)
B Brain and spinal cord (Central nervous system)	**I** Concentrates and stores bile (Gallbladder)	**N** Female egg (Ovum)	**G** Vertebrae between coccyx and lumbar vertebrae (Sacrum)	**O** Fleshy mass hanging at back of throat (Uvula)
B Lower or back brain (Cerebellum)	**I** Excretory organ (Gland)	**N** Kneecap (Patella)	**G** Glands producing saliva (Salivary glands)	**O** Excretory duct of the testes (Vas Deferens)
B Outer layer of cerebrum (Cerebral cortex)	**I** Head of penis (Glans)	**N** Cranial and spinal nerves (Peripheral nervous system)	**G** Shoulder blade (Scapula)	**O** Carries blood towards the heart (Vein)
B Largest portion of brain (Cerebrum)	**I** Large muscle of buttocks (Gluteous maximus)	**N** Bones of fingers and toes (Phalanges)	**G** White-outer coat of eye (Sclera)	**O** Large vein emptying into the right atrium of heart (Vena cava)

(Continues)

B Membrane lining eyelids and covering sclera (Conjunctiva)	**I** Hormone secreted by pancreas (Insulin)	**N** Hormone secreted by corpus luteum (Progesterone)	**G** Extends from pyloric sphincter to large intestine (Small intestine)	**O** Cheek bones (Zygomatic arch)
B Transparent film in front of pupil (Cornea)	**I** Skin (Integumentary)	**N** Male reproductive gland that surrounds part of urethra (Prostate gland)	**G** Male gamete (Spermatozoa)	**O** Cell produced when egg and sperm unite (Zygote)
B Band of fibers connecting two brain hemispheres (Corpus callosum)	**I** Colored part of eye (Iris)	**N** Artery connecting heart and lungs (Pulmonary Artery)	**G** Circular muscle constricting an opening (Sphincter)	**O**
G Space between axon and neuron (Synapse)	**G** Part of autonomic nervous system (Sympathetic Nerves)	**N** Opening into inner eye (Pupil)	**G** Nerves running from brain down vertebrae (Spinal cord)	**O**
G Holds and digests food (Stomach)	**G** Breastbone (Sternum)	**G** Stirrup (Stapes)	**G** Ductless gland below diaphragm (Spleen)	**O**

Prompts And Correct Questions For Anatomy Challenge Game

Integumentary System

Points	Prompt	Question
100	The fluid secreted through the pores to help cool the body	What is perspiration? OR What is sweat?
200	A burn that may be painless because the nerves have been destroyed	What is a third degree burn?
300	The second innermost layer of skin that contains hair follicles and sweat and oil glands	What is the dermis?
400	The substance that gives skin its color	What is melanin?
500	Innermost layer of skin that contains fatty and connective tissue	What is subcutaneous tissue?

Skeletal System

Points	Prompt	Question
100	Contains the cranium and facial bones	What is the skull?
200	Type of joint that moves in only one plane, backward and forward	What is a hinge joint?
300	Condition in which the bones lose their density and weaken	What is osteoporosis?
400	The only moveable bone in the face	What is the mandible?
500	Movement toward the body's midline	What is adduction?

Muscular System

Points	Prompt	Question
100	Type of muscle that moves without conscious effort	What is involuntary muscle?
200	Type of muscle that moves internal organs	What is smooth muscle?
300	Point where muscle attaches to the bone that does not move when the muscle contracts	What is the origin?
400	Tissue that attaches muscle to bone	What is a tendon?
500	Circular band of muscle fibers that constricts a natural body opening	What is a sphincter?

Nervous System

Points	Prompt	Question
100	Largest and uppermost part of the brain	What is the cerebrum?
200	Recurring seizures in the brain caused by excessive irregular electrical activity	What is epilepsy?
300	The outer three layers of membrane covering the brain and spinal cord	What is the dura mater?
400	Part of the brain that controls appetite, temperature, and sleep	What is the hypothalamus?
500	Special capillaries that prevent drugs in the bloodstream from entering the brain	What is the blood-brain barrier?

Special Senses

Points	Prompt	Question
100	Third innermost layer of the eye that contains light-sensitive nerve cells	What is the retina?
200	A decrease in ability to focus on close objects	What is presbyopia?
300	Responsible for maintaining equilibrium	What is the inner ear? OR What are the semicircular canals?
400	Eye disorder caused by increase in intraocular pressure	What is glaucoma?
500	Inflammation of the lining of the nose	What is rhinitis?

Endocrine System

Points	Prompt	Question
100	Gland that produces insulin	What is the pancreas?
200	Hormone that makes it possible for sugar to pass from the blood to be used for energy	What is insulin?
300	Gland that maintains the body's normal level of metabolism	What is the thyroid?
400	Condition in which blood sugar level is less than normal	What is hypoglycemia?
500	Hormone that prepares the uterus for pregnancy	What is progesterone?

(Continues)

Circulatory System

Points	Prompt	Question
100	Procedure that measures the electrical activity of the heart	What is an EKG? OR What is an ECG?
200	The one vein in the body that carries oxygen-rich blood	What is the pulmonary vein?
300	Condition in which blood does not clot normally	What is hemophilia?
400	Pressure in arteries when the heart is contracting and pushing blood into the aorta	What is systolic? OR What is systolic blood pressure?
500	Red pigment in blood	What is hemoglobin?

Respiratory System

Points	Prompt	Question
100	Structure commonly known as the throat	What is the pharynx?
200	Muscular partition that aids in the process of breathing	What is the diaphragm?
300	Thin, moist membrane that covers the lungs	What is the pleura?
400	Small flap of cartilage that prevents food from entering the respiratory tract	What is the epiglottis?
500	Rapid breathing that causes the body to lose carbon dioxide too quickly	What is hyperventilation?

Digestive System

Points	Prompt	Question
100	Another name for digestive canal	What is the alimentary canal?
200	Muscular tube that connects the pharynx and stomach	What is the esophagus?
300	Part that absorbs most of the water from the body's waste material	What is the colon? OR What is the large intestine?
400	Organ that produces bile and removes poisons from the blood	What is the liver?
500	Enlargement or inflammation of the rectal column veins	What are hemorrhoids?

(Continues)

Urinary and Reproductive Systems

Points	Prompt	Question
100	Hollow muscular organ that stores urine	What is the urinary bladder? OR What is the bladder?
200	Use of a mechanical device to serve as a kidney substitute	What is dialysis?
300	Basic structural and functional unit of the kidney	What is a nephron?
400	Human egg immediately after being fertilized by a sperm	What is a zygote?
500	Absence of the menstrual cycle	What is amenorrhea?

Mini-Dissection Picture Guide

1. Bones.   Examine the bones to see their shape and structure. Look for where they attach to ligaments. If you have neck bones, look for the spinal cavity and spinal process. Break or cut a long bone to examine the marrow.

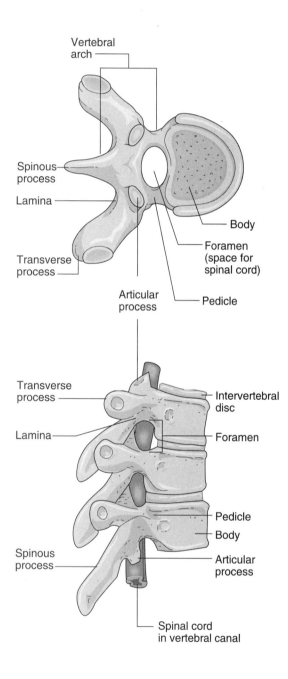

Vertebral arch
Spinous process
Lamina
Transverse process
Articular process
Body
Foramen (space for spinal cord)
Pedicle

Transverse process
Lamina
Spinous process
Intervertebral disc
Foramen
Pedicle
Body
Articular process
Spinal cord in vertebral canal

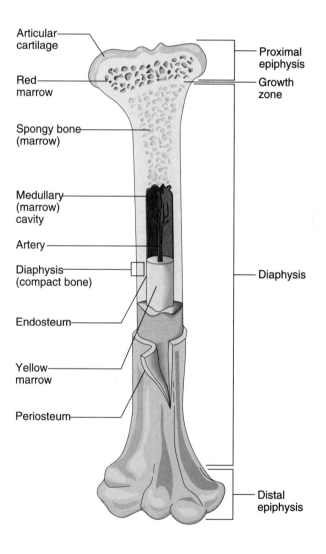

Articular cartilage
Red marrow
Spongy bone (marrow)
Medullary (marrow) cavity
Artery
Diaphysis (compact bone)
Endosteum
Yellow marrow
Periosteum
Proximal epiphysis
Growth zone
Diaphysis
Distal epiphysis

2. Turkey leg.   Cut through the layers of the leg and look for muscles, membranes, sheaths, ligaments, and tendons.

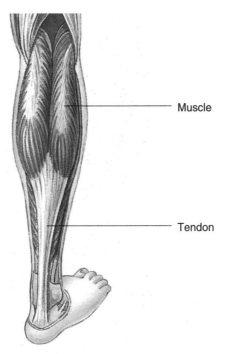

Muscle

Tendon

3. Beef heart.   Observe the arteries on the surface and the openings for the vena cava and aorta. Note the pericardium. Cut the heart down the center and note the thickness of the walls, septum, atria, ventricles, valves, and papillary muscles.

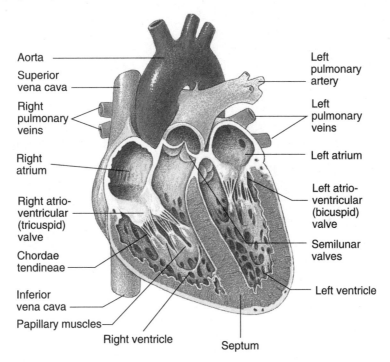

Aorta

Superior vena cava

Right pulmonary veins

Right atrium

Right atrio-ventricular (tricuspid) valve

Chordae tendineae

Inferior vena cava

Papillary muscles

Right ventricle

Left pulmonary artery

Left pulmonary veins

Left atrium

Left atrio-ventricular (bicuspid) valve

Semilunar valves

Left ventricle

Septum

4. **Kidneys.** Cut lengthwise and look for the outer and inner layers (cortex and medulla) and internal system of cavities, including the renal pelvis in the center.

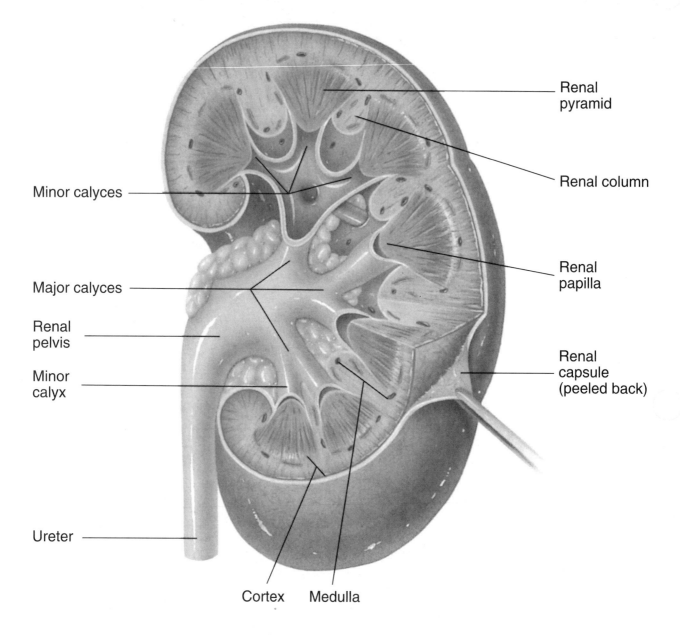

Renal pyramid

Renal column

Minor calyces

Renal papilla

Major calyces

Renal pelvis

Minor calyx

Renal capsule (peeled back)

Ureter

Cortex   Medulla

5. Cow eye.   Examine the outer surface (sclera, choroid coat, cornea, iris) before cutting the eye in half to view the interior structure.

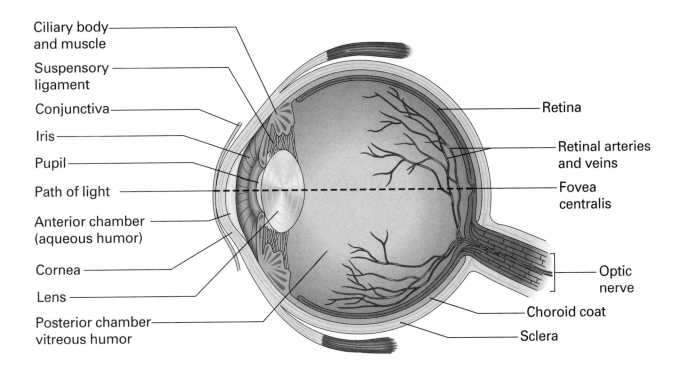

Ciliary body and muscle

Suspensory ligament

Conjunctiva

Iris

Pupil

Path of light

Anterior chamber (aqueous humor)

Cornea

Lens

Posterior chamber vitreous humor

Retina

Retinal arteries and veins

Fovea centralis

Optic nerve

Choroid coat

Sclera

Human Body Scavenger Hunt I

Working with your partner, write in a body part or list of related items for each number. Then write a brief description of the part, including its function.

Number	Part	Function	Source of Information
1			
2			
3			
4			
5			
6			
7			
8			
9			
10			
11			

Human Body Scavenger Hunt II

Working with your partner, write in a body part or list of related items for each number. Then write a brief description of the part, including its function.

Number	Part	Function	Source of Information
6			
7			
8			
9			
10			
11			
12			
13			
14			
15			
16			
17			

Diseases and Disorders

1. Alzheimer's disease
2. anemia
3. aneurysm
4. arteriosclerosis
5. arthritis
6. asthma
7. Bell's palsy
8. bronchitis
9. carpal tunnel syndrome
10. cataracts
11. cerebral vascular accident
12. conjunctivitis
13. diabetes mellitus
14. eczema
15. emphysema
16. epilepsy
17. fibromyalgia
18. glaucoma
19. gout
20. hemophilia
21. hepatitis B
22. hypertension
23. impetigo
24. leukemia
25. macular degeneration
26. melanoma
27. Ménière's disease
28. meningitis
29. multiple sclerosis
30. muscular dystrophy
31. myocardial infarction
32. osteoporosis
33. otitis media
34. Parkinson's disease
35. pneumonia
36. psoriasis
37. shingles
38. tetanus
39. tinnitus
40. tuberculosis

Bingo Cards

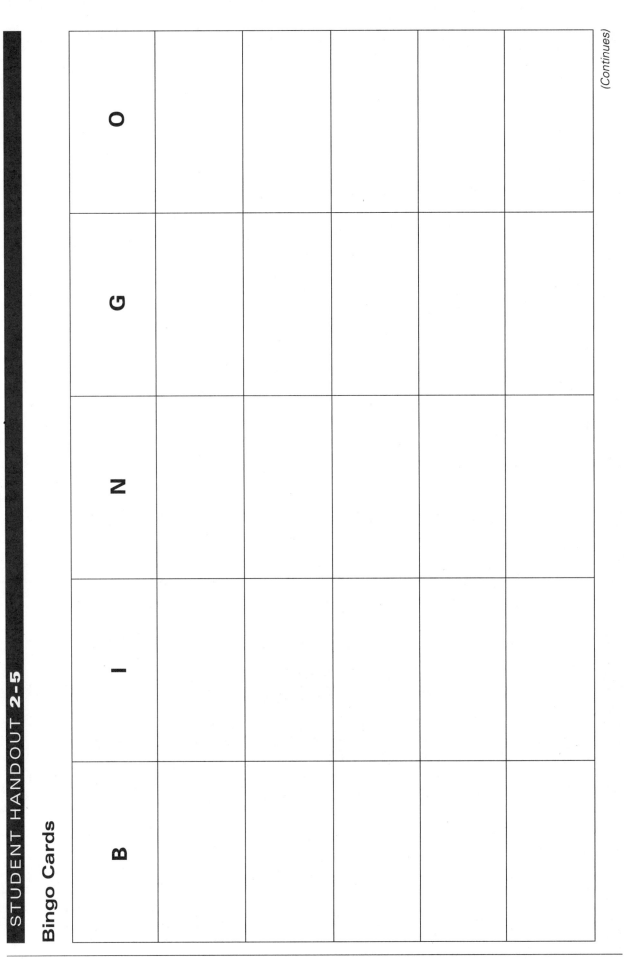

B	I	N	G	O

(Continues)

B	I	N	G	O
Bronchiole	Estrogen	Kidney	Radius	Tympanic Membrane
Breasts	Eustachian Tube	Neuron	Rectum	Ulna
Atrium	Fallopian Tubes	Occipital Bone	Red Blood Cells	Ureter
Bronchus	Epidermis	Optic Nerve	Stomach	Urethra
Capillary	Fibula	Ovary	RH Factor	Thymus

(Continues)

B	I	N	G	O
Aqueous Humor	Epidermis	Mandible	Peritoneum	Tibia
Artery	Dendrite	Kidney	Pericardium	Testes
Atrium	Dermis	Larynx	Parasympathetic Nerves	Zygote
Auricle	Diaphram	Liver	Parathyroid	Thalamus
Aveoli	Diaphysis	Lymph	Parietal	Thymus

(Continues)

B	I	N	G	O
Artery	Diaphragm	Metacarpal	Parathyroid	Thalamus
Atrium	Diaphysis	Lymph	Pericardium	Thymus
Auricle	Endometrium	Malleus	Parietal Lobe	Thyroid
Alveoli	Epidermis	Mandible	Perineum	Tibia
Biceps	Epididymus	Medulla Oblongata	Peritoneum	Tonsils

(Continues)

B	I	N	G	O
Atrium	Diaphysis	Lymph	Parietal Lobe	Thymus
Auricle	Endometrium	Malleus	Retina	Thyroid
Alveoli	Epidermis	Mandible	Perineum	Tibia
Biceps	Epididymus	Medulla Oblongata	Pharynx	Tonsils
Bladder	Epiglottis	Melanin	Peritoneum	Trachea

(Continues)

B	I	N	G	O
Auricle	Endometrium	Malleus	Parietal Lobe	Thyroid
Alveoli	Epiglottis	Mandible	Perineum	Tibia
Biceps	Esophagus	Medulla Oblongata	Peritoneum	Tonsils
Bladder	Epidermis	Melanin	Pharynx	Trachea
Brain Stem	Epididymus	Metacarpal	Pineal Gland	Trapezius

(Continues)

B	I	N	G	O
Alveoli	Epidermis	Medulla Oblongata	Peritoneum	Trachea
Biceps	Epididymus	Melanin	Perineum	Trapezius
Bladder	Epiglottis	Metacarpal	Pineal Gland	Tricuspid Valve
Brain Stem	Esophagus	Mitral Valve	Pharynx	Tympanic Membrane
Breasts	Estrogen	Nephron	Quadracep	Ulna

(Continues)

B	I	N	G	O
Biceps	Epididymus	Melanin	Pharynx	Tibia
Bladder	Epiglottis	Metacarpal	Pineal Gland	Tonsils
Brain Stem	Esophagus	Mitral Valve	Quadracep	Trachea
Breasts	Estrogen	Nephron	Radius	Trapezius
Bronchiole	Eustachian Tube	Neuron	Rectum	Tricuspid Valve

(Continues)

B	I	N	G	O
Bladder	Fallopian Tubes	Metacarpal	Pineal Gland	Tonsils
Brain Stem	Esophagus	Mitral Valve	Quadracep	Trachea
Breasts	Estrogen	Nephron	Radius	Tricuspid Valve
Bronchiole	Eustachian Tube	Neuron	Rectum	Trapezius
Bronchus	Tricuspid Valve	Occipital Bone	Red Blood Cells	Tympanic Membrane

(Continues)

B	I	N	G	O
Brain Stem	Esophagus	Mitral Valve	Quadracep	Trapezius
Breasts	Estrogen	Nephron	Radius	Tricuspid Valve
Bronchiole	Eustachian Tube	Neuron	Rectum	Tympanic Membrane
Bronchus	Fallopian Tubes	Occipital Bone	Red Blood Cells	Ulna
Bursa	Femer	Optic Nerve	Retina	Ureter

(Continues)

B	I	N	G	O
Bronchiole	Estrogen	Nephron	Radius	Tympanic Membrane
Breasts	Eustachian Tube	Neuron	Rectum	Ulna
Bursa	Fallopian Tubes	Occipital Bone	Red Blood Cells	Ureter
Bronchus	Femer	Optic Nerve	Retina	Urethra
Capillary	Fibula	Ovary	RH Factor	Urinary Meatus

(Continues)

B	I	N	G	O
Bronchiole	Fallopian Tubes	Neuron	Rectum	Ulna
Bronchus	Femer	Occipital Bone	Red Blood Cells	Ureter
Bursa	Fibula	Optic Nerve	Retina	Urethra
Capillary	Foreskin	Ovary	RH Factor	Urinary Meatus
Carpal	Gallbladder	Ovum	Sacrum	Uvula

(Continues)

B	I	N	G	O
Bursa	Femer	Occipital Bone	Red Blood Cells	Ureter
Bronchus	Fibula	Optic Nerve	Retina	Urethra
Carpal	Foreskin	Ovary	RH Factor	Urinary Meatus
Capillary	Gallbladder	Ovum	Sacram	Uvula
Central Nervous System	Gland	Patella	Salivary Glands	Vas Deferens

(Continues)

B	I	N	G	O
Capillary	Foreskin	Ovary	RH Factor	Urinary Meatus
Carpal	Gallbladder	Ovum	Sacrum	Uvula
Central Nervous System	Gluteous Maximus	Patella	Salivary Glands	Vas Deferens
Cerebellum	Glans	Plasma	Scapula	Vein
Cerebral Cortex	Gland	Phalanges	Sclera	Vena Cava

(Continues)

B	I	N	G	O
Carpal	Gallbladder	Patella	Sacram	Vas Deferens
Central Nervous System	Gland	Plasma	Salivary Glands	Vein
Cerebellum	Glans	Phalanges	Scapula	Vena Cava
Cerebral Cortex	Gluteous Maximus	Pinna	Sclera	Ventricle
Cerebrum	Hemoglobin	Pituitary	Scrotum	Vertibrae

(Continues)

B	I	N	G	O
Central Nervous System	Gland	Pinna	Scapula	Vein
Cerebellum	Glans	Pituitary	Sclera	Vena Cava
Cerebral Cortex	Gluteous Maximus	Plasma	Scrotum	Ventricle
Cerebrum	Hemoglobin	Pleura	Sebaceous Glands	Vertibrae
Choroid	Hormone	Pons	Semi-circular Canals	Viscera

(Continues)

B	I	N	G	O
Cerebellum	Glans	Phalanges	Sclera	Vas Deferens
Cerebral Cortex	Gluteous Maximus	Pinna	Scrotum	Vein
Cerebrum	Hemoglobin	Pituitary	Sebaceous Glands	Vena Cava
Choroid	Hormone	Plasma	Semi-circular Canals	Ventricle
Clavicle	Hyoid	Pleura	Nasal Septum	Vertibrae

(Continues)

B	I	N	G	O
Cerebral Cortex	Hemoglobin	Pinna	Scrotum	Vein
Cerebrum	Hormone	Pituitary	Sebaceous Glands	Vena Cava
Choroid	Hyoid	Plasma	Semi-circular Canals	Ventricle
Clavicle	Hypothalamus	Pleura	Nasal Septum	Vertibrae
Cochlea	Incus	Pons	Sinoatrial (SA) Node	Viscera

(Continues)

B	I	N	G	O
Cerebrum	Gallbladder	Optic Nerve	RH Factor	Vein
Choroid	Hormone	Pituitary	Sebaceous Glands	Vena Cava
Clavicle	Hyoid	Plasma	Semi-circular Canals	Ureter
Cochlea	Hypothalamus	Pleura	Nasal Septum	Vertibrae
Colon	Incus	Pons	Sympathetic Nerves	Viscera

(Continues)

B	I	N	G	O
Choroid	Gallbladder	Optic Nerve	RH Factor	Vein
Clavicle	Hormone	Pituitary	Sebaceous	Vena Cava
Cochlea	Gluteous Maximus	Plasma	Semi-circular Canals	Tricuspid Valve
Colon	Hypothalamus	Nephron	Red Blood Cells	Tympanic Membrane
Cones	Incus	Pons	Retina	Viscera

(Continues)

B	I	N	G	O
Clavicle	Hormone	Pituitary	Sinoatrial (SA) Node	Vena Cava
Cochlea	Hyoid	Plasma	Small Intestine	Ventricle
Colon	Hypothalamus	Pleura	Spermatozoa	Vertibrae
Cones	Incus	Pons	Sphincter	Viscera
Conjunctiva	Insulin	Progesterone	Sternum	Vulva

(Continues)

B	I	N	G	O
Cochlea	Hyoid	Plasma	Small Intestine	Ventricle
Colon	Hypothalamus	Pleura	Spermatozoa	Vertibrae
Cones	Incus	Pons	Sphincter	Viscera
Conjunctiva	Insulin	Progesterone	Spinal Cord	Vulva
Cornea	Integumentary	Prostate Gland	Spleen	White Blood Cells

(Continues)

B	I	N	G	O
Colon	Incus	Pons	Sphincter	Viscera
Cones	Insulin	Progesterone	Spinal Cord	Vulva
Conjunctiva	Integumentary	Prostate Gland	Spleen	White Blood Cells
Cornea	Iris	Pulmonary Artery	Stapes	Zygomatic Arch
Corpus Callosum	Hypothalamus	Pupil	Sternum	Zygote

(Continues)

B	I	N	G	O
Bursa	Incus	Pons	Synapse	Viscera
Capillary	Insulin	Keratin	Spinal Cord	Testosterone
Carpal	Epiglottis	Kidney	Spleen	Thalamus
Cornea	Esophagus	Larynx	Stapes	Thymus
Corpus Callosum	Estrogen	Pupil	Sternum	Zygote

(Continues)

B	I	N	G	O
Bursa	Incus	Mandible	Sphincter	Tendon
Capillary	Insulin	Keratin	Pons	Testes
Carpal	Epiglottis	Kidney	Spleen	Thalamus
Cornea	Esophagus	Larynx	Stapes	Thymus
Corpus Callosum	Estrogen	Melanin	Scapula	Zygote

(Continues)

B	I	N	G	O
Bursa	Incus	Metacarpal	Sphincter	Tendon
Artery	Dermis	Mitral Valve	Pons	Ulna
Atrium	Diaphragm	Kidney	Quadracep	Ureter
Auricle	Esophagus	Larynx	Radius	Thymus
Corpus Callosum	Estrogen	Melanin	Pupil	Zygote

(Continues)

Location of Taste Buds

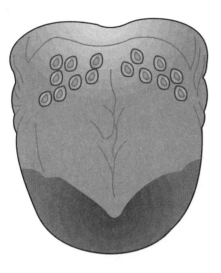

Sweet

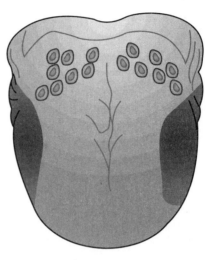

Sour

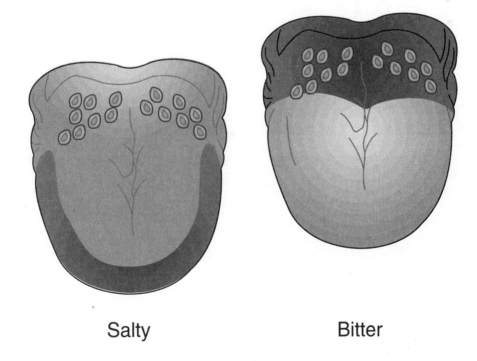

Salty

Bitter

Diagram of a Taste Bud

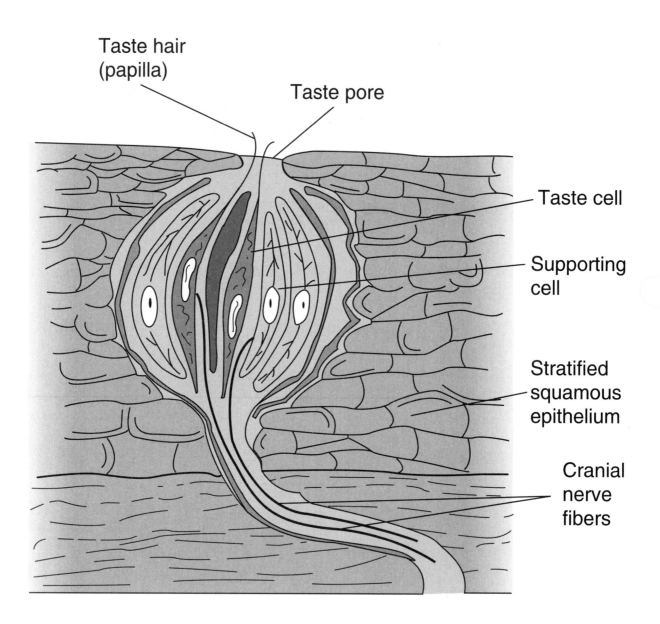

Taste hair (papilla)

Taste pore

Taste cell

Supporting cell

Stratified squamous epithelium

Cranial nerve fibers

Light Rays and Vision

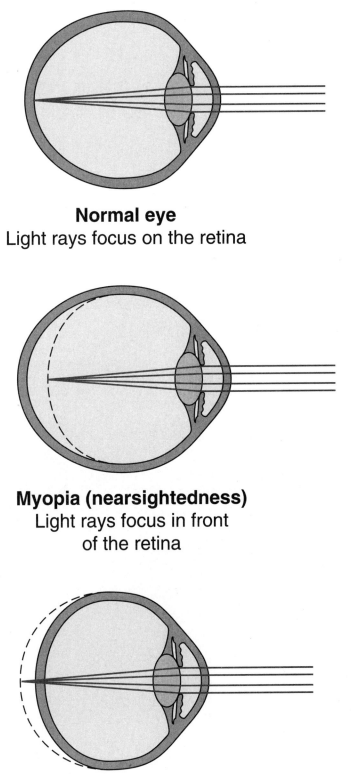

Normal eye
Light rays focus on the retina

Myopia (nearsightedness)
Light rays focus in front
of the retina

Hyperopia (farsightedness)
Light rays focus beyond
the retina

Structures of the Eye

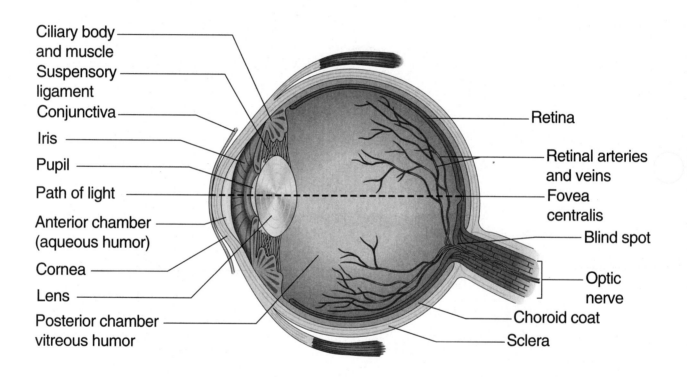

Ciliary body and muscle

Suspensory ligament

Conjunctiva

Iris

Pupil

Path of light

Anterior chamber (aqueous humor)

Cornea

Lens

Posterior chamber vitreous humor

Retina

Retinal arteries and veins

Fovea centralis

Blind spot

Optic nerve

Choroid coat

Sclera

Pathway of Urine

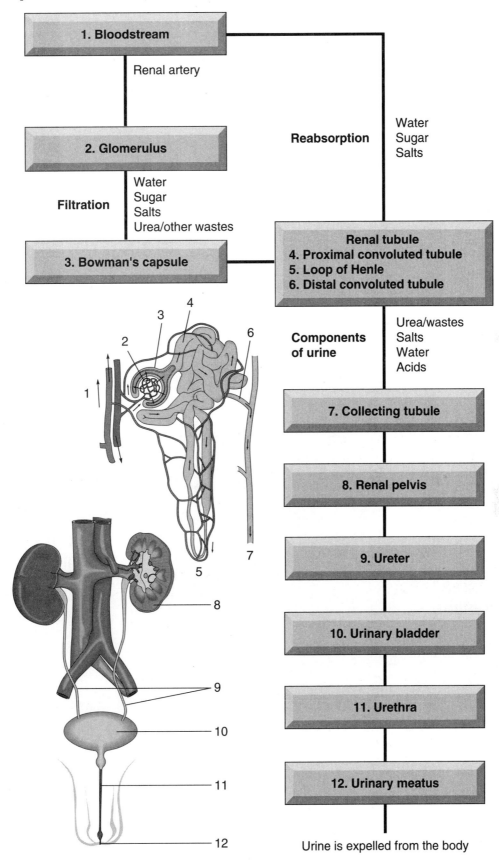

```
1. Bloodstream
      |
   Renal artery
      |
2. Glomerulus                    Reabsorption    Water
      |                                          Sugar
   Filtration  Water                             Salts
              Sugar
              Salts
              Urea/other wastes
      |
3. Bowman's capsule ──── Renal tubule
                         4. Proximal convoluted tubule
                         5. Loop of Henle
                         6. Distal convoluted tubule
                                |
                         Components    Urea/wastes
                         of urine      Salts
                                       Water
                                       Acids
                                |
                         7. Collecting tubule
                                |
                         8. Renal pelvis
                                |
                         9. Ureter
                                |
                         10. Urinary bladder
                                |
                         11. Urethra
                                |
                         12. Urinary meatus
                                |
                    Urine is expelled from the body
```

Pathway of Food

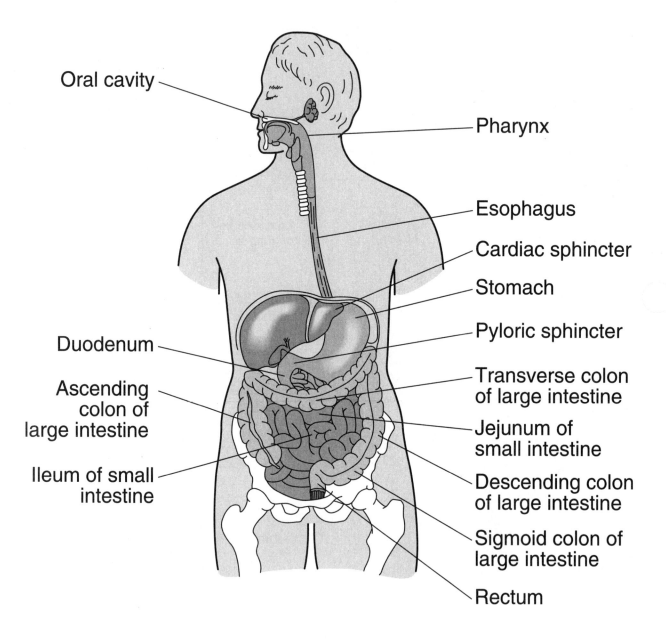

Oral cavity

Pharynx

Esophagus

Cardiac sphincter

Stomach

Pyloric sphincter

Transverse colon
of large intestine

Duodenum

Jejunum of
small intestine

Ascending
colon of
large intestine

Descending colon
of large intestine

Ileum of small
intestine

Sigmoid colon of
large intestine

Rectum

Pathway of Respiration

Pathway of Respiration
Air enters through the
1. Nasal cavity
2. Pharynx
3. Larynx
4. Trachea
5. Bronchial tree
6. Bronchus
7. Bronchiole
8. Alveoli

Nasal cavity

Larynx

Pharynx

Trachea ⎤
Right lung
Bronchus ⎦

Bronchial tree

Alveoli

Bronchiole

Pathway of Hearing

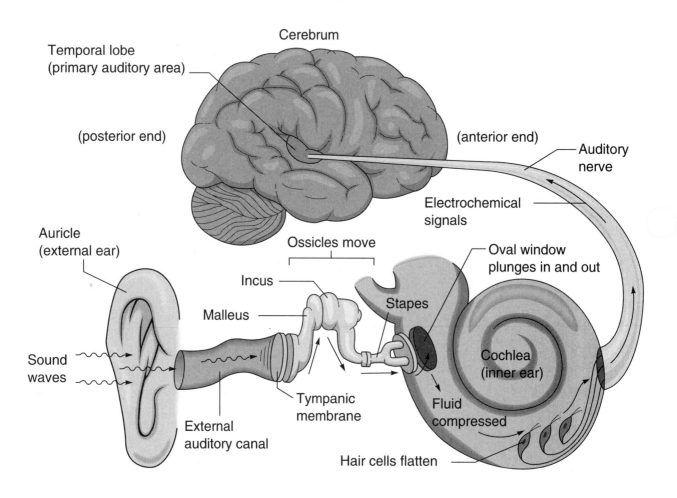

Pathway of Vision

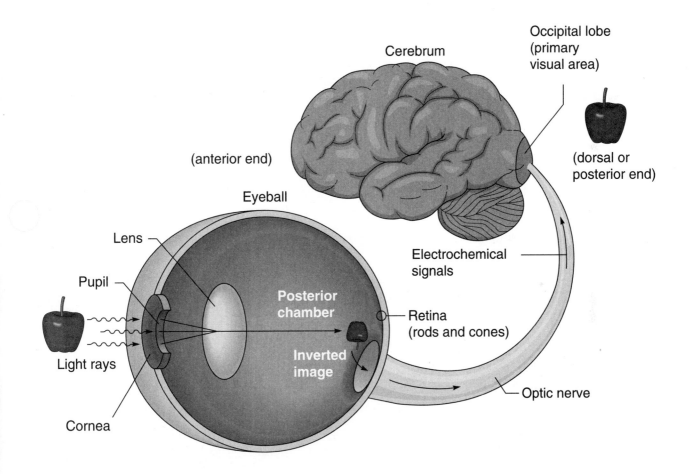

Anatomy Challenge Categories I

Integumentary System	Skeletal System	Muscular System	Nervous System	Special Senses
100	100	100	100	100
200	200	200	200	200
300	300	300	300	300
400	400	400	400	400
500	500	500	500	500

Anatomy Challenge Categories II

Endocrine System	Circulatory System	Respiratory System	Digestive System	Urinary and Reproductive Systems
100	100	100	100	100
200	200	200	200	200
300	300	300	300	300
400	400	400	400	400
500	500	500	500	500

Vital Signs, Wellness, and Prevention

INTRODUCTION

Tasks connected with vital signs are often difficult for new students to master, yet are some of the most important skills they must learn. Taking an accurate pulse or blood pressure, counting respirations, and reading a thermometer accurately are essential to providing quality health care. The activities in this chapter provide students with opportunities to improve their skill in taking vital signs, learn facts about what they measure, and provide meaningful information about health status.

In addition to vital signs, students will learn about wellness and disease prevention. Chronic conditions are today's major health problems. Many can be prevented or decreased in severity by lifestyle changes. Knowledge and practice of wellness and prevention strategies are vital to good health. With longer life spans, quality of life and taking responsibility for one's own health are increasingly important concerns for us all. Mastering skills in these areas will enable students to be positive role models and healthier, more effective caregivers.

ACTIVITY 3-1
MONITORING VITAL SIGNS

What Students Will Learn

- The effect of activities of daily living on vital signs.
- How to proficiently chart vital signs.

What You Will Need

- Aneroid sphygmomanometer for each student.
- Stethoscope for each student.
- Digital thermometer for each student.
- Supplies for cleaning thermometers.

What To Do

1. Have each student choose a classmate or a close friend or relative they see frequently to act as a patient.
2. Give students the following instructions:
   a. Begin by taking vital signs on the patient after rest (sitting or lying down quietly for 10–15 minutes). If possible, take vital signs first thing in the morning before the patient gets out of bed.

    b. Chart the results.

    c. Over the next several days, take vital signs after various activities such as eating, climbing the stairs or other physical activity, before and after a major exam or stressful day at work, at the end of a regular class, and the like. Chart each of these results.

3. If students are able to and have access to Excel software or a similar program, have them type in results and run a line chart. You can put a few of these charts on overheads to show the class (without names, of course).

4. Have students analyze what has been charted and summarize their observations of the effect of activities of daily living on temperature, pulse, and blood pressure.

Follow-up Discussion

1. Do the vital signs all fluctuate?

2. Is time of day significant?

3. Is activity level significan?

4. Are persons who are more active and who maintain a normal body weight different in their vital sign fluctuations than those who are sedentary or overweight?

ACTIVITY 3-2
VITAL FACTS

What Students Will Learn

- Facts about vital signs.
- The significance of various vital signs.

What You Will Need

- Instructor Sheet 3-1, True/False Statements About Vital Signs.

What To Do

1. Divide the class into two teams and have each team count off to determine the order in which students respond.

2. Flip a coin to determine which team starts.

3. Read aloud a fact from Instructor Sheet 3-1. Player number 1 on the starting team is given the opportunity to state whether the fact is true or false. If the answer is correct, the team scores a point. If it is incorrect, the team loses a point.

Instructor Sheet **3-1**   Instructor Sheet **3-1**   Instructor Sheet **3-1**

                                    (Continued)   *(Continued)*

4. After each statement, briefly discuss the correct answer.
5. Play alternates between the teams until all facts have been used, all students have had a chance to play, or the time allotted for the game runs out. The winner is the team with the most points/highest score.

Follow-up Discussion

1. Why is it important for the health care worker to learn more about vital signs than simply how to take and record them?
2. What do vital signs tell us about the health status of a patient?

ACTIVITY 3-3
WELLNESS CROSSWORD PUZZLE

What Students Will Learn

- Wellness vocabulary.

What You Will Need

- A copy of Student Handout 3-1, Wellness Crossword Puzzle, for each student.
- Transparency 3-1, Wellness Crossword Puzzle.
- Transparency 3-2, Wellness Crossword Puzzle Solution.
- Instructor Sheet 3-2, Wellness Crossword Puzzle Solution.

What To Do

1. Distribute a copy of the crossword puzzle (Student Handout 3-1 to each student. Tell students that some answers consist of more than one word. These are run together without spaces on the puzzle.
2. Students can work on the puzzle in class or as a homework assignment.
3. When students have completed the puzzle, use the overhead to show the answers (Transparency 3-2) so students can correct their work.
4. Alternate activity: Display Transparency 3-1 and have the class solve the puzzle as a group.

Follow-up Discussion

1. Why is a knowledge of wellness important for today's health care worker?
2. When might you apply wellness knowledge in your future occupation?

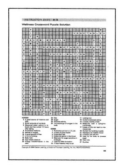
Instructor Sheet **3-2**

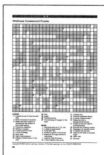
Student Handout **3-1**

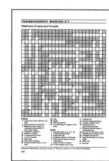
Transparency Master **3-1**

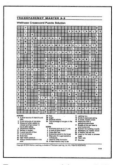
Transparency Master **3-2**

ACTIVITY 3-4
WELLNESS WORD SEARCH

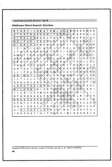

Instructor Sheet **3-3**

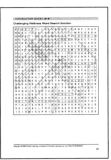

Instructor Sheet **3-4**

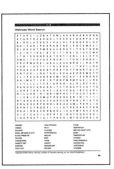

Student Handout **3-2**

What Students Will Learn

- Wellness vocabulary.

What You Will Need

- A copy of Student Handout 3-2, Wellness Word Search, or Student Handout 3-3, Challenging Wellness Word Search, for each student. Tell students that some answers consist of more than one word. These are run together without spaces on the puzzle.
- Transparencies 3-3, Wellness Word Search, or 3-5, Challenging Wellness Word Search.
- Transparencies 3-4 Wellness Word Search Solutions, or 3-6 Challenging Wellness Word Search Solutions.
- Instructor Sheet 3-3, Wellness Word Search Solution or 3-4, Challenging Wellness Word Search Solutions.

What To Do

1. Assign the wellness word search or challenging wellness word search for a classroom or homework activity.
2. If the activity is done in class, you can have a contest and award a prize (such as extra points, certificates, small trinkets) to the student who successfully completes the assignment first.
3. See Instructor Sheets 3-3 and 3-4 for the solutions, and use the corresponding transparencies to show the solutions, which are the same for both puzzles, to the class. Note that the challenging word search is difficult and might be frustrating for some students. This is actually a two-part activity in that the student must first identify the word from its definition before searching for it in the puzzle.

Follow-up Discussion

1. Ask review questions about the words on the puzzle to check for student understanding of the terms. Ask students how the terms relate to wellness and disease prevention.

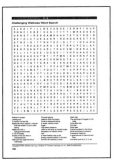

Student Handout **3-3**

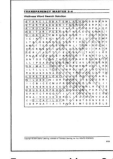

Transparency Master **3-3**

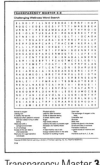

Transparency Master **3-4**

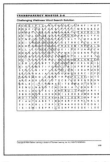

Transparency Master **3-5**

Transparency Master **3-6**

ACTIVITY 3-5
WELLNESS POSTERS

What Students Will Learn
- Positive lifestyle habits.

What You Will Need
- A list of topics related to wellness, such as alcohol, physical exercise, proper nutrition and weight control, safe sex, smoking, stress management.
- Supplies for groups to make posters: posterboard, marking pens, glue, old magazines, colored paper, and so on.
- Access to reference materials about wellness, such as journals, books, and the Internet.

What To Do
1. Divide the class into groups of three to five students.
2. Assign each group—or let them choose—a wellness topic.
3. Instruct the groups to research and discuss wellness strategies and good habits related to their topics and then make posters to illustrate them.
4. Ask students to present their completed posters to the class along with good health habits to the class.

Follow-up Discussion
1. What did you learn from making your poster?
2. What did you learn from listening to the presentations from the other groups?
3. How might the lifestyle and health status of the health care worker serve as a model for patients?

ACTIVITY 3-6
WELLNESS PROJECTS

What Students Will Learn
- Positive lifestyle habits.

What You Will Need
- A copy of Student Handout 3-4, Wellness Projects, for each student.

What To Do
1. Distribute Student Handout 3-4 to students and ask them to choose one of the projects.
2. Give students one week to complete their projects.
3. Have students present their project results to the class.

Follow-up Discussion
1. What did you learn from the projects that you might apply to your own life?
2. What did you learn that might help in your work with patients?

Student Handout **3-4**

ACTIVITY 3-7
PERSONAL WELLNESS PLAN

Student Handout **3-5**

Student Handout **3-6**

Student Handout **3-6**
(Continued)

What Students Will Learn

- How to apply wellness strategies to their own lives.

What You Will Need

- A copy of Student Handout 3-5, Personal Wellness Inventory, for each student.
- A copy of Student Handout 3-6, Personal Wellness Plan, for each student.

What To Do

1. Distribute Student Handout 3-5 and ask students to fill out the inventory either in class or as homework. Because the questions are personal, the inventories should *not* be collected. This should be announced before the students begin.

Instructor's Note: If some of the questions—for example, the ones about tobacco and alcohol use—are inappropriate for your class, you may delete them. They have been placed as the last items on the inventory and wellness plan for easy removal.

2. When completed, conduct a class discussion about wellness strategies and distribute Student Handout 3-6 for the students to use in creating a personal wellness plan. The wellness plans should also remain confidential.
3. After 1 or 2 weeks, conduct a follow-up discussion, either in small groups or as a whole class.

Follow-up Discussion

1. Have you been successful carrying out your plan?
2. What has been the most difficult in following your plan?
3. What suggestions do you have about incorporating wellness habits in daily life?
4. If you followed your plan, do you feel any different? Explain.

Instructor's Note: Do not press students to discuss anything they are not comfortable sharing.

ACTIVITY 3-8
HOW HEALTHY ARE MY EATING HABITS?

What Students Will Learn

- How to read food labels.
- The amount of fat, fiber, and nutrients they consume in their daily diets.
- How to plan menus for weight loss and healthy eating.

What You Will Need

- Cans of food with nutrition labels that students bring to class.
- A copy of Student Handout 3-7, Food Diary, for each student.
- A copy of Student Handout 3-8, Food Exchanges and Guidelines for Healthy Eating, for each student.

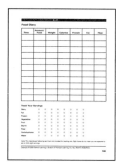

Student Handout **3-7**

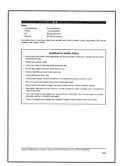

Student Handout **3-8**

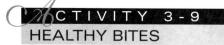

Student Handout **3-8**
(Continued)

What To Do

1. Explain or review how labels present contents and percentages of nutrients.
2. Have students work in pairs or small groups to compare the nutrients in the products they have brought to class.
3. Distribute Student Handouts 3-7 and 3-8.
4. Instruct students to eat as usual and write down what they eat for several days.
5. If you wish, ask them to track calories, fats, carbohydrates, and fiber.
6. After meals have been tracked for several days, ask the students to evaluate their eating habits and discuss in class or write a paper about what they have learned about themselves.
7. Instruct students to write a plan for healthier eating.

Follow-up Discussion

1. What did you learn about your eating habits?
2. Is there a time of day or day of the week that you find yourself eating in a less healthy way?
3. Do mood or stress level affect your eating? How?
4. What would you have to change to be a healthy eater?
5. Is it possible to eat in restaurants or fast food places and still eat a healthy diet?
6. What strategies can you use for healthy eating when eating out?
7. How can you change the way (rather than what) you cook so it is healthier?
8. What strategies can you use to be sure you drink at least 64 ounces of water each day?
9. What is the best healthy meal you ate during the past week?
10. Give some ideas for healthy desserts.
11. Do you skip meals? If so, how do you feel during the day?

ACTIVITY 3-9
HEALTHY BITES

What Students Will Learn

- How to plan food that is easy to prepare and nutritious.

What You Will Need

- No special materials are required for this activity.

What To Do

1. Plan a healthy snack day and ask students to volunteer, individually or in small groups, to bring snacks to share that fulfill the following requirements: taste good, are low in fat, have moderate sodium content, and contain some nutritive value.
2. You may want to have the class vote and award a small prize for the best snack.

3. Suggest that students look for recipe ideas in the many health-oriented cookbooks that are currently available, in magazines such as *Cooking Light*, and on the Internet.

Follow-up Discussion

1. What impact do eating habits have on health?
2. Do you think it is possible to change eating habits and still enjoy foods?
3. How might people incorporate more healthy selections in their diet?

ACTIVITY 3-10
THE BENEFITS OF EXERCISE

What Students Will Learn

- Physical activity is a major factor in establishing and maintaining good health.
- How exercise can be incorporated into daily life without the need to work out or join a gym.

What You Will Need

- Transparencies 3-7, Benefits of Exercise, 3-8, Why People Don't Exercise, and 3-9, No Need to Join a Gym.
- Blank transparencies and pens *or* butcher paper and pens.

What To Do

1. Divide the class into three groups to brainstorm ideas about exercise.
2. Assign one of the following topics to each group: benefits of exercise, reasons why people don't exercise, or how to incorporate exercise into daily life (no need to join a gym).
3. Give groups 10 or 15 minutes to list as many ideas as possible. Each group needs a recorder who will write its list on the transparencies or butcher paper to use later for presenting the ideas to the rest of the class.
4. You can use Transparencies 3-7, 3-8, and 3-9 for follow-up discussion after the groups have completed their reports to the class.

Follow-up Discussion

1. Why is it difficult for Americans in particular to get enough exercise?
2. What effect does physical activity have on health?
3. What changes can people make in their lives to increase their level of physical activity?

Transparency Master **3-7**

Transparency Master **3-8**

Transparency Master **3-9**

ACTIVITY 3-11
THE EFFECTS OF EXERCISE

Instructor's Note: This activity is meant to be done over the length of the entire term or module.

What Students Will Learn

- The benefits of moderate exercise on cardiovascular health.

What You Will Need

- Students who will commit to participating in and conducting this study for the length of the term.
- Sphygmomanometer and stethoscope.
- Scale.

What To Do

1. Divide the class into two groups.
2. Assign one group a routine of moderate exercise for 30 minutes a day, 4 days per week. Suggest that students walk, bicycle, swim, jump rope (if they are in relatively good shape), and the like. They might meet each day after classes to do some form of aerobic exercise, such as dance routines, or to take a walk together. It will be important to motivate the group to stay with the program for the entire term.
3. Do not assign an exercise routine to the second group. Ask them to change their lifestyle a little by taking the stairs when possible, parking in a spot far from the store, walking when they can (rather than driving), and so on.
4. Before students begin exercise routines, have them weigh each other and take vital signs. Ask them to chart these data.
5. Have students check vitals and weight once per week, or wait until the end of the term to check them.

Follow-up Discussion

1. Did any individual show changes in weight or vital signs?
2. Do you feel any different than you did at the beginning of the project? Explain.
3. Was it difficult to stick with an exercise program?
4. How did you motivate yourself?
5. Did one group show more differences than the other group?
6. How much exercise is "enough?"

ACTIVITY 3-12
RELAX!

What Students Will Learn

- How to use muscle relaxation to reduce stress and promote a sense of well-being.*

---

*Source: Adapted from M. E. Milliken, (1998). *Understanding human behavior: A guide for health care providers* (6th ed.). Clifton Park, NY: Delmar Learning.

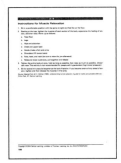

Student Handout **3-9**

What You Will Need

- A copy of Student Handout 3-9, Instructions for Muscle Relaxation, for each student.

What To Do

1. Explain the concept of muscle relaxation and how it can promote wellness as well as help health care workers perform more efficiently and with less stress. Relaxation, as used here, refers to the deliberate release of tension in the muscles. This technique reduces stress by improving blood circulation and allowing the release of blood lactate, a substance associated with anxiety (Milliken, 1998). Using relaxation techniques also produces the sensation of being rested. With practice, it is possible to quickly identify and release muscle tension when it begins to occur.

2. Conduct a simple muscle relaxation exercise in class using Student Handout 3-9.

3. Give each student a copy of Student Handout 3-9 to take home. Encourage them to practice the technique.

Follow-up Discussion

1. Have you tried doing the muscle relaxation exercises at home?
2. If so, did you find them helpful? Explain.
3. How can relaxation exercises benefit health care workers?
4. How can the exercises benefit patients?

ACTIVITY 3-13
MEDITATION

What Students Will Learn

- How to practice meditation as a way to reduce stress and promote a sense of well-being.*

What You Will Need

- A copy of Student Handout 3-10, Instructions for Meditation, for each student.

What To Do

1. Explain the concept of meditation and how it can promote wellness as well as help health care workers perform more efficiently and with less stress. When individuals are awake, the mind is continually engaged in thinking. Meditation is a process for quieting the mind by clearing it of thoughts. It slows the rate of brain waves experienced during normal activity. The regular practice of meditation has been shown to bring about physiological changes that result in both psychological and physiological (such as lowering the blood pressure) well-being (Mitchell & Haroun, 2001). An increasing number of health care professionals are recommending meditation as a therapeutic technique, even for serious illnesses such as cancer.

Source: Adapted from M. E. Milliken, (1998). *Understanding human behavior: A guide for health care providers* (6th ed.). Clifton Park, NY: Delmar Learning, and J. Mitchell & L. Haroun (2001). *Introduction to health care.* Clifton Park, NY: Delmar Learning.

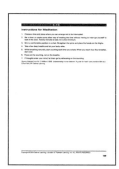

Student Handout **3-10**

2. Explain to students that meditation, when used in this way, is *not* associated with any religion.
3. There are a number of meditation methods (see Student Handout 3-10).
4. Give each student a copy of Student Handout 3-10. Encourage them to try meditation at home.

Follow-up Discussion

1. Have you tried doing the meditation exercise at home? If so, describe your experience with it.
2. Did you find the exercise helpful? If so, in what way?
3. How might meditation benefit health care workers?

Instructor's Note: You might want to invite a yoga instructor, acupuncturist, or other professional to talk to the class and assist with this activity.

ACTIVITY 3-14
RACE FOR PREVENTION

What Students Will Learn

- The value of positive lifestyle habits in preventing or decreasing the severity of many diseases and conditions.

What You Will Need

- A list of diseases and conditions, such as the following:
  AIDS
  brain injury
  cancer: lung, skin
  carpal tunnel syndrome
  diabetes
  emphysema
  heart disease
  hepatitis B
  hypertension
  osteoporosis
  stroke

What To Do

1. Divide the class into two teams. Each team should have as many members as the number of diseases or conditions you have listed so that everyone will have a turn. (You may have more teams if the class is large.)
2. As you or a student call out a disease or condition, the team members confer and then send a student to the board who writes as many preventive measures for that disease as possible in a given time, such as 30 seconds for both the team huddle and writing on the board.
3. Scoring may be done in either of two ways: award one point to the team that lists the most correct measures; or award each team a point for each correct measure they list.

Follow-up Discussion

1. Are you surprised at how many serious diseases and conditions are affected by lifestyle choices?
2. What are some ways people can develop healthier lifestyles?
3. Why is knowledge about prevention important for health care workers?
4. How do you think you will apply this knowledge in your own life and work?

REFERENCES

Milliken, M. E. (1998). *Understanding human behavior: A guide for health care providers* (6th ed.). Clifton Park, NY: Delmar Learning.

Mitchell, J., & Haroun, L. (2002). *Introduction to health care.* Clifton Park, NY: Delmar Learning.

True/False Statements About Vital Signs

Fact	Correct Answer	Comments
1. When checking vital signs, if the previous readings were normal, it is okay to assume that current readings will be normal.	FALSE	Vital signs change, and comparing new with previous measurements provides important information about patients' status.
2. Sweating usually indicates an abnormal condition or disease.	FALSE	Sweating is part of the body's normal cooling system.
3. Normal body temperature varies with the method used to obtain it.	TRUE	Normal adult ranges: Aural: 97.6°F to 99.6°F (36.5°C to 37.5°C) Axillary: 96.6°F to 98.6°F (36°C to 37°C) Oral: 97.6°F to 99.6°F (36.5°C to 37.5°C) Rectal: 98.6°F to 100.6°F (37°C to 38°C)
4. The temperature taken rectally tends to be lower than that taken orally.	FALSE	Rectal temperatures are about 1° higher than those taken orally.
5. Body temperature is typically lowest in the early morning.	TRUE	Body temperature varies throughout the day, being slightly higher in the evening than in the morning.
6. During pregnancy, body temperature may be higher.	TRUE	This is true. Normal body temperature can actually be influenced by a variety of factors, such as age, time of day, and physical exercise.
7. When using a mercury thermometer, it must be shaken down to below 90° in order to obtain an accurate reading.	FALSE	Although most thermometers are now electronic, mercury thermometers are still used. Shaking the mercury to below 96° is low enough.
8. A body temperature that is below normal is known as "afebrile."	FALSE	"Afebrile" refers to a normal body temperature. From the Greek *a-*, not + Latin *febris*, fever.
9. A fever indicates that the body is unable to defend itself against invading microorganisms.	FALSE	A rise in body temperature, measured as a fever, is actually a natural defense mechanism against invading microorganisms.
10. A health care worker should not use his or her thumb to take a pulse.	TRUE	The thumb has a pulse of its own that can be misinterpreted as the patient's.
11. There are several pulse points on the body.	TRUE	Temporal, carotid, brachial, antecubital, radial, femoral, popliteal, dorsalis. (*Note:* caution students against pressing on the carotid artery.)

(Continues)

Fact	Correct Answer	Comments
12. "Tachycardia" refers to an adult pulse of less than 60 beats per minute.	FALSE	"Tachycardia" refers to an adult pulse of 100 or more beats per minute, which is abnormally rapid. "Bradycardia" refers to the abnormally low rate.
13. Average pulse rates decrease with age.	TRUE	Average for newborns = 140 Average for adults = 80
14. "Apnea" means irregular heartbeat.	FALSE	"Apnea" means absence of respirations. Irregular heartbeat is called arrhythmia.
15. Always advise patients when you are measuring their respiration rate.	FALSE	Respirations can be consciously altered, so don't tell patients when you are measuring them.
16. Hypotension in an adult refers to blood pressure below 90/60.	TRUE	"Hypo-" means abnormally decreased, beneath, or under. The average BP range in an adult is 90/60 to 140/90.
17. If a patient is having difficulty breathing, this is known as "dyspnea."	TRUE	From the Greek *dys*, bad, and *pnoē*, breathing.
18. Average respiration rate increases with age.	FALSE	Average for newborns = 30–60 per minute Average for adults = 16–20 per minute
19. Hypertension can go undetected because in many cases there are no symptoms.	TRUE	Undetected hypertension can lead to heart disease, stroke, and major organ damage.
20. The diastolic phase of heart activity is when the muscle relaxes and the chambers refill with blood.	TRUE	"Systolic" refers to the phase when the heart chambers contract and push blood out.
21. An individual's blood pressure is pretty stable throughout the day.	FALSE	BP is extremely variable and changes with factors such as time of day, level of exercise, and consumption of food and drink.
22. More than 60% of Americans over age 65 develop hypertension.	TRUE	Hypertension is common in older Americans. It usually has no symptoms. High blood pressure over time contributes to heart disease, strokes, and other serious health conditions.
23. Body weight can indicate edema before it is visible.	TRUE	Water is relatively heavy, weighing 8 pounds per gallon. Therefore, even small amounts would result in weight gain.

(Continues)

Fact	Correct Answer	Comments
24. A person's height does not change once he or she has finished growing.	FALSE	Height can decrease with conditions such as osteoporosis.
25. The axillary route for measuring temperature will result in the lowest reading.	TRUE	It is about 1° lower than the oral and aural.
26. Body temperature is not affected by the amount of clothing worn.	FALSE	Clothing can retain heat.
27. An adult pulse of over 100 beats per minute is considered higher than normal.	TRUE	The average pulse for an adult is 80 beats per minute. The normal range is 60–100 beats per minute.
28. The shivering that takes place during a fever increases the metabolism through muscular action.	TRUE	The muscles are tensed during shivering and this increases the metabolism (process that produces energy for the body).
29. Intermittent fevers, in which the temperature rises and falls, occur most commonly in the early morning hours.	FALSE	They occur most commonly at night.
30. Monitoring the height of healthy children is an important part of their routine health care.	TRUE	Height is an important indicator of physical development.

Wellness Crossword Puzzle Solution

ACROSS

3 A good source of vitamins and fiber
5 Small amounts of nutrients
8 Measured when patient is relaxed and has waited 12 hours after eating
9 Preventive medicine
12 Bathed in oxygen
16 A good source of fiber
17 A Unit of energy
19 Body heat
20 High blood pressure
23 Energy transformation in the cells
25 Fats
28 Sugar
29 Physical activity
30 The exchange of oxygen in the body

DOWN

1 Nutrients such as A, C, E, etc.
2 A state of good health
4 Pulse after rest
5 Endocrine gland in the throat
6 Meal plan for sugar-sensitive individuals
7 Used for DNA formation
10 A heart-healthy way to eat
11 Lacking iron
13 Guide to balanced eating
14 A sweet, healthy snack
15 Measured with a sphygmomanometer
17 Excess of this can lead to arteriosclerosis
18 Nutrient for building muscle
21 Necessary for healthy blood
22 A healthy life has this
24 Used by the body to process sugar
26 Heart rate
27 Slumber

Wellness Word Search Solution

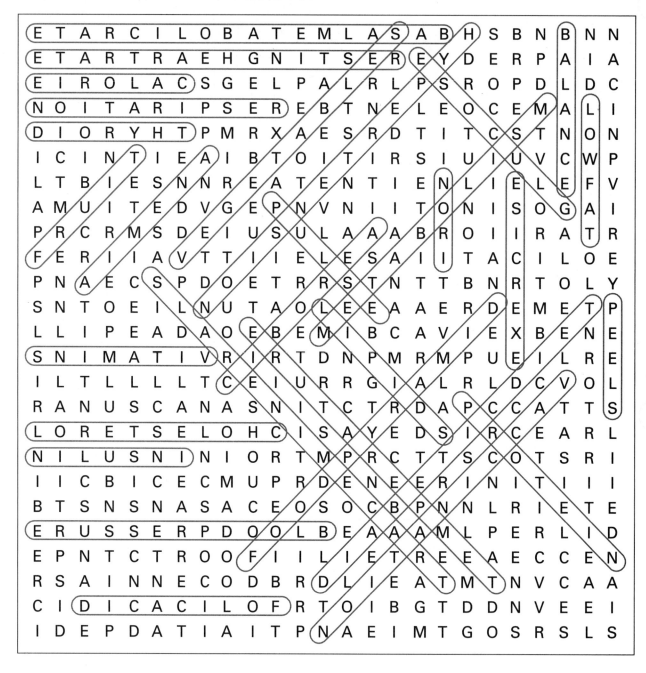

Challenging Wellness Word Search Solution

```
E L S D I P I L L N E V S D O E I E R N F I H U P
R O G C I E D E I E S I F T T I M R E S S E A
U R N S T I R E D G A M D A A A T E T H Y R O I D
S E I O L E T U E S A E R I R O N O S R E C T F O
S T N E I O I T T R H T E C I D L T I I O C A O A
E S I T R S A D Y A R A I E E T R R C P C U L A F
R E R P O B N P C A R L T R A C E M I N E R A L S
P L L I L F D E E I O E G E I I V O P U A A E C A
D O O E A O X H T B T I P P M N I D O E N N F X S
O H S A O E G F A R C E R M D G T E I L U F E I E
O C I F C N T T S R E I B I E N A B A L A N C E S
L S R I I S E B P T I P C A O T M C C E L E G I L
B I V T E M E T I F O A Y I I R I S P R F H L A E
S F S I L B I V T L C A T H L D N I E D A R U S E
E E I A R H A I A I N A O E A N S S S R C I C F P
R A S E M E O I L B R E T R P N P U L S E I O T E
A A E A S R I O F I O T O C S I E R B E N S S U N
B N L E I I F I P M R A E I T S B M A O T D E D I
R E N U L N A S O T C A I H N I A I B A U S I I
A H C L O E E T E C I E R F R U I T X A F A R Y I
S B E O B R R L O E H R O I L E O E S U W O C S B
N O I T A N I C C A V O L N I L U S N I O N T H F
P I A U T S A B E T I B A R S R F E R R L N S L E
S S I A E B L L T R P I C R A A R O D S R O O H I
I E I S M I E E P R I C S S N F R E S G E I L O E
```

Wellness Crossword Puzzle

ACROSS

3 A good source of vitamins and fiber
5 Small amounts of nutrients
8 Measured when patient is relaxed and has waited 12 hours after eating
9 Preventive medicine
12 Bathed in oxygen
16 A good source of fiber
17 A Unit of energy
19 Body heat
20 High blood pressure
23 Energy transformation in the cells
25 Fats
28 Sugar
29 Physical activity
30 The exchange of oxygen in the body

DOWN

1 Nutrients such as A, C, E, etc.
2 A state of good health
4 Pulse after rest
5 Endocrine gland in the throat
6 Meal plan for sugar-sensitive individuals
7 Used for DNA formation
10 A heart-healthy way to eat
11 Lacking iron
13 Guide to balanced eating
14 A sweet, healthy snack
15 Measured with a sphygmomanometer
17 Excess of this can lead to arteriosclerosis
18 Nutrient for building muscle
21 Necessary for healthy blood
22 A healthy life has this
24 Used by the body to process sugar
26 Heart rate
27 Slumber

Wellness Word Search

```
E T A R C I L O B A T E M L A S A B H S B N B N N
E T A R T R A E H G N I T S E R E Y D E R P A I A
E I R O L A C S G E L P A L R L P S R O P D L D C
N O I T A R I P S E R E B T N E L E O C E M A L I
D I O R Y H T P M R X A E S R D T I T C S T N O N
I C I N T I E A I B T O I T I R S I U I U V C W P
L T B I E S N N R E A T E N T I E N L I E L E F V
A M U I T E D V G E P N V N I I T O N I S O G A I
P R C R M S D E I U S U L A A A B R O I I R A T R
F E R I I A V T T I I E L E S A I I T A C I L O E
P N A E C S P D O E T R R S T N T T B N R T O L Y
S N T O E I L N U T A O L E E A A E R D E M E T P
L L I P E A D A O E B E M I B C A V I E X B E N E
S N I M A T I V R I R T D N P M R M P U E I L R E
I L T L L L T C E I U R R G I A L R L D C V O L
R A N U S C A N A S N I T C T R D A P C C A T T S
L O R E T S E L O H C I S A Y E D S I R C E A R L
N I L U S N I N I O R T M P R C T T S C O T S R I
I I C B I C E C M U P R D E N E E R I N I T I I I
B T S N S N A S A C E O S O C B P N N L R I E T E
E R U S S E R P D O O L B E A A A M L P E R L I D
E P N T C T R O O F I I L I E T R E E A E C C E N
R S A I N N E C O D B R D L I E A T M T N V C A A
C I D I C A C I L O F R T O I B G T D D N V E E I
I D E P D A T I A I T P N A E I M T G O S R S L S
```

AEROBIC	FOOD PYRAMID	PULSE
ANEMIA	FRUIT	RESPIRATION
BALANCE	GLUCOSE	RESTING HEART RATE
BASAL METABOLIC RATE	HYPERTENSION	SLEEP
BLOOD PRESSURE	INSULIN	TEMPERATURE
CALORIE	IRON	THYROID
CHOLESTEROL	LIPIDS	TRACE MINERALS
DIABETIC DIET	LOWFAT	VACCINATION
EXERCISE	METABOLISM	VEGETABLES
FOLIC ACID	PROTEIN	VITAMINS

Challenging Wellness Word Search

```
E L S D I P I L L N E V S D O E I E R N F I H U P
R O G C I E D E I E E S I F T T T I M R E S S E A
U R N S T I R E D G A M D A A A T E T H Y R O I D
S E I O L E T U E S A E R I R O N O S R E C T F O
S T N E I O I T T R H T E C I D L T I I O C A O A
E S I T R S A D Y A R A I E E T R R C P C U L A F
R E R P O B N P C A R L T R A C E M I N E R A L S
P L L I L F D E E I O E G E I I V O P U A A E C A
D O O E A O X H T B T I P P M N I D O E N N F X S
O H S A O E G F A R C E R M D G T E I L U F E I E
O C I F C N T T S R E I B I E N A B A L A N C E S
L S R I I S E B P T I P C A O T M C C E L E G I L
B I V T E M E T I F O A Y I I R I S P R F H L A E
S F S I L B I V T L C A T H L D N I E D A R U S E
E E I A R H A I A I N A O E A N S S S R C I C F P
R A S E M E O I L B R E T R P N P U L S E I O T E
A A E A S R I O F I O T O C S I E R B E N S S U N
B N L E I I F I P M R A E I T S B M A O T D E D I
R E N U L N A S O T C A I H N I A I I B A U S I I
A H C L O E E T E C I E R F R U I T X A F A R Y I
S B E O B R R L O E H R O I L E O E S U W O C S B
N O I T A N I C C A V O L N I L U S N I O N T H F
P I A U T S A B E T I B A R S R F E R R L N S L E
S S I A E B L L T R P I C R A A R O D S R O O H I
I E I S M I E E P R I C S S N F R E S G E I L O E
```

Bathed in oxygen
Lacking iron
A healthy life has this
Measured when patient is relaxed and has waited 12 hours after eating
Measured with a sphygmomanometer
A unit of energy
Excess of this can lead to arteriosclerosis
Meal plan for sugar-sensitive individuals

Physical activity
Used for DNA formation
Guide to balanced eating
A sweet, healthy snack
Sugar
High blood pressure
Used by the body to process sugar
Necessary for healthy blood
Fats
A heart-healthy way to eat
Energy transformation in the cells
Nutrient for building muscle

Heart rate
The exchange of oxygen in the body
Pulse after rest
Slumber
Body heat
Endocrine gland in the throat
Small amounts of nutrients
Preventive medicine
A good source of vitamins and fiber
Nutrients such as A, C, E, etc.

Wellness Projects

Choose one of the following to prepare and present to the class:

1. Write a 3-day meal plan for someone on a weight-loss diet. Use your meal plans to create a poster that includes photos and recipes.

2. Gather recipes for several favorite holiday foods. Adjust the recipes to make healthier versions. Examples: use broth to replace some or all of the butter when making giblet dressing for turkey; use egg whites in place of whole eggs. Present old and new recipes to the class with a sample of one dish for everyone to taste.

3. Create a 3-day meal plan for someone who needs a special diet due to illness or disease. An example would be a diabetic diet. Use your meal plans to create a poster that includes photos and recipes.

4. Collect a few restaurant menus (be sure to ask before you take them). Use the menus to show healthy food choices while eating out.

5. Create a healthy exercise plan for the following three people:
   - 25-year-old healthy active female
   - 45-year-old healthy nonactive male
   - 60-year-old male who has had bypass surgery

6. Make a poster that shows at least five stress reduction techniques.

7. Develop a smoking cessation plan.

8. Give up smoking for one week. Keep a diary and talk with the class about what you learned, how you did, what was hardest, easiest, and so on.

Personal Wellness Inventory

Respond to the following statements by checking the "YES" or "NO" box.

1. I exercise or do some form of physical activity for at least 20 minutes every day.

   ☐ YES   ☐ NO

2. I eat a balanced diet.

   ☐ YES   ☐ NO

3. I avoid eating lots of high-fat foods.

   ☐ YES   ☐ NO

4. I maintain a healthy weight for my height.

   ☐ YES   ☐ NO

5. I eat breakfast every day.

   ☐ YES   ☐ NO

6. I sleep at least seven hours a night.

   ☐ YES   ☐ NO

7. I get routine medical tests appropriate for my age and gender.

   ☐ YES   ☐ NO

8. I visit the dentist on a regular basis.

   ☐ YES   ☐ NO

9. I avoid the use of tobacco.

   ☐ YES   ☐ NO

10. If I drink alcohol, I do so in moderation.

    ☐ YES   ☐ NO

Personal Wellness Plan

To maintain optimal wellness, your response to each statement on the Personal Wellness Inventory should be answered "YES." For any item you responded to with a "NO," think about ways you can improve that aspect of your personal wellness and note your ideas here.

1. **If you don't exercise:**   The latest research shows that physical activity may be the single most important factor in determining overall health. What kinds of activities do you enjoy? Is there anyone among your family members or friends with whom you could walk, swim, or enjoy some other form of physical activity?

   _____

   _____

   _____

   _____

   _____

2. **If you don't eat a balanced diet:**   Start by learning all you can about the types of foods that provide good nutrition. If time is a problem, there are easy ways to prepare healthy foods so you can avoid the high-calorie fast-food trap. For example, fruits, cut-up vegetables, and healthy sandwiches can be carried along and eaten on the run. What are some other ways to improve your eating habits?

   _____

   _____

   _____

   _____

3. **If you eat lots of high-fat foods:**   Avoiding high-fat foods can be difficult because fat makes food taste good and we've become accustomed to eating high-fat foods in restaurants. Using oils like olive and safflower, while still high in calories, is more healthy than using animal fats and hydrogenated oils (margarine). Herbs and spices add flavor without fat. Look for foods that taste good on their own and don't need lots of extra fat to give them flavor. What are some ways you can change your cooking and eating habits?

   _____

   _____

   _____

   _____

4. **If you weigh too much—or too little:**   (If you are significantly underweight, you may have an eating disorder that can lead to serious health problems. It is suggested that you consult a health care professional.) At least 61% of Americans weigh more than they should. Many methods promise to help us lose that extra weight, but research shows that the only way to lose and keep off the pounds is to cut calories and increase physical activity. (If you are underweight, you may have an eating disorder that can lead to serious health problems. It would be a good idea to seek professional help.) What can you do to manage your weight?

   _____

   _____

   _____

   _____

5. **If you don't eat breakfast:**   An interesting study of almost 30,000 people in California found that not eating breakfast increases the risk of premature death by 50%. Eating in the morning provides energy the body needs to get the day going. How can you make time to start the day with breakfast? What foods do you think would be most appealing to you?

_____

_____

_____

6. **If you don't get enough sleep:**   The demands of modern life, especially for adult students, can make sleep seem like a luxury. Look and see if there is anything—perhaps a television program that isn't really *that* good—that you can trade for additional sleep. People who are well rested are actually more efficient and get more done during their waking hours. Are there ways you can reorganize your life to free up more time for rest?

_____

_____

_____

7. **If you don't get medical tests:**   Many serious conditions, if caught early, can be successfully treated. Taking time now may save both time and discomfort later. If lack of health insurance or money is a problem, investigate low-cost screening tests often offered as a public service by clinics, pharmacies, and community health fairs.

_____

_____

_____

8. **If you don't visit the dentist regularly:**   Dental heath affects much more than just appearance. Gum infections can cause tooth loss and the bacteria from infection in the mouth can spread throughout the body. If money is a problem, see if your area has a dental school that offers low-cost care or dentists who set up payment plans. Record what you find out.

_____

_____

_____

9. **If you smoke:**   Tobacco is the leading cause of avoidable deaths in the United States. There are many groups and products available to help people quit this difficult habit. Do some research to see what might work for you. Record your findings.

_____

_____

_____

10. **If you drink a lot of alcohol:**   There are many groups and organizations that offer help to those who have problems with alcohol. Overuse of alcohol can jeopardize your life and the lives of others, as well as interfere with carrying out the responsibilities you will have as a health care worker. What might you do now about your use of alcohol?

_____

_____

_____

_____

Food Diary

Time	Amount/Food	Weight	Calories	Protein	Fat	Fiber

Track Your Servings

Dairy	☐	☐	☐	☐	☐	☐	☐	☐
Fat	☐	☐	☐	☐	☐	☐	☐	☐
Protein	☐	☐	☐	☐	☐	☐	☐	☐
Vegetables	☐	☐	☐	☐	☐	☐	☐	☐
Fruit	☐	☐	☐	☐	☐	☐	☐	☐
Starch	☐	☐	☐	☐	☐	☐	☐	☐
Fiber	☐	☐	☐	☐	☐	☐	☐	☐
Carbohydrates	☐	☐	☐	☐	☐	☐	☐	☐
Water	☐	☐	☐	☐	☐	☐	☐	☐

Note: The checkboxes following each item are provided for tracking only. Eight boxes do not mean you are expected to eat or drink eight servings.

Food Exchanges and Guidelines for Healthy Eating

Fat Group

Carbohydrates	0 grams/portion
Protein	0 grams/portion
Fat	5 grams/portion
Calories	45 per portion

Examples: butter, margarine, mayonnaise, oils, salad dressings, nuts, olives, coconut, avocado, peanut butter, cream cheese.

Dairy

Carbohydrates	12 grams/portion
Protein	8 grams/portion
Fat	0–4 grams/portion
Calories	90–100 per portion

Examples: milk, yogurt, cottage cheese.

Starch

Carbohydrates	15 grams/portion
Protein	3 grams/portion
Fat	1 gram/portion
Calories	80 per portion

Examples: bagels, bread, hamburger or hot dog buns, cereal, bran, crackers, baked beans, dried beans, peas, lentils, lima beans, corn, pasta, potatoes, yams, winter squash, English muffins, rice, pretzels, rice cakes, tortillas, popcorn, pancakes, waffles, muffins.

Fruit

Carbohydrates	15 grams/portion
Protein	0 grams/portion
Fat	0 grams/portion
Calories	60 per portion

Examples: apple, applesauce, apricots, banana, blueberries, cantaloupe, cherries, dates, figs, fruit cocktail, grapefruit, grapes, honeydew melon, kiwi, mango, orange, papaya, peach, pear, pineapple, plums, prunes, raisins, strawberries, tangerines, watermelon, cranberry, juices, fruit juice bars.

Vegetables

Carbohydrates	5 grams/portion
Protein	2 grams/portion
Fat	0 grams/portion
Calories	25 per portion

Examples: artichoke, asparagus, bean sprouts, beans (green, wax, or Italian), beets, broccoli, Brussels sprouts, cabbage, carrots, cauliflower, eggplant, peppers (green), okra, onions, peapods, tomato, sauerkraut, spinach, squash (summer), turnips, water chestnuts, bamboo shoots, tomato or vegetable juice, greens (collard, kale, mustard, turnip), tomato paste, rhubarb, spaghetti sauce, mushrooms, celery, cucumber, green onions, radishes, salad greens (endive, lettuce, romaine, spinach), zucchini.

Meats

Carbohydrates	0 grams/portion
Protein	7 grams/portion
Fat	38 grams/portion
Calories	55–100 per portion

Examples: lean or extra lean meats (such as beef, pork, lamb, chicken, turkey), egg whites, fish, low-fat cheeses, veal, peanut butter.

Guidelines for Healthy Eating

- Eat at least three fruits, three vegetables, six ounces protein, 3 starches, two fats, and two dairy products each day.

- Watch your calorie intake.

- Limit your intake of fats, especially saturated fats.

- Do not skip meals. Eat every three hours or so.

- Drink at least 64 ounces of water each day.

- Limit caffeine and diet colas.

- Limit alcohol intake. Alcohol contains a lot of calories and little nutritional value.

- Be sure to exercise at least three to four times each week.

- Flavor foods with spices, vinegar, soy sauce, salsa, and the like for healthier eating.

- Use healthy fats such as nuts, olive oil, nut oils, canola oil, olives, avocado, and nut butters for most of your fats.

- If you are trying to lose weight and you go off your food plan, don't be too hard on yourself. Just begin eating in a healthy way again.

- Think of a weight-loss program as a healthy change in eating habits rather than a diet.

Instructions for Muscle Relaxation

1. Sit in a comfortable position with the spine straight and feet flat on the floor.

2. Starting at the toes, tighten the muscles of each section of the body, experience the feeling of tension, and then relax. Move up as follows:

   a. Toes (flex)

   b. Legs

   c. Hips and abdomen

   d. Chest and upper back

   e. Hands (make a fist) and arms

   a. Shoulders (lift toward ears)

   b. Face, head, and neck (be sure to relax the jaw afterward)

   c. Raise and lower eyebrows, pull together and release

3. Tighten the entire body at once, hold as long as possible, then relax as much as possible. (*Important note:* This activity is not recommended for people with hypertension [high blood pressure].)

4. Sit for several minutes and experience the lack of tension. If you become aware of any areas of tension, tighten and then release the muscles in that area.

Source: Adapted from M. E. Milliken (1998). *Understanding human behavior: A guide for health care providers* (6th ed.). Clifton Park, NY: Delmar Learning.

Instructions for Meditation

1. Choose a time and place where you can arrange not to be interrupted.

2. Set a timer or create some other way of tracking the time without having to interrupt yourself to look at the clock. Twenty minutes is best; ten is the minimum.

3. Sit in a comfortable position in a chair. Straighten the spine and place the hands on the thighs.

4. Take a few deep breaths and let your body relax.

5. While breathing naturally, start counting each time you exhale. When you reach four (four breaths), start over.

6. Focus on the counting, not on the breaths.

7. If thoughts enter your mind, let them go by refocusing on the counting.

Source: Adapted from M. E. Milliken (1998). *Understanding human behavior: A guide for health care providers* (6th ed.). Clifton Park, NY: Delmar Learning.

Wellness Crossword Puzzle

ACROSS

3 A good source of vitamins and fiber
5 Small amounts of nutrients
8 Measured when patient is relaxed and has waited 12 hours after eating
9 Preventive medicine
12 Bathed in oxygen
16 A good source of fiber
17 A Unit of energy
19 Body heat
20 High blood pressure
23 Energy transformation in the cells
25 Fats
28 Sugar
29 Physical activity
30 The exchange of oxygen in the body

DOWN

1 Nutrients such as A, C, E, etc.
2 A state of good health
4 Pulse after rest
5 Endocrine gland in the throat
6 Meal plan for sugar-sensitive individuals
7 Used for DNA formation
10 A heart-healthy way to eat
11 Lacking iron
13 Guide to balanced eating
14 A sweet, healthy snack
15 Measured with a sphygmomanometer
17 Excess of this can lead to arteriosclerosis
18 Nutrient for building muscle
21 Necessary for healthy blood
22 A healthy life has this
24 Used by the body to process sugar
26 Heart rate
27 Slumber

Wellness Crossword Puzzle Solution

The crossword grid contains the following solution words:

- VITAMINS (vertical, top left)
- WELLNESS (vertical, right)
- VEGETABLES
- TRACE MINERALS
- THYROID
- BASAL METABOLIC RATE
- VACCINATION
- AEROBIC
- WHOLE GRAIN
- CALORIE
- TEMPERATURE
- HYPERTENSION
- METABOLISM
- LIPIDS
- GLUCOSE
- EXERCISE
- RESPIRATION
- (plus intersecting words including CALORIES, CHOLESTEROL, DIABETES, FAT, NUTRIENTS, DIET, ANEMIA, INSULIN, etc.)

ACROSS

3 A good source of vitamins and fiber
5 Small amounts of nutrients
8 Measured when patient is relaxed and has waited 12 hours after eating
9 Preventive medicine
12 Bathed in oxygen
16 A good source of fiber
17 A Unit of energy
19 Body heat
20 High blood pressure
23 Energy transformation in the cells
25 Fats
28 Sugar
29 Physical activity
30 The exchange of oxygen in the body

DOWN

1 Nutrients such as A, C, E, etc.
2 A state of good health
4 Pulse after rest
5 Endocrine gland in the throat
6 Meal plan for sugar-sensitive individuals
7 Used for DNA formation
10 A heart-healthy way to eat
11 Lacking iron
13 Guide to balanced eating
14 A sweet, healthy snack
15 Measured with a sphygmomanometer
17 Excess of this can lead to arteriosclerosis
18 Nutrient for building muscle
21 Necessary for healthy blood
22 A healthy life has this
24 Used by the body to process sugar
26 Heart rate
27 Slumber

Wellness Word Search

```
E T A R C I L O B A T E M L A S A B H S B N B N N
E T A R T R A E H G N I T S E R E Y D E R P A I A
E I R O L A C S G E L P A L R L P S R O P D L D C
N O I T A R I P S E R E B T N E L E O C E M A L I
D I O R Y H T P M R X A E S R D T I T C S T N O N
I C I N T I E A I B T O I T I R S I U I U V C W P
L T B I E S N N R E A T E N T I E N L I E L E F V
A M U I T E D V G E P N V N I I T O N I S O G A I
P R C R M S D E I U S U L A A A B R O I I R A T R
F E R I I A V T T I I E L E S A I I T A C I L O E
P N A E C S P D O E T R R S T N T T B N R T O L Y
S N T O E I L N U T A O L E E A A E R D E M E T P
L L I P E A D A O E B E M I B C A V I E X B E N E
S N I M A T I V R I R T D N P M R M P U E I L R E
I L T L L L T C E I U R R G I A L R L D C V O L
R A N U S C A N A S N I T C T R D A P C C A T T S
L O R E T S E L O H C I S A Y E D S I R C E A R L
N I L U S N I N I O R T M P R C T T S C O T S R I
I I C B I C E C M U P R D E N E E R I N I T I I I
B T S N S N A S A C E O S O C B P N N L R I E T E
E R U S S E R P D O O L B E A A A M L P E R L I D
E P N T C T R O O F I I L I E T R E E A E C C E N
R S A I N N E C O D B R D L I E A T M T N V C A A
C I D I C A C I L O F R T O I B G T D D N V E E I
I D E P D A T I A I T P N A E I M T G O S R S L S
```

AEROBIC	FOOD PYRAMID	PULSE
ANEMIA	FRUIT	RESPIRATION
BALANCE	GLUCOSE	RESTING HEART RATE
BASAL METABOLIC RATE	HYPERTENSION	SLEEP
BLOOD PRESSURE	INSULIN	TEMPERATURE
CALORIE	IRON	THYROID
CHOLESTEROL	LIPIDS	TRACE MINERALS
DIABETIC DIET	LOWFAT	VACCINATION
EXERCISE	METABOLISM	VEGETABLES
FOLIC ACID	PROTEIN	VITAMINS

Wellness Word Search Solution

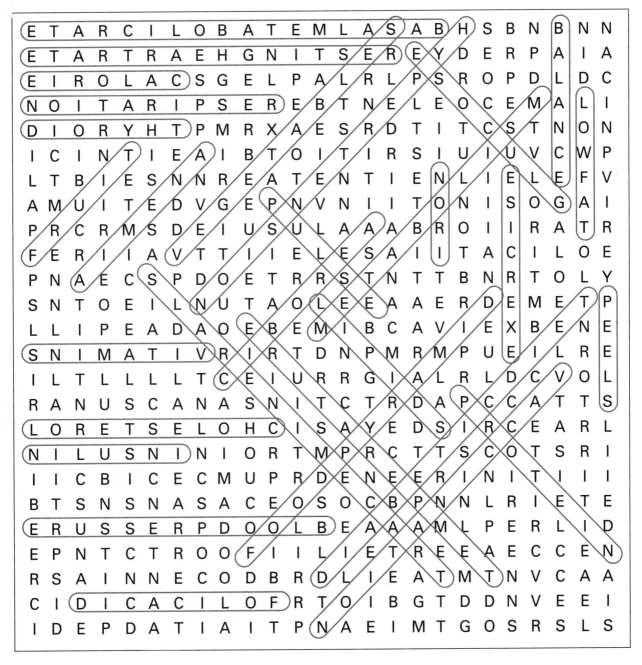

Challenging Wellness Word Search

```
E L S D I P I L L N E V S D O E I E R N F I H U P
R O G C I E D E I E E S I F T T T I M R E S S E A
U R N S T I R E D G A M D A A A T E T H Y R O I D
S E I O L E T U E S A E R I R O N O S R E C T F O
S T N E I O I T T R H T E C I D L T I I O C A O A
E S I T R S A D Y A R A I E E T R R C P C U L A F
R E R P O B N P C A R L T R A C E M I N E R A L S
P L L I L F D E E I O E G E I I V O P U A A E C A
D O O E A O X H T B T I P P M N I D O E N N F X S
O H S A O E G F A R C E R M D G T E I L U F E I E
O C I F C N T T S R E I B I E N A B A L A N C E S
L S R I I S E B P T I P C A O T M C C E L E G I L
B I V T E M E T I F O A Y I I R I S P R F H L A E
S F S I L B I V T L C A T H L D N I E D A R U S E
E E I A R H A I A I N A O E A N S S S R C I C F P
R A S E M E O I L B R E T R P N P U L S E I O T E
A A E A S R I O F I O T O C S I E R B E N S S U N
B N L E I I F I P M R A E I T S B M A O T D E D I
R E N U L N A S O T C A I H N I A I I B A U S I I
A H C L O E E T E C I E R F R U I T X A F A R Y I
S B E O B R R L O E H R O I L E O E S U W O C S B
N O I T A N I C C A V O L N I L U S N I O N T H F
P I A U T S A B E T I B A R S R F E R R L N S L E
S S I A E B L L T R P I C R A A R O D S R O O H I
I E I S M I E E P R I C S S N F R E S G E I L O E
```

Bathed in oxygen
Lacking iron
A healthy life has this
Measured when patient is relaxed and has waited 12 hours after eating
Measured with a sphygmomanometer
A unit of energy
Excess of this can lead to arteriosclerosis
Meal plan for sugar-sensitive individuals

Physical activity
Used for DNA formation
Guide to balanced eating
A sweet, healthy snack
Sugar
High blood pressure
Used by the body to process sugar
Necessary for healthy blood
Fats
A heart-healthy way to eat
Energy transformation in the cells
Nutrient for building muscle

Heart rate
The exchange of oxygen in the body
Pulse after rest
Slumber
Body heat
Endocrine gland in the throat
Small amounts of nutrients
Preventive medicine
A good source of vitamins and fiber
Nutrients such as A, C, E, etc.

Challenging Wellness Word Search Solution

```
E L S D I P I L L N E V S D O E I E R N F I H U P
R O G C I E D E I E E S I F T T T I M R E S S E A
U R N S T I R E D G A M D A A A T E T H Y R O I D
S E I O L E T U E S A E R I R O N O S R E C T F O
S T N E I O I T R H T E C I D L T I I O C A O A
E S I T R S A D Y A R A I E E T R R C P C U L A F
R E R P O B N P C A R L T R A C E M I N E R A L S
P L L I L F D E E I O E G E I I V O P U A A E C A
D O O E A O X H T B T I P P M N I D O E N N F X S
O H S A O E G F A R C E R M D G T E I L U F E I E
O C I F C N T T S R E I B I E N A B A L A N C E S
L S R I I S E B P T I P C A O T M C C E L E G I L
B I V T E M E T I F O A Y I R I S P R F H L A E
S F S I L B I V T L C A T H L D N I E D A R U S E
E E I A R H A I A I N A O E A N S S S R C I C F P
R A S E M E O I L B R E T R P N P U L S E I O T E
A A E A S R I O F I O T O C S I E R B E N S S U N
B N L E I I F I P M R A E I T S B M A O T D E D I
R E N U L N A S O T C A I H N I A I I B A U S I I
A H C L O E E T E C I E R O F R U I T X A F A R Y I
S B E O B R R L O E H R O I L E O E S U W O C S B
N O I T A N I C C A V O L N I L U S N I O N T H F
P I A U T S A B E T I B A R S R F E R R L N S L E
S S I A E B L L T R P I C R A A R O D S R O O H I
I E I S M I E E P R I C S S N F R E S G E I L O E
```

Benefits of Exercise

- Promotes the body's production of endorphins that help relieve stress and improve one's mental outlook.

- Improves the quality of sleep.

- Helps with weight control.

- Increases physical and mental energy.

- Increases the strength of the heart muscle and helps prevent heart disease.

- May raise the body's resistance to disease, including certain types of cancer.

- If weight-bearing, builds bone strength and aids in the prevention of osteoporosis.

Source: Adapted from J. Mitchell & L. Haroun (2002). *Introduction to health care.* Clifton Park, NY: Delmar Learning.

Why People Don't Exercise

- Not interested in active recreational exercise.

- Spend many hours watching television or using the computer.

- Use the car for most transportation.

- Don't do as much manual labor because of increased use of technology.

- Unsafe to walk on many streets and parking areas that are designed mainly for cars.

- Believe it is too much work, inconvenient, too time-consuming.

Source: Adapted from J. Mitchell & L. Haroun (2002). *Introduction to health care.* Clifton Park, NY: Delmar Learning.

No Need to Join a Gym

- Whenever possible, leave the car at home.

- Park at the far end of the mall or grocery store parking lot.

- Use the stairs instead of elevators.

- Wash the car by hand instead of using the car wash.

- Do jobs yourself that require physical effort, such as mowing the lawn and washing windows.

- Find a sport or activity you enjoy.

- Substitute activity for a few hours of television each week.

Source: Adapted from J. Mitchell & L. Haroun (2002). *Introduction to health care.* Clifton Park, NY: Delmar Learning.

CHAPTER 4

Standard Precautions and Emergency Procedures

INTRODUCTION

All healthcare workers who might come into contact with body fluids must have a thorough understanding of standard precautions intended to minimize the spread of infections. The purpose of the activities in this chapter is to help students understand the importance of infection control and standard precautions and learn about safe practices for lab and clinic settings.

First aid is another important skill for health care workers. Emergencies can happen anywhere—in the workplace, at home, or at school. Students will learn the reasons why specific emergency procedures are performed. This knowledge will help them make good decisions if they are confronted with an emergency situation.

ACTIVITY 4-1
CROSSWORD PUZZLE

What Students Will Learn

- Standard precautions and emergency procedures vocabulary

What You Will Need

- A copy of Student Handout 4-1, Standard Precautions and Procedures Emergency Vocabulary Crossword Puzzle, for each student.
- Transparency 4-1, Standard Precautions and Emergency Procedures Vocabulary Crossword Puzzle.
- Transparency 4-2, Standard Precautions and Emergency Procedures Vocabulary Crossword Puzzle Solution.
- Instructor Sheet 4-1, Standard Precautions and Emergency Procedures Vocabulary Crossword Puzzle Solution.

What To Do

1. Distribute Student Handout 4-1 and ask students to complete the crossword puzzle.
2. The puzzle may be worked as an individual assignment, in small groups, or as a large group using Transparency 4-1.
3. See Instructor Sheet 4-1 for puzzle solution.

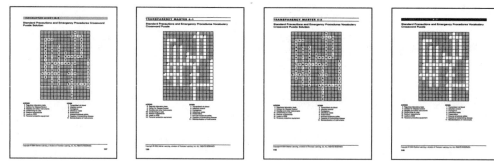

Instructor Sheet **4-1** Transparency Master **4-1** Transparency Master **4-2** Student Handout **4-1**

Follow-up Discussion

1. Why is knowing the vocabulary of health care procedures important for the health care worker?

ACTIVITY 4-2
BREAK THAT CHAIN!

What Students Will Learn

- The chain of infection model.
- How infectious diseases are spread.
- Various practices and procedures that health care workers can use to break the chain and stop the spread of disease.

What You Will Need

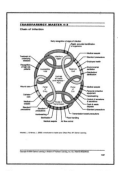

Transparency Master **4-3**

- Transparency 4-3, Chain of Infection
- A copy of Student Handout 4-2, Breaking the Chain, for each student.

What To Do

1. Use Transparency 4-3 to discuss or review the chain of infection and practices that can break the chain.
2. Following the presentation, turn off the overhead projector and distribute Student Handout 4-2 to the students. Allow about 10 minutes for the students to list as many of the chain-breaking practices as they can remember.
3. Ask students to share their answers. They may come up with correct answers that differ from what was shown or discussed. These should be counted as correct.
4. The student with the most correct responses may be awarded a small prize.
5. Alternate Activity: Have small groups work on creating the lists.

Student Handout **4-2**

Follow-up Discussion

1. Why is it essential that health care workers practice infection control?
2. What are the possible consequences of carelessness in the presence of infectious disease?
3. What are ways that health care workers in various occupations practice infection control?

ACTIVITY 4-3
COLLECT THOSE CARDS!

Instructor Sheet **4-2**

Instructor Sheet **4-2**
(*Continued*)

Student Handout **4-3**

Student Handout **4-3**
(*Continued*)

What Students Will Learn

- Information about the transmission and control of infection.
- Standard precautions facts and procedures.

What You Will Need

- Enough sets of playing cards made from the statements on Instructor Sheet 4-2, Instructions for Making Playing Cards, for each group of six or seven students. (Each set contains the same cards.)
- A copy of Student Handout 4-3, Answer Sheet for Checker, for each group.
- A die for each group (or some other method of determining which player in each group begins the game).

What To Do

1. Divide class into groups of six or seven students.
2. Give each group a set of cards and explain the rules of the game:
   - Students play as individuals.
   - The object of the game is to collect as many cards as possible.
   - The cards are shuffled and placed face down where all students can reach them.
   - One group member is selected to be the checker and receives a copy of Student Handout 4-3, which is not shown to the other students. The checker does not play the game, but has the job of determining if the answers given by the players are correct, using Student Handout 4-3 as a guide. If there is disagreement, the group may discuss an answer and then consult with the instructor for a final judgment.
   - The player to go first is chosen at random (players can roll a die for the highest number) and selects a card from the pile. If the card contains a question, the player may give an answer. If the answer is correct, he or she keeps the card and play moves to the next player (counterclockwise). If the answer is incorrect, the card is passed to the next player to try to answer. If the card contains instructions ("Pass the card to the player on your left"), these must be followed and the player receiving the card keeps that card and also draws from the pile. Play continues until all cards are used or until the allotted time for the game runs out.

Follow-up Discussion

1. Ask students if there were questions they answered incorrectly. If so, review any necessary material.
2. After reviewing, ask questions to check on students' understanding of this important topic.

ACTIVITY 4-4
SAFETY FASHION SHOW

What Students Will Learn
- Purpose, types, and availability of personal protective equipment.

What You Will Need
- Students: Access to the Internet, telephone books, and a telephone.
- Access to the school's supply of personal protective equipment.

What To Do
1. Divide the class into groups of about five students each. This activity can be as simple or complex as you like. Let the students have fun with it!
2. Instruct the students to put together a fashion show with personal protective equipment including various types of gowns, gloves, face masks, goggles, safety needles, and so on.
3. Tell the students they must research the various types of personal protective equipment, to their purposes. Tell when they are used, and the like.
4. Have the students locate doctors' offices, hospitals, sales reps, and so on, who will donate samples of items to be used; or borrow items from the school lab supplies.
5. Instruct the students to write a script and practice their presentations.
6. Present the show to classmates or to students in other classes.
7. Alternate activity: If a fashion show is too complicated, students can make posters to present to the class and then display in the classroom.

Follow-up Discussion
1. Review the material presented in the show by asking students to summarize the purpose and use of the various types of personal protective equipment.
2. How are clothing and equipment handled after they are worn?
3. What types of personal protective equipment do you anticipate using in your occupation?

ACTIVITY 4-5
RATIONALE, PLEASE

What Students Will Learn
- Rationale for first aid and emergency procedures.
- The importance of thinking about the purpose of their actions when they are performing procedures.

What You Will Need
- Instructor Sheet 4-3, First Aid and Emergency Procedures (includes the rationale for each procedure).

What To Do
1. Divide the class into two teams and have each team count off. Students will take turns in numerical order supplying rationale.
2. Flip a coin to determine which team starts.

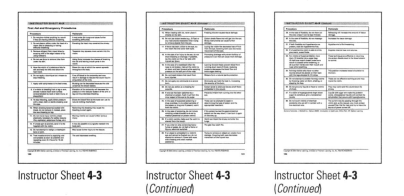

Instructor Sheet **4-3**   Instructor Sheet **4-3**
                            (*Continued*)

Instructor Sheet **4-3**
(*Continued*)

3. Read aloud a first aid or emergency procedure from Instructor Sheet 4-3.
4. Player number one on the starting team is given the opportunity to supply the correct rationale. (*Note:* there may be correct answers in addition to those listed on the sheet. The instructor is the final judge.)
5. If the answer is correct, the team scores a point. If it is incorrect, the team loses a point, and the other team has an opportunity to supply the rationale.
6. After each statement, briefly discuss the rationale for the answer to reinforce the information for the whole class.
7. Play alternates between the teams until all procedures have been used or until the allotted time for playing the game is finished.

Follow-up Discussion

1. Why is it essential for health care workers to understand the reasons for the procedures they perform?
2. What are possible consequences of taking action without knowing why the action is appropriate?

ACTIVITY 4-6
EMERGENCY MATCH

What Students Will Learn

- First aid procedures for various medical emergencies.*

What You Will Need

- Signs for posting on the walls. These must be large enough to be seen around the classroom. Write one of the following emergency situations on each sign:
  1. Severe allergic reaction—victim has difficulty breathing
  2. Severe bleeding from deep cut on arm
  3. Sucking wound in chest
  4. Suspected broken leg
  5. Suspected muscle strain in leg
  6. 2nd degree burn from heat source
  7. Hypothermia
  8. Fainting—no injury suspected
- Instructor Sheet 4-4, Emergency Conditions and Corresponding First Aid Procedures, for making sets of cards to distribute to students. You can make stur-

Instructor Sheet **4-4**

---

*Source of procedures: J. Mitchell & L. Haroun (2002). *Introduction to health care*. Clifton Park, NY: Delmar Learning.

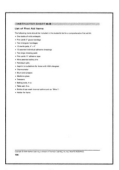

Instructor Sheet **4-4**
(*Continued*)

Instructor Sheet **4-4**
(*Continued*)

dier cards for reuse by copying the procedures onto 3 × 5 index cards or copying the page onto light card stock before cutting.

What To Do

1. Before class starts, put up the signs with the emergency conditions around the classroom.
2. When it is time for the activity, distribute one first aid procedure card to each student.
3. Give students a few minutes to go to the sign that lists the condition for which their procedure is most appropriate.
4. Instruct the class that if two students with the same procedure go to the same sign, the one who arrives second needs to look for another condition that requires the same procedure. (For example, "Do not give anything by mouth.")
5. When students have formed groups under the signs, ask them to discuss the condition and appropriate first aid, and then determine the best order to be followed for the procedures.
6. When the groups have finished discussing and ordering the procedures, have them line up and present the procedures to the rest of the class.

Follow-up Discussion

1. In an emergency situation, what should be done first? Second?
2. Why is it important to perform first aid steps in a certain order?
3. Are there any procedures presented by the groups that you didn't understand?

ACTIVITY 4-7
BUILDING A FIRST AID KIT

What Students Will Learn

- How to put together a useful basic first aid kit.

What You Will Need

- Instructor Sheet 4-5, List of First Aid Items.

What To Do

1. Either as a class or individually, have students create a list of items for a first aid kit for school, office, or home.
2. You can also ask students to list items needed for a first aid kit for the car.
3. Once the lists are created, use the following suggestions to complete the activity:
   - Each student puts together a first aid kit for the home or auto.
   - Each student in the class volunteers to supply one item for a classroom first aid kit.
   - Each student creates a poster showing the items needed for a good first aid kit. (Remember to include something to hold the kit.)

Follow-up Discussion

1. Why is it important to be prepared to handle emergencies?
2. Why should health care workers learn to gather equipment and other necessary supplies before beginning clinical procedures and administrative tasks?

Instructor Sheet **4-5**

ACTIVITY 4-8
HOW WELL DO I FOLLOW DIRECTIONS?

What Students Will Learn

- The importance of following directions.
- How well they follow directions.

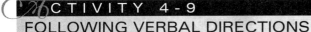

Instructor Sheet **4-6**

What You Will Need

- Student Handout 4-4, How Well Can You Follow Directions?
- Instructor Sheet 4-6, "How Well Can You Follow Directions" Answer Key.
- Students: Each will need a pencil and an 8½ × 11 piece of paper.

What To Do

1. Distribute Student Handout 4-4 and read the following instructions to the class:
   - "You have a 5-minute time limit to complete this test. Be sure that you carefully read the instructions. Begin the test when I tell you to start. Good luck!" Then tell the students to start.
2. At the end of 5 minutes, ask students to put their pencils down. See Instructor Sheet 4-6 for the answers to the test.

Follow-up Discussion

1. Why is it important to follow directions in the health care workplace?
2. What are some possible consequences of failing to follow directions in the laboratory? When performing invasive procedures on patients?
3. Why do we sometimes not hear instructions correctly?

Student Handout **4-4**

ACTIVITY 4-9
FOLLOWING VERBAL DIRECTIONS

What Students Will Learn

- The importance of listening carefully and following instructions.

What You Will Need

- Students: A plain piece of paper and a pen or pencil.
- Transparency 4-4, Answer Key for Verbal Instructions.
- Instructor Sheet 4-7.

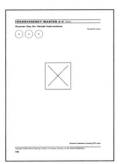 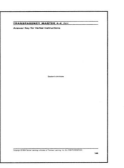 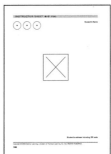 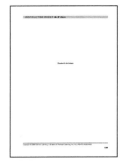

Transparency Master **4-4**

Transparency Master **4-4**
(*Continued*)

Instructor Sheet **4-7**

Instructor Sheet **4-7**
(*Continued*)

What To Do

1. Tell students they will have only 2 minutes to follow the directions you will give verbally.
2. Give the following directions:
   - Do not pick up your pencil.
   - Listen to all directions before you do anything.
   - Print your name in the upper right-hand corner of your paper.
   - Place three circles, approximately the size of dimes, in the upper left hand corner of your paper.
   - Put a smaller circle inside each of the three circles that you have just made.
   - In the center of your paper, draw a box with an "X" in it.
   - In the center of the back of your paper, write your date of birth.
   - In the bottom right-hand corner of your paper, write your home address, including your zip code.
   - Pick up your pencil and follow the directions you just heard.
3. Display Transparency 4-4 to show the results of following the directions correctly and have the students compare their results.

Follow-up Discussion

1. Was it difficult to remember all the directions?
2. Why is it important to be able to follow verbal directions?
3. Why do you think health care workers must be able to follow verbal directions?

REFERENCES

Mitchell, J., & Haroun, L. (2002). *Introduction to health care.* Clifton Park, NY: Delmar Learning.

Standard Precautions and Emergency Procedures Crossword Puzzle Solution

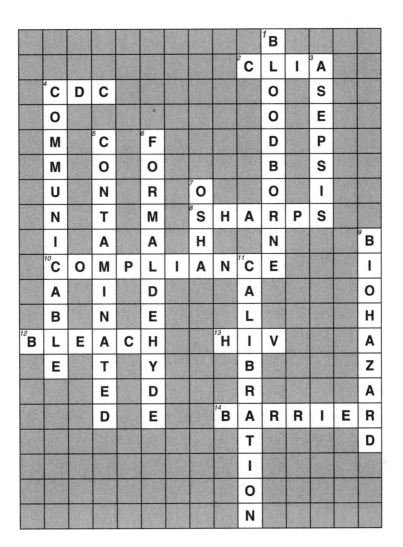

ACROSS
- **2** Regulates laboratory tests
- **4** Centers for Disease Control
- **8** Needles and other instruments
- **10** Conforming to rules
- **12** Sodium hypochlorite
- **13** Leads to AIDS
- **14** Personal protective equipment

DOWN
- **1** Transmitted via blood
- **3** Infection control
- **4** Contagious
- **5** Infectious waste
- **6** Preservative
- **7** Ensures employee safety
- **9** Capable of transmitting disease
- **11** Standardization of instruments

Instructions for Making Playing Cards
(Infection Control and Standard Precautions)

1. Use 3 × 5 cards to make the playing cards.

2. Write one question from the following list on each card. Include the corresponding letter with the question so the student checker can quickly find the answer on Student Handout 4-3.

3. Prepare the five instruction cards for each set (these are found at the end of the list of questions).

4. Each set should contain 30 different cards. *Hint:* If you use different colored cards for each set, it will help keep them from getting mixed up.

Questions

(A)   What is the most effective way to destroy most bacterial infections?

(B)   For which serious infectious disease are health care workers most at risk?

(C)   What is produced by the body's immune system to fight infection?

(D)   What problem can result when patients fail to take the full course of a drug prescribed to fight an infection?

(E)   Why are diseases caused by viruses more difficult to treat than diseases caused by bacteria?

(F)   What is the difference between medical and surgical asepsis?

(G)   What is the single most important way that the individual health care worker can help control the spread of infection?

(H)   What is the correct way to handle a needle after giving an injection to a healthy patient?

(I)   When should standard precautions be followed by health care workers who are in direct contact with patients?

(J)   What is an opportunistic infection?

(K)   Why is the common cold difficult to treat?

(L)   What is the difference between antiseptics and disinfectants?

(M)   Why should the hands be washed both before putting on gloves and after removing them?

(N)   What should you do if after washing your hands you accidentally touch the faucet with your bare hands?

(O)   Why should the hands be held lower than the arms during handwashing?

(P)   What are three examples of personal protective equipment for health care workers?

(Q)   If a health care worker receives an accidental needle stick while performing a procedure, what does OSHA require the employer to provide?

(R)   What must be worn, at a minimum, by the health care worker when wiping up a spill of blood?

(S)   Which types of accidental needle sticks received by health care workers must be reported to their employer?

(T)   When might it be necessary to change gloves when working on only one patient?

(U)   When are airborne precautions used?

(V)   When bodily fluids are involved, with which types of patients should health care workers use standard precautions?

(W)   What is a nosocomial infection?

(X)   When should gloves be worn by health care workers?

(Y)   When would a health care worker use a mask and eye protection?

Instruction Cards

Pass this card to the player on your right.

Pass this card to the player on your left.

Pass this card to the second player on your right.

Pass this card to the second player on your left.

Give this card to the player of your choice.

First Aid and Emergency Procedures

Procedure	Rationale
1. Do not give victims anything by mouth if they are having difficulty breathing.	It may enter the lungs and cause further breathing difficulties.
2. Do not place a pillow under the head of a victim who is wheezing or having difficulty breathing	Elevating the head may constrict the airway.
3. Remove stingers from insect bites by scraping with a flat edge instead of by using tweezers.	Tweezers may squeeze more venom into the victim.
4. Do not use force to remove ticks from under the skin.	Using force increases the chance of breaking the tick and leaving mouth parts in the victim.
5. Have the victim of a poisonous bite lie still and keep the bite area below the heart level.	Slows the rate at which the venom spreads throughout the body.
6. Do not apply a tourniquet as a means to stop bleeding.	Cuts off blood to the extremity and may result in damage to tissues that could require amputation of the limb.
7. Apply cold compresses to bruised areas.	Bruising can be decreased because the cold constricts the blood vessels.
8. If a victim is bleeding from a leg or arm, elevate it above heart level (unless contraindicated by neck or back injury, or discomfort).	Elevation of the extremity will decrease the pressure in the vascular system of the arm or leg and thus decrease bleeding.
9. To stop bleeding, apply direct pressure with a clean cloth or sterile dressing over the area.	Slows the blood flow so the body can use its natural clotting mechanism.
10. When dressing becomes soaked with blood, do not remove it; instead, place the new dressing on top.	Removing the dressing may cause the bleeding to start again.
11. Do not move injury victims unless absolutely necessary for safety reasons (fire, explosion, poisonous fumes, etc.).	Moving victims can cause further serious injury.
12. If a body part is severed, send it to the hospital with the victim.	It may be possible to surgically reattach the body part.
13. Do not attempt to realign a misshapen bone or joint.	May cause further injury to the tissues.
14. Treat muscle strains by applying cold compresses as soon as possible and repeating every 3–4 hours for 15–20 minutes.	The cold decreases swelling.

Procedure	Rationale
15. When treating with ice, never place it directly on the skin.	Freezing the skin causes tissue damage.
16. Do not use cotton swabs (e.g., Q-Tips) or any instruments (tweezers) when trying to remove objects from the eye.	Cotton sheds fibers that will get into the eye. Sharp instruments can cause further damage.
17. If there has been a blow to the eye, lay the victim flat and cover both eyes.	Laying the victim flat decreases loss of fluid from the eye. Covering both eyes decreases movement of the eyes.
18. In the case of an injury to the ear, do not block bleeding or drainage. If possible, lay the victim on his or her side with injured ear down.	Promoting drainage will prevent buildup of pressure in ear that can cause more damage.
19. In the case of a nosebleed when the nose is not broken, instruct the victim to sit down and lean forward while applying pressure on the soft part of the nose.	Leaning forward helps prevent blood from running down back of throat. Applying pressure decreases the blood flow and encourages clotting.
20. Do not break blisters that result from burn injuries.	Blisters form a natural sterile protection.
21. Do not apply any ointments to a severe burn.	Ointments can hold the heat in, increasing the severity of the burn.
22. Do not use cotton as a dressing for wounds.	Cotton tends to stick and leaves small fibers embedded in the wound.
23. If one eye has been splashed by a chemical or poison, flush it out from the inner aspect of the eye to the outer.	Prevents irritant from running into the other eye.
24. In the case of suspected poisoning or drug overdose, try to collect samples of the poison or drug and if present, vomit from the victim.	These can be analyzed to assist in determining the type of poison and the appropriate treatment.
25. In the case of poisoning, do not induce vomiting unless directed to do so by medical personnel or poison control.	If the poison burned the gastrointestinal system on the way down, it can burn it again on the way up.
26. If a victim vomits, make sure the vomit is cleared from the mouth.	Vomit can block the airway and enter the lungs.
27. If you enter an area containing heavy fumes or gases, do not light a flame or flip any electrical switches.	The gas may catch fire.
28. If an object is embedded in a victim's eye and cannot be flushed out, do not attempt to remove it. Cover both eyes with dressing and await medical assistance.	Trying to remove an object can create more damage. Covering both eyes decreases movement of the injured eye.

Procedure	Rationale
29. In the case of frostbite, do not thaw out the area unless it can be kept thawed.	Refreezing will increase the amount of tissue damage.
30. In the case of frostbite, do not massage the area.	Increases the tissue damage.
31. If both frostbite and hypothermia are present, treat the hypothermia first.	Hypothermia is life threatening.
32. If a hypothermia victim is able to drink, give warm, sweet fluids.	Supplies internal heat and calories.
33. For victims of hyperventilation, have them (1) breathe into a paper bag; (2) hold one nostril closed (make sure mouth is closed) while breathing; or (3) cup their hands over their mouth and nose while breathing.	These techniques are effective in returning the carbon dioxide level in the blood stream to normal.
34. Fainting victims who have no other injuries should be placed on their back with the legs elevated 8–12 inches.	This position increases blood circulation to the brain.
35. Do not attempt to awaken fainting victims by throwing water on them, shaking, or slapping the face.	These are not effective techniques and may injure the victim.
36. Do not give any liquids or food to victims of shock.	They may vomit and this could block the airway.
37. If a victim of hyperglycemia (high blood sugar) is conscious, give unsweetened liquids.	Liquids with sugar will make the problem worse. Unsweetened liquids will combat the dehydration that occurs with hyperglycemia.
38. Do not touch victims of electrical accidents who are still in contact with a live electrical wire.	The current may be passing through the victim and, as the rescuer, you must protect yourself first. Call for help and try to have the source of power turned off.

Source of rationale: J. Mitchell & L. Haroun (2002). *Introduction to health care.* Clifton Park, NY: Delmar Learning.

Emergency Conditions and Corresponding First Aid Procedures

Copy and cut out the procedures along the dotted lines to distribute to students. (Do not include the name of the emergency conditions when making the cards. These are simply headings for the groups of procedures and for checking student performance.)

Severe Allergic Reaction—Victim Has Difficulty Breathing

Try to determine what caused the problem.

Ask victim if he/she has emergency medication.

Do not give anything by mouth.

Do not place a pillow or anything else under the victim's head.

Severe Bleeding from Deep Cut on Arm

Elevate the limb above heart level.

Apply direct pressure with a clean cloth.

Continue to add dressings on top of old ones as needed.

Sucking Wound in Chest

Apply an airtight dressing as quickly as possible.

Leave one edge of the dressing unsealed.

Do not give anything by mouth.

Do not move victim unless absolutely necessary.

Suspected Broken Leg

Immobilize the limb.

After immobilization, check for circulation below the injury.

Do not attempt to realign the limb.

Do not give anything by mouth.

Suspected Muscle Strain in Leg

Apply cold compresses as soon as possible.

Elevate the limb.

Contact physician—may recommend antiinflammatory medication.

Rest injured area for at least 24 hours.

2nd Degree Burn from Heat Source

Run cool water over the affected area for several minutes.

Do not break blisters.

Cover affected area with a clean cloth or apply a loose bandage.

Prevent chilling, a common condition with this type of injury.

Hypothermia

Condition may affect breathing—if respirations are below 6 per minute, give rescue breathing.

Remove any wet clothing and replace with dry clothing, blanket, as available.

Apply warm packs to the neck, chest, and groin.

If victim is able to drink, give warm, sweet fluids.

Wrap victim in blankets or use own body to provide warmth.

Fainting—No Injury Suspected

If you're present at time of incident, help prevent patient from falling.

Place victim on back.

Elevate the legs 8–12 inches.

Do not attempt to awaken with water in face, shaking, or slapping.

List of First Aid Items

The following items should be included in the student's list for a comprehensive first aid kit:

- One bottle of mild antiseptic
- Five yards 2" gauze bandage
- Two triangular bandages
- 12 sterile pads, 4" × 4"
- 12 assorted individual adhesive dressings
- Two large dressing pads
- Five yards ½" adhesive tape
- Nine assorted safety pins
- Petroleum jelly
- Aspirin (or substitute for those with ASA allergies)
- Thermometer
- Blunt-end scissors
- Medicine glass
- Tweezers
- Baking soda, 4 oz.
- Table salt, 8 oz.
- Bottle of eye wash (normal saline such as "Blinx")
- Holder for items

"How Well Can You Follow Directions?"
Answer Key

The only writing students should have on their test papers is the date in the top right-hand corner and the name of the health care occupation they are interested in pursuing in the top center of their test papers. Item #13 contains the test instructions.

The directions given in item #1 state to **read** all parts before doing anything. If students didn't do this, suggest they do it now.

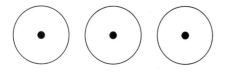

Student's Name

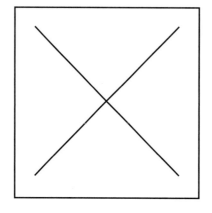

Student's address including ZIP code

Student's birthdate

Standard Precautions and Emergency Procedures Vocabulary Crossword Puzzle

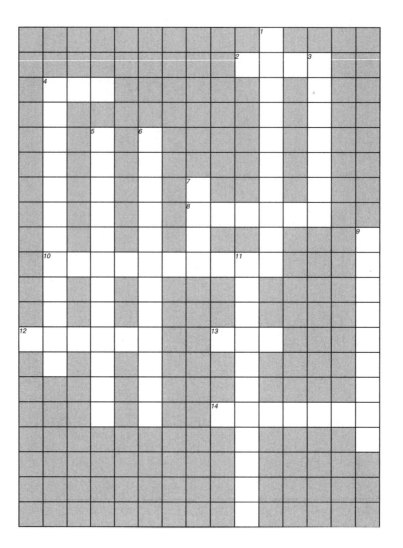

ACROSS

 2 Regulates laboratory tests
 4 Centers for Disease Control
 8 Needles and other instruments
 10 Conforming to rules
 12 Sodium hypochlorite
 13 Leads to AIDS
 14 Personal protective equipment

DOWN

 1 Transmitted via blood
 3 Infection control
 4 Contagious
 5 Infectious waste
 6 Preservative
 7 Ensures employee safety
 9 Capable of transmitting disease
 11 Standardization of instruments

Breaking the Chain

Under each link in the chain, list as many practices as you can that will help break the chain and prevent the spread of infectious disease.

Link #1   **Infectious Agent** _____

_____

_____

_____

Link #2   **Reservoir Host** _____

_____

_____

_____

Link #3   **Portal of Exit** _____

_____

_____

_____

Link #4   **Route of Transmission** _____

_____

_____

_____

Link #5   **Portal of Entry** _____

_____

_____

_____

Link #6   **Susceptible Host** _____

_____

_____

_____

Answer Sheet for Checker

Question	Answer
(A) What is the most effective way to destroy most bacterial infections?	Antibiotics
(B) For which serious infectious disease are health care workers most at risk?	Hepatitis B
(C) What is produced by the body's immune system to fight infection?	Antibodies
(D) What problem can result when patients fail to take the full course of a drug prescribed to fight an infection?	The drug becomes ineffective because the organisms/pathogens/germs become resistant to it
(E) Why are diseases caused by viruses more difficult to treat than diseases caused by bacteria?	Viruses cannot be killed by antibiotics
(F) What is the difference between medical and surgical asepsis?	Medical asepsis decreases pathogens and surgical asepsis eliminates them; or medical asepsis is used for nonsterile procedures and interaction with patients, and surgical asepsis is used for surgical and invasive procedures
(G) What is the single most important way that the individual health care worker can help control the spread of infection?	Frequent handwashing
(H) What is the correct way to handle a needle after giving an injection to a healthy patient?	Dispose of it immediately in a puncture-resistant container
(I) When should standard precautions be followed by health care workers who are in direct contact with patients?	At all times
(J) What is an opportunistic infection?	One that occurs when the body is in a weakened condition and unable to effectively fight infection
(K) Why is the common cold difficult to treat?	It is a virus and therefore cannot be cured with antibiotics
(L) What is the difference between antiseptics and disinfectants?	Antiseptics kill bacteria; disinfectants kill bacteria and most viruses
(M) Why should the hands be washed both before putting on gloves and after removing them?	To remove microorganisms/pathogens/germs that may get on the hands during the process
(N) What should you do if after washing your hands you accidentally touch the faucet with your bare hands?	Wash them again—they are contaminated

Question	Answer
(O) Why should the hands be held lower than the arms during handwashing?	To prevent contaminated water from running up the arms (which may run down and contaminate the washed hands)
(P) What are three examples of personal protective equipment for health care workers?	Gloves, gowns, lab coats, masks, face shields, goggles
(Q) If a health care worker receives an accidental needle stick while performing a procedure, what does OSHA require the employer to provide?	A confidential medical evaluation, any necessary treatment, and follow-up attention
(R) What must be worn, at a minimum, by the health care worker when wiping up a spill of blood?	Gloves
(S) Which type of accidental needle sticks received by health care workers must be reported to their employer?	All needle sticks must be reported
(T) When might it be necessary to change gloves when working on only one patient?	If you touch something considered to be contaminated; if you are performing different procedures or touching different parts of the body so that infection can be transported from one area to another
(U) When are airborne precautions used?	When working with patients who have diseases that are spread by tiny particles that move through the air; tuberculosis is an example
(V) When bodily fluids are involved, with which types of patients should health care workers use standard precautions?	With all patients
(W) What is a nosocomial infection?	Infection acquired by a patient while being cared for in a health care facility
(X) When should gloves be worn by health care workers?	When there is any possibility of contact with blood, body fluids, mucous, or skin that is not intact (cuts, wounds, and so on)
(Y) When would a health care worker use a mask and eye protection?	When there is a possibility of being splashed with blood, mucus, or other bodily fluids

How Well Can You Follow Directions?

1. Read carefully through all the test items.

2. Write today's date—month/day/year in the top right-hand corner of your test paper.

3. Write the name of the health care occupation you are interested in pursuing in the top center of your test paper.

4. Write the name of your school in the top left-hand corner of your test paper.

5. Count the number of students in your class and write this number in the bottom right-hand corner of your test paper.

6. In the lower left-hand corner of your test paper, write the names of the subjects or classes you are taking now.

7. Just above your answer to item 5, write "This test is very easy."

8. In the center of your test paper, draw a rectangle and inside the rectangle write the words "HEALTH CARE." The size of the rectangle and words is not important.

9. Directly above your answer to item 8, draw a row of three small circles. Once again, size is not important.

10. Write one reason you are interested in health care at the top of the page on the back of your test paper.

11. Answer the question: Will you have to take a certifying exam before you can work in your chosen occupation? (If you don't know, write "I don't know"). Write the answer in the center on the back of your test paper.

12. It is recommended that between 20% and 35% of our daily intake of calories be from fats. What is the maximum number of calories recommended from fats for a person who consumes a total of 1800 calories per day? Write the answer below your answer to 10.

13. Now that you have carefully read all the test items so far, and you have not carried out any of the actual work, skip the next question, go back to the beginning, and complete only test items 2 and 3.

14. What is the name of a group of body organs that work together to perform a related function? (You shouldn't be reading this far! Go back to 13.)

Standard Precautions and Emergency Procedures Vocabulary Crossword Puzzle

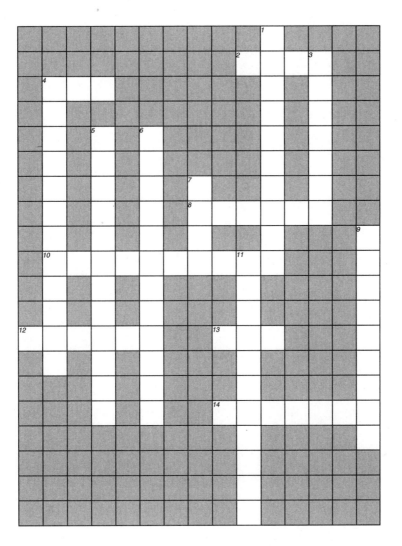

ACROSS

2 Regulates laboratory tests
4 Centers for Disease Control
8 Needles and other instruments
10 Conforming to rules
12 Sodium hypochlorite
13 Leads to AIDS
14 Personal protective equipment

DOWN

1 Transmitted via blood
3 Infection control
4 Contagious
5 Infectious waste
6 Preservative
7 Ensures employee safety
9 Capable of transmitting disease
11 Standardization of instruments

Standard Precautions and Emergency Procedures Vocabulary Crossword Puzzle Solution

								¹B			
							²C	L	I	³A	
⁴C	D	C						O		S	
O								O		E	
M		⁵C		⁶F				D		P	
M		O		O				B		S	
U		N		R		⁷O		O		I	
N		T		M		⁸S	H	A	R	P	S
I		A		A		H		N			⁹B
¹⁰C	O	M	P	L	I	A	N	¹¹C	E		I
A		I		D		L		A			O
B		N		E				L			H
¹²B	L	E	A	C	H		¹³H	I	V		A
E		T		Y			B				Z
		E		D			R				A
		D		E		¹⁴B	A	R	R	I	E	R
							T				D
							I				
							O				
							N				

ACROSS

2 Regulates laboratory tests
4 Centers for Disease Control
8 Needles and other instruments
10 Conforming to rules
12 Sodium hypochlorite
13 Leads to AIDS
14 Personal protective equipment

DOWN

1 Transmitted via blood
3 Infection control
4 Contagious
5 Infectious waste
6 Preservative
7 Ensures employee safety
9 Capable of transmitting disease
11 Standardization of instruments

Chain of Infection

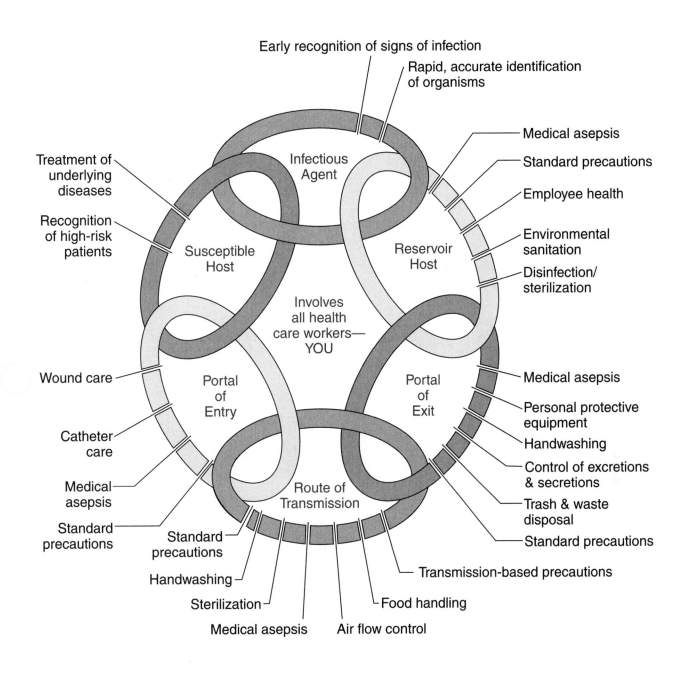

Mitchell, J., & Haroun, L. (2002). *Introduction to health care.* Clifton Park, NY: Delmar Learning.

Answer Key for Verbal Instructions

Student's name

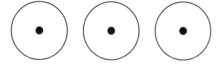

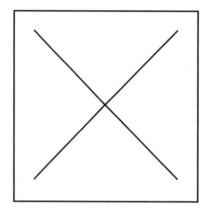

Student's address including ZIP code

Answer Key for Verbal Instructions

Student's birthdate

Math Review

INTRODUCTION

Many students suffer from math anxiety, an emotional reaction causing them to doubt their ability to understand and perform mathematical computations. When students believe they "can't do math," their attitudes can inhibit their actual abilities. As experts who have studied math anxiety point out, learning math is really a question of "attitude rather than aptitude" (Kogelman and Warren, 1978). Some of the activities in this chapter are designed to help students confront their fears, decide if their fears really make sense, and think about ways to develop more positive attitudes about math.

In addition to math anxiety, students may lack math skills because they avoided math classes in the past or because over the years they have forgotten many math operations. Fractions, decimals, percentages, and the metric system are common problem areas addressed in this chapter. Many of the activities in this chapter are visual and hands-on to help students review and understand concepts they may have found difficult in the past. The activities represent only a few operations and are intended only to supplement, not substitute for, more comprehensive explanations and exercises.

It is important to carefully assess the levels of students. Nothing is to be gained from assigning activities that are too basic or too advanced. Also, be sure to explain to students whom you believe could benefit from such exercises that manipulative and seemingly simple activities such as paper folding and arranging cards are not childish, as some may think, but are strategies designed to help visual and kinesthetic learners.

ACTIVITY 5-1
SHARING FEARS

What Students Will Learn
- Acknowledging commonly held misperceptions about math is the first step to overcoming them.
- Lacking *confidence* in one's math abilities is not the same as actually lacking the *ability* to learn or do math.

What You Will Need
- A copy of Student Handout 5-1, Sharing Fears, for each student.

What To Do

1. Divide the class into groups of three to five students. Distribute Student Handout 5-1. Ask the groups to share their experiences with math, using the questions as a discussion guide.
2. When the groups have finished their discussions, collect the lists of fears they have written for use in Activity 5-2.

Follow-up Discussion

1. Did many members of the groups have the same fears?
2. Where do you think these fears come from?
3. How can our negative beliefs affect our performance?

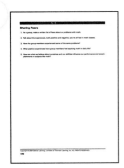

Student Handout **5-1**

ACTIVITY 5-2
FEAR NOT!

What Students Will Learn

- Many people have negative beliefs about learning and performing math operations.
- These beliefs, while widely held, are generally false.

What You Will Need

- The lists of fears that the groups wrote for Activity 5-1.

What To Do

1. Divide the class into two teams.
2. Have the students on each team count off.
3. Students play a game in numerical order starting with student number one.
4. Read a fear from the group lists.
5. Student number one from each team races to the front of the room or rings a buzzer or bell. The first student to reach the front or ring the buzzer wins the opportunity to refute the statement by saying, "That's not true!" and giving a plausible example that demonstrates it to be false. Doing so earns a point for his or her team. (For example, if the fear is "I'm not smart enough to learn math," a plausible answer would be, "Any student who is in this program has the ability. He or she may simply have to spend a little more time studying math.")
6. The second round is played by students number two, and so on.
7. The team that gives the most examples refuting the fears is the winner.

Follow-up Discussion

1. Why do you think so many people doubt their ability to do math?
2. How do negative beliefs about ability affect students?
3. How can facing these fears help students decrease their negative influence?

ACTIVITY 5-3
OVERCOMING MATH ANXIETY

What Students Will Learn

- How to overcome math anxiety.

What You Will Need

- A copy of Student Handout 5-2, Overcoming Math Anxiety, for each student.
- A copy of Student Handout 5-3, Overcoming Math Anxiety Discussion Questions, for each group.

What To Do

1. Divide class into groups of three to five students.
2. Each group should choose a facilitator who reads the statement and questions and keeps the group discussion moving, if necessary; a recorder; and a presenter.
3. Assign each group one of the statements about overcoming math anxiety from Student Handout 5-2.
4. Give the groups approximately 10 minutes to discuss the statements and answer the questions listed on Student Handout 5-3.
5. The recorder should write the group's answers.
6. When the groups are finished, ask the presenters to share their group's ideas with the class.

Follow-up Discussion

1. Conduct a follow-up discussion wrapping up the topic of math anxiety by drawing on the ideas and examples the groups shared with the class.

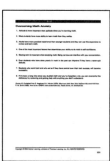

Student Handout **5-2**

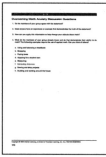

Student Handout **5-3**

ACTIVITY 5-4
WHEN WILL I USE MATH?

What Students Will Learn

- Basic math skills are used in many health care occupations.
- Accuracy in performing math operations on the job is important to ensure patient safety and facility efficiency.

What You Will Need

- A copy of Student Handout 5-4, Heath Care Occupations, for each student. (*Note:* If all students are studying the same occupation, such as medical assisting, you may choose to focus on that occupation and not use the list.)
- A copy of Student Handout 5-5, Questions for Group Discussion, for each student.

What To Do

1. Working with the whole class, ask students to think of examples of how math would be applied in their future occupation or in occupations on the list.
2. Alternate activity: Divide the class into groups and assign each group part of the list of occupations to discuss and suggest examples of on-the-job applications.

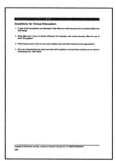

Student Handout **5-4**

Student Handout **5-5**

Follow-up Discussion

1. Use the questions in Student Handout 5-5, Questions for Group Discussion, to lead discussions.

---

*A*CTIVITY 5-5
FORMING FRACTIONS

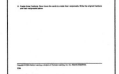

Instructor Sheet **5-1**

What Students Will Learn*

- The relationships of numerators and denominators.
- The concept of lowest common denominator.

What You Will Need

- A set of cards, each containing one of the digits 1 through 8, for each student or a copy of Student Handout 5-6, Number Cards, for each student and scissors for students to cut out the squares along the dotted lines.
- A copy of Student Handout 5-7, Forming Fractions, for each student.
- Instructor Sheet 5-1, Forming Fractions—Answers for Student Handout 5-7.

Student Handout **5-6**

What To Do

1. Review the following concepts with students:
   - *Improper fraction:* One in which the numerator is larger than the denominator; for example, $\%_5$ and $\frac{3}{2}$.
   - *Mixed number:* One that contains both a whole number and a fraction; for example, $1\frac{4}{5}$ and $1\frac{1}{2}$. *Note:* Point out that mixed numbers are the correct way to express what would be an improper fraction; for example, $\%_5 = 1\frac{4}{5}$.
   - *Reciprocal:* A fraction "turned upside down." Reciprocals are used when dividing fractions; for example, the reciprocal of $\frac{3}{4}$ is $\frac{4}{3}$ and the reciprocal of $\frac{7}{8}$ is $\frac{8}{7}$.
   - *Lowest terms:* Fraction has lowest possible denominator; fraction in which numerator and denominator cannot be evenly divided by the same number. For example, $\frac{50}{100} = \frac{10}{20} = \frac{1}{2}$; $\frac{4}{6} = \frac{2}{3}$.
2. Distribute the sets of cards or Student Handout 5-6 and instruct the students to cut out the cards.
3. Distribute Student Handout 5-7 and instruct the students to complete the exercises.
4. Correct exercises in class using Instructor Sheet 5-1 as a guide.

Student Handout **5-7**

Follow-up Discussion

1. Discuss with students when multiplying and dividing fraction skills may be useful in their day to day lives.

---

*Source: Adapted from M. Sobel & E. Maletsky (1988). *Teaching mathematics: A sourcebook of aids, activities, and strategies* (2nd ed.). Englewood Cliffs, NJ: Prentice Hall.

ACTIVITY 5-6
PLAYING WITH FRACTIONS

What Students Will Learn

- Use of the fractions ½, ¼, ⅛, ¹⁄₁₆, ⅓, ⅕ and how they relate to a whole.
- Relationship of fractions to decimals and percentages.

What You Will Need

- A copy of Student Handout 5-8, Fraction Flash Cards I, for each student.
- A pair of scissors for each student.
- Heavy cardstock or graph paper for students to make their own manipulatives.

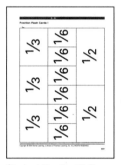

Student Handout **5-8**

What To Do

1. Copy Student Handout 5-8 onto heavy cardstock (using the heavier weight paper makes the pieces easier to work with). If you have the resources, you can copy onto regular paper and then laminate each page before cutting.
2. Give each student a copy of Student Handout 5-8 and have him or her use a pair of scissors to cut the page into parts.
3. Working with the whole class, give students equivalency problems using fractions and have them arrange their cut-out pieces to calculate the answers:
   - ⅓ = ˣ⁄₆
   - ½ = ˣ⁄₆
   - ⁴⁄₆ = ˣ⁄₃
   - ⅔ = ˣ⁄₆
   - ⁴⁄₆ = ˣ⁄₃
   - ²⁄₆ = ˣ⁄₃
4. Point out to the students that the number on the bottom of the fraction (the denominator) equals the number of that fraction that equals a whole (for example, it takes eight pieces of ⅛ to make one whole).
5. Alternate activity: Give students graph paper and have them draw their own parts to cut out. If using graph paper, have students draw four boxes that are each 32 squares wide and 10 squares long. On one box, draw vertical lines every eight boxes. On a second box, draw vertical lines every four boxes. On the third box, draw vertical lines every two boxes. Students should now have one whole box, one with four quarters, one with eight eighths, and one with sixteen sixteenths.

Follow-up Discussion

1. How helpful is it to be able to visualize basic math problems?
2. How can you use this approach for more difficult problems?

ACTIVITY 5-7
COMPARING FRACTIONS

What Students Will Learn

- Concept of fraction equivalencies.
- Concept of lowest common denominator.

What You Will Need

- A copy of Student Handouts 5-8, Fraction Flash Cards I, 5-9, Fraction Flash Cards II, and 5-10, Comparing Fractions, for each student.
- Transparencies 5-1, Fraction Flash Cards I, and 5-2, Fraction Flash Cards II.
- Instructor Sheet 5-2, Comparing Fractions—Answers for Student Handout 5-10.

What To Do

1. Review the concepts of fraction equivalencies and lowest common denominator.
   - *Fraction equivalencies:* Fractions that have the same value; for example, $\frac{1}{2} = \frac{2}{4} = \frac{3}{6} = \frac{4}{8}$ etc.
   - *Lowest common denominator:* The smallest number that all the denominators of two or more fractions can be divided into evenly; for example, the lowest common denominator for $\frac{1}{7}$ and $\frac{1}{3}$ is 21 because this is the smallest number into which both 7 and 3 can be divided evenly, and the lowest common denominator for $\frac{4}{9}$ and $\frac{5}{18}$ is 18.
2. Use Transparency 5-1 to demonstrate the relationships between thirds, sixths, and halves as they appear on the number lines. For example, $\frac{1}{3} = \frac{2}{6}$ and $\frac{1}{2} = \frac{3}{6}$. Point out that $\frac{1}{3}$ cannot be expressed in halves but that $\frac{1}{2}$ and $\frac{1}{3}$ can each be expressed in sixths: $\frac{1}{2} = \frac{3}{6}$ and $\frac{1}{3} = \frac{2}{6}$.
3. Distribute a copy of Student Handouts 5-8, 5-9, and 5-10 to each student and instruct the students to complete the exercises.
4. Allow about 15 minutes for them to complete the activity, which involves examining the relationships between fractions and using visuals to review the concepts of relationships between fractions and the lowest common denominator.
5. Use Instructor Sheet 5-2 as a guide for correcting Student Handout 5-10.

Follow-up Discussion

1. How comfortable are you with fractions after completing this exercise?

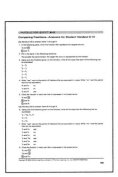

Instructor Sheet **5-2**

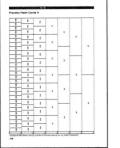

Student Handout **5-8**

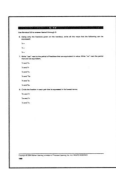

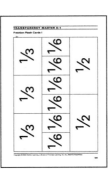

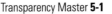

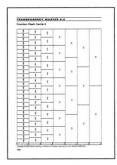

Student Handout **5-9**   Student Handout **5-10**   Student Handout **5-10**
(Continued)   Transparency Master **5-1**   Transparency Master **5-2**

ACTIVITY 5-8
MULTIPLICATION MODELS FOR FRACTIONS

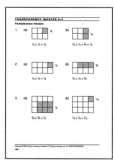

Student Handout **5-11**

Transparency Master **5-3**

Transparency Master **5-4**

What Students Will Learn

- The concept that multiplication involving fractions results in answers that are smaller than either number being multiplied, instead of larger as with whole numbers.*

What You Will Need

- Four or five sheets of 8½ × 11 paper for each student.
- A copy of Student Handout 5-11, Using Paper Models to Show Multiplication of Fractions, for each student.†
- A pair of scissors for each student.
- Transparencies 5-3, Multiplying Fractions, and 5-4, Multiplication Models.

What To Do

1. Discuss with students that multiplication can be confusing with fractions because we are accustomed to the concept of *times* or increasing when performing multiplication with whole numbers in which the result is always larger than either of the numbers in the problem.
2. Use Transparency 5-3 to demonstrate the concept of multiplication as groups of numbers. Point out that multiplying with fractions actually means to "take a part of," and, therefore, to reduce rather than to make a quantity larger. (The actual multiplication comes when the numerators and denominators are multiplied by each other.)
3. Give each student several sheets of paper, a pair scissors, and a copy of Student Handout 5-11. Instruct the students to complete the exercises.
4. After 10 minutes, when most students have completed the exercises, discuss the answers using Transparency 5-4.

Follow-up Discussion

1. How helpful did you find the pictures in understanding multiplication of fractions?

Source: Adapted from L. H. Charles & M. R. Brummett (1989). *Connections: Grade 6.* Mt. View, CA: Creative Publications.

†*Source:* Adapted from M. Sobel & E. Maletsky (1988). *Teaching mathematics: A sourcebook of aids, activities, and strategies* (2nd ed.). Englewood Cliffs, NJ: Prentice Hall.

ACTIVITY 5-9
ACTING IT OUT—DIVIDING FRACTIONS

What Students Will Learn

- The concept that division involving fractions results in answers that are larger than either number being divided, instead of smaller as with whole numbers.
- The process of inverting and multiplying to solve division problems with fractions.

What You Will Need

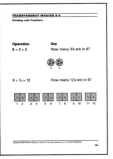

Transparency Master **5-5**

- Transparency 5-5, Dividing with Fractions.
- A card or sheet of paper for each student, each card or sheet containing one digit (0–9) that is large enough for all students to see.

What To Do

1. Begin with the following:
   - Discuss with students that division with fractions can be confusing because the numbers are actually multiplied rather than divided.
   - Also, point out that the answers are larger than either number in the problem, rather than smaller as they are when dividing two whole numbers.
   - Finally, explain that remembering that one fraction must be inverted before multiplying makes the whole process difficult for many people.
2. Give each student a card and ask four students at a time to step to the front of the classroom and "act out" a division problem as follows:
   - Each pair forms a fraction by one student holding his or her card over the card of the other. You or another student can say the problem out loud ("One half divided by one third").
   - The students who are playing the divisor then invert it by changing the placement of their cards. They then say the next step out loud (*Note:* The divisor is the fraction that is "dividing into" the other one. In the problem $\frac{1}{2} \div \frac{1}{3}$, $\frac{1}{3}$ is the divisor: $\frac{1}{2} \div \frac{1}{3} = \frac{1}{2} \times \frac{3}{1} = \frac{3}{2} = 1\frac{1}{2}$)
3. Alternate activity: Students use their cards from Student Handout 5-6 (or set of cards on which the digits 1 through 8 are written; see Activity 5-5) to create division problems with fractions in which they move about the cards on their desks to invert the divisor. Have them write out the problems they create and solve.

Follow-up Discussion

1. Why are the answers in a fraction division problem larger than either of the numbers in the problem?
2. What are some ways to explain what happens when fractions are divided?

ACTIVITY 5-10
VISUALIZING DECIMALS

What Students Will Learn

- An understanding of the place values of decimals.

What You Will Need

- Graph paper (at least 25 × 40 squares per sheet) for each student.
- Variety of colored pencils.

What To Do

1. On the graph paper, have students draw a square that is 25 squares wide and 40 squares long, resulting in a block with 1,000 small squares.
2. Review with students the concept of one tenth (.1), one hundredth, (.01), and one thousandth (.001). Remind them that the farther to the right of the decimal the number is, the smaller the decimal unit is.
3. Using the graph paper square, have students color in one thousandth of the block (one box), one hundredth (ten boxes), and one tenth (100 boxes or four rows of 25 boxes) using a different color pencil for each quantity.
4. You can expand on this activity by using other numbers such as 0.8, 0.03, 0.007, and so on. Students can use more than one graph paper square to illustrate mixed numbers such as 1.03, 1.8, and so on.
5. Alternate activity: You can also use the graph paper square to illustrate decimal multiplication. Instruct the students as follows:
   - Draw a box 10 squares by 10 squares.
   - Give a multiplication problem such as 0.6×0.3.
   - Have students shade three boxes across and six boxes down. Count how many boxes are shaded (0.18) (eighteen hundredths). This is the answer to the problem: $0.6 \times 0.3 = 18$ hundredths, or 0.18.

Follow-up Discussion

1. Do you find decimals more difficult than fractions to work with? Why or why not?

ACTIVITY 5-11
WHAT A DIFFERENCE A DECIMAL POINT MAKES!

What Students Will Learn

- How the position of the decimal point determines the value of a number.*

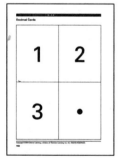

What You Will Need

- A set of cards for each group of three to five students. The set contains four cards that have one of the following written on each: 1, 2, 3, and a decimal point. (The set can be created from Student Handout 5-12, Decimal Cards. Either cut in advance or have students cut up their copy to make the cards.)
- Transparency 5-6, Decimal Point Combinations.

Student Handout **5-12**

What To Do

1. Divide the class into groups of three to five students and give each group a set of the four cards (all sets contain the same cards).
2. Allow them 5 to 10 minutes to come up with all the numbers that can be formed using any number of the cards in any order.
3. Remind the students that whole numbers have a decimal point following the last digit, understood to be there even when not actually written in; for example, 2 = 2.0 and 837 = 837.0.
4. Use Transparency 5-6, Decimal Point Placement, to show all the possible combinations. The group that forms the most numbers is the winner.

TRANSPARENCY MASTER 5-6
Decimal Point Placement

The following numbers can be formed using the four cards created from Student Handout 5-12:

.1	.12	.123	.13	.132	.2
.21	.213	.23	.231	.3	.31
.312	.32	.321	1	1.2	1.23
1.3	1.32	2	2.1	2.13	2.3
2.31	3	3.1	3.12	3.2	3.21
12	12.3	13	13.2	21	21.3
23	23.1	31	31.2	32	32.1
123	132	213	231	312	321

Transparency Master **5-6**

*Source: Adapted from M. Sobel & E. Maletsky (1988). *Teaching mathematics: A sourcebook of aids, activities, and strategies* (2nd ed.). Englewood Cliffs, NJ: Prentice Hall.

Follow-up Discussion

1. Have students share what numbers they were able to create.

ACTIVITY 5-12
ORDERING DECIMALS

What Students Will Learn

- Recognition of the numerical values of decimals.

What You Will Need

- Enough cards with a variety of decimals written on them (you can use the decimals from Activity 5-11) so that each student will get a card. These should be large enough for the students to see when they are held up in the front of the room. (Students can make the cards, using decimals of their choice, if given cardstock and marking pens.)

What To Do

1. Divide the class into groups of 6 to 10 students.
2. Distribute the decimal cards to each group, one per student.
3. Allow a few minutes for groups to put the decimals in order. Then have each group come to the front of the room and stand in the correct order in terms of value.
4. Ask the class to determine whether the group has ordered the decimals correctly.
5. Alternate version for small classes: Give each student a decimal card. Then call on students at random to come to the front of the room and line up in the correct order in relation to the decimals already being displayed.

Follow-up Discussion

1. Discuss with students again the place values of decimals (tenths, hundredths, etc.).

ACTIVITY 5-13
DECIMAL NUMBER LINE

What Students Will Learn

- Recognition of the numerical values of decimals.

What You Will Need

- A 4×6 size sticky note or other sticker for each student with a different decimal number on each. Be sure to use whole numbers and numbers with unneeded zeroes following the decimal point in them as well.

What To Do

1. Place one of the sticky notes or stickers on each student's forehead.
2. Do not let the students see what numbers are on their own stickers.
3. Ask students to arrange themselves in order from smallest to largest number (or largest to smallest) without speaking to each other.

Follow-up Discussion

1. What did you learn from this activity?

Activity 13 is adapted from an online site.

ACTIVITY 5-14
PERCENTAGE GRIDS

What Students Will Learn*

- Concept that percentages are fractions expressed in hundredths.
- Relationship of percentages, fractions, and decimals.

What You Will Need

- A copy of Student Handouts 5-13, Percentage Grids, and 5-14, Create Your Own Percentage Grids, for each student.
- Colored pencils for each student.
- Transparency 5-7, Percentage Grids Answers.
- Instructor Sheet 5-3, Percentage Grids—Answers for Student Handout 5-13.

What To Do

1. Discuss the concept that a percentage is a fraction—part of a whole—with a denominator of 100, meaning that percentages are always expressed in parts per hundred.
2. Distribute copies of Handouts 5-13 and 5-14 to each student.
3. Allow the students about 10 minutes time to complete the activity.
4. Have students pair up to exchange and check each other's original grids.
5. When students have completed working in pairs, discuss the answers using Instructor Sheet 5-3 and Transparency 5-7.
6. Ask students to share their own examples with the class.

Follow-up Discussion

1. Discuss the answers that the students have arrived at.

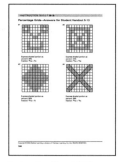
Instructor Sheet **5-3**

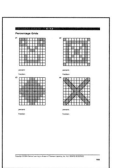
Student Handout **5-13**

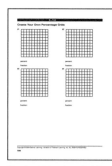
Student Handout **5-14**

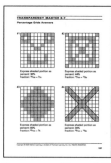
Transparency Master **5-7**

Source: Adapted from J. Akers, C. Tierney, C. Evans & M. Murray (1998). *Name that portion: Fractions, percents, and decimals.* White Plains, NY: Dale Seymour Publications.

ACTIVITY 5-15
LEARNING THE METRIC SYSTEM

Student Handout **5-15**

Student Handout **5-15**
(Continued)

Instructor Sheet **5-4**

What Students Will Learn

- The quantities expressed by metric measurements.
- How metric and Celsius measurements compare to English and Fahrenheit measurements.

What You Will Need

- Containers with metric measures for each group of three to four students (medicine spoons or cups work well).
- An eye dropper.
- A thermometer with Celsius measurement.
- A thermometer with Fahrenheit measurement.
- Teaspoon, tablespoon, and liquid measuring cups with standard measures.
- A metric ruler at least one meter long.
- An outdoor thermometer.
- Graph paper or other notepaper for charting results.
- A copy of Student Handout 5-15, Measuring, for each student.
- Instructor Sheet 5-4, Measuring—Answers for Student Handout 5-15.

What To Do

1. Divide students into groups of three or four.
2. Give each student a copy of Student Handout 5-15.
3. Give each group a set of measuring cups, spoons, thermometer, etc.
4. Ask students to determine the metric equivalent of standard English measurements such as 1 teaspoon, 1 tablespoon, normal body temperature, the ambient temperature of the room, the size of a floor tile in standard English and metric measurement, each person's height in metric, etc.
5. Have students use an outdoor thermometer to track the outdoor temperature in Fahrenheit and Celsius for at least 1 week.
6. Correct exercises on Student Handout 5-15 using Instructor Sheet 5-4.

Follow-up Discussion

1. What are some of the metric equivalents you discovered?
2. How might having an understanding of the equivalencies help you in your health care career?

ACTIVITY 5-16
CONVERSION SAYINGS

Student Handout **5-16**

What Students Will Learn

- Use of metric measurements in place of English measurements.

What You Will Need

- A copy of Student Handout 5-16, Conversions Please! for each student.
- Instructor Sheet 5-5, Conversion Sayings—Answers for Student Handout 5-16.

Instructor Sheet **5-5**

What To Do

1. Distribute Student Handout 5-16 and have the students convert the sayings to use metric words. For example, "Give him an inch and he'll take a mile." ("Give him 2.5 centimeters and he'll take 1.6 kilometers.")

2. Supply correct answers using Instructor Sheet 5-5.

Follow-up Discussion

1. How will knowing the metric system help you in a healthcare setting?

2. What are some other ways to become familiar with the weights, lengths, and volumes expressed in metric units?

ACTIVITY 5-17
FUN WITH NUMBERS

What Students Will Learn

- Some fun tricks that demonstrate interesting number characteristics and patterns.

What You Will Need

- A copy of Student Handouts 5-17, Fun with Numbers, and 5-18, Fun with Numbers Worksheet, for each student.
- Instructor Sheet 5-6, Fun with Numbers Worksheet—Answers for Student Handout 5-18.

What To Do

1. Distribute Student Handouts 5-17 and 5-18 and instruct the students to complete the worksheet using Student Handout 5-17 as a guide.

2. Give correct answers using Instructor Sheet 5.6.

Follow-up Discussion

1. Ask students to share any hints for working with numbers that they may have learned through experience or while in school.

Instructor Sheet **5-6**   Student Handout **5-17**   Student Handout **5-17** *(Continued)*   Student Handout **5-18**

ACTIVITY 5-18
MATH BASEBALL

What Students Will Learn

- Solving math problems.

What You Will Need

- Something to represent the bases and home plate.
- A list of math problems. An excellent source for all types of problems is *Practical problems in mathematics for health occupations*, by L. Simmers (Clifton Park, NY: Delmar Learning, 1996).

What To Do

1. Divide the students into two teams.
2. Choose a "pitcher" for each team.
3. Have pitcher choose a math question from the list you give him or her.
4. The "batter" must answer the question correctly to make it to first base.
5. Unless you use very difficult questions, batters should be "out" after getting one math problem wrong.
6. Play like real baseball so that second batter goes to first base after answering a question correctly and first batter goes to second, etc.
7. Keep track of "runs" and the team with the most runs wins.
8. You can play by having students actually move around the room to different bases you have set up, or by just keeping track as everyone sits in their seat.

Follow-up Discussion

1. Which type of math problems do you find most difficult?
2. What are some ways, in addition to games, to improve math skills?

REFERENCES

Akers, J., Tierney, C., Evans, C., & Murray, M. (1998). *Name that portion: Fractions, percents, and decimals.* White Plains, NY: Dale Seymour Publications.

Charles, L. H. & Brummett, M. R. (1989). *Connections: Grade 6.* Mt. View, CA: Creative Publications.

Math Activities: http://online.edfac.unimelb.edu.au/485129/DecProj/teaching/lessons.

Kogelman, S. & Warren, J. (1978). *Mind over math.* New York: McGraw-Hill.

Pappas, T. (1998). *More joy of mathematics: Exploring mathematics all around you.* San Carlos, CA: Wide World Publishing.

Simmers, L. (1996). *Practical problems in mathematics for health occupations.* Clifton Park, NY: Delmar Learning.

Smith, R. M. (1998). *How to be a GREAT math student* (3rd ed.). Pacific Grove, CA: Brooks/Cole.

Sobel, M. & Maletsky, E. (1988). *Teaching mathematics: A sourcebook of aids, activities, and strategies* (2nd ed.). Englewood Cliffs, NJ: Prentice Hall.

Forming Fractions—Answers for Student Handout 5-7

1. Arrange the cards to form as many fractions as possible. Write your list below. (The fractions do not have to be in their lowest terms.)

$\frac{1}{2}$ $\frac{1}{3}$ $\frac{1}{4}$ $\frac{1}{5}$ $\frac{1}{6}$ $\frac{1}{7}$ $\frac{1}{8}$

$\frac{2}{3}$ $\frac{2}{4}$ $\frac{2}{5}$ $\frac{2}{6}$ $\frac{2}{7}$ $\frac{2}{8}$

$\frac{3}{4}$ $\frac{3}{5}$ $\frac{3}{6}$ $\frac{3}{7}$ $\frac{3}{8}$

$\frac{4}{5}$ $\frac{4}{6}$ $\frac{4}{7}$ $\frac{4}{8}$

$\frac{5}{6}$ $\frac{5}{7}$ $\frac{5}{8}$

$\frac{6}{7}$ $\frac{6}{8}$

$\frac{7}{8}$

2. Which fraction on your list has

   a. the greatest value? $\frac{7}{8}$

   b. the least value? $\frac{1}{8}$

3. Arrange cards to create two examples of improper fractions. Write them below.

   Answers will vary. The numerator must be larger than the denominator.

4. Arrange cards to create two examples of mixed numbers. Write them below.

   Answers will vary. Must have both a whole number and a fraction.

5. Create two fractions that are equivalent in value. Write them below.

   Possible correct answers:

   $\frac{1}{2} = \frac{3}{6} = \frac{4}{8}$ $\frac{1}{3} = \frac{2}{6}$ $\frac{1}{4} = \frac{2}{8}$

6. Create three fractions. Now move the cards to create their reciprocals. Write the original fractions and their reciprocals below.

   Answers will vary. The reciprocal must be the inverse of the original fraction.

Comparing Fractions—Answers for Student Handout 5-10

Use Handout 5-8 to answer items 1 through 5:

1. In the following pairs, circle the fraction that represents the largest amount:

   $\frac{1}{6}$ and ⟨$\frac{1}{3}$⟩

   ⟨$\frac{1}{2}$⟩ and $\frac{1}{6}$

2. Fill in the blank in the following sentence:

   The smaller the denominator, the *larger* the amount represented by the fraction.

3. Using only the fractions given on the handout, write all the ways that each of the following can be expressed:

   $\frac{1}{3} = \frac{2}{6}$

   $\frac{3}{6} = \frac{1}{2}$

   $\frac{2}{3} = \frac{4}{6}$

   $\frac{1}{2} = \frac{3}{6}$

   $\frac{2}{6} = \frac{1}{3}$

4. Write "yes" next to the pair(s) of fractions that are equivalent in value. Write "no" next the pair(s) that are not equivalent.

   $\frac{5}{6}$ and $\frac{2}{3}$ no

   $\frac{1}{3}$ and $\frac{4}{6}$ no

   $\frac{1}{2}$ and $\frac{3}{6}$ yes

5. Circle the fraction in each pair that is expressed in its lowest terms.

   $\frac{2}{6}$ and ⟨$\frac{1}{3}$⟩

   ⟨$\frac{2}{3}$⟩ and $\frac{4}{6}$

   ⟨$\frac{1}{2}$⟩ and $\frac{3}{6}$

Use Handout 5-9 to answer items 6 through 8:

6. Using only the fractions given on the handout, write all the ways that the following can be expressed:

   $\frac{1}{2} = \frac{14}{28}, \frac{7}{14}, \frac{2}{4}$

   $\frac{1}{3} = \frac{7}{21}$

   $\frac{1}{4} = \frac{7}{28}$

7. Write "yes" next to the pair(s) of fractions that are equivalent in value. Write "no" next the pair(s) that are not equivalent.

   $\frac{1}{7}$ and $\frac{2}{14}$ yes

   $\frac{1}{2}$ and $\frac{2}{7}$ no

   $\frac{1}{3}$ and $\frac{3}{14}$ no

   $\frac{1}{2}$ and $\frac{14}{28}$ yes

   $\frac{1}{4}$ and $\frac{7}{28}$ yes

   $\frac{1}{3}$ and $\frac{8}{28}$ no

8. Circle the fraction in each pair that is expressed in its lowest terms.

   $\frac{3}{21}$ and ⟨$\frac{1}{7}$⟩

   $\frac{7}{28}$ and ⟨$\frac{1}{4}$⟩

   ⟨$\frac{1}{2}$⟩ and $\frac{7}{14}$

Percentage Grids—Answers for Student Handout 5-13

#1

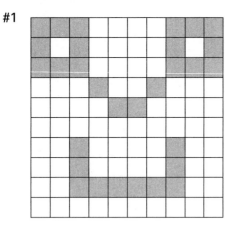

Express shaded portion as
percent: 30%
fraction: $^{30}/_{100} = ^{3}/_{10}$

#2

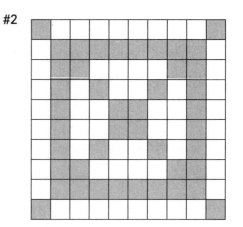

Express shaded portion as
percent: 44%
fraction: $^{44}/_{100} = ^{22}/_{50}$

#3

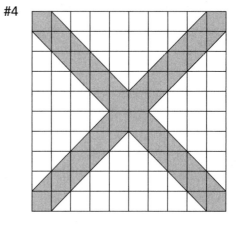

Express shaded portion as
percent: 60%
fraction: $^{60}/_{100} = ^{3}/_{5}$

#4

Express shaded portion as
percent: 36%
fraction: $^{36}/_{100} = ^{18}/_{50}$

Measuring—Answers for Student Handout 5-15

Measurement Sizes

What is the average number of drops it takes to fill 5 ml? *approximately 60*

How many teaspoons does it take to equal 5 ml? *approximately 1*

How many teaspoons does it take to equal 15 ml? *approximately 3*

If you have containers that are large enough, calculate how a liter compares to a quart. Is it more or less than one quart? *more than a quart*

Linear Measurements

Answers will vary.

Temperature

Answers will vary. Check to see if the equivalencies are calculated correctly.

Conversion Sayings—Answers for Student Handout 5-16

1. "He demanded .45 kilograms of flesh."

2. "A miss is as good as 1.6 kilometers." (Or it could be converted to feet: "A miss is as good as 5,280 feet.")

3. "Every 2.5 centimeters a king."

4. "157 centimeters, eyes of blue . . . ."

5. "28.4 grams of prevention are worth .45 kilograms of cure."

6. "First down and 914.4 centimeters (or 9.144 meters) to go."

7. "Give him 2.5 centimeters and he'll take 1.6 kilometers."

Fun With Numbers Worksheet—Answers for Student Handout 5-18

Without actually doing the math, determine which of the following numbers is evenly divisible by 2:

28	367	*98,064*	3	*2,584,756*
44,449	*54,690*	*258*	437	395

Without actually doing the math, determine which of the following numbers is evenly divisible by 3:

2,970	107	*375*	385

Without actually doing the math, determine which of the following numbers is evenly divisible by 9:

3,204	29	*2,304*	*43,101*	5,419

Without actually doing the math, determine which of the following numbers is evenly divisible by 6:

168	1,018	*1,008*	*21,942*	3,655

Without actually doing the math, determine which of the following numbers is evenly divisible by 8:

2,045	*4,712*	*456*	*29,184*	1,538

Sharing Fears

1. As a group, make a written list of fears about or problems with math.

2. Talk about the experiences, both positive and negative, you've all had in math classes.

3. Have the group members experienced some of the same problems?

4. What positive experiences have group members had applying math in daily life?

5. How can what we believe about ourselves and our abilities influence our performance and accomplishments in subjects like math?

Overcoming Math Anxiety

1. *Attitude* is more important than *aptitude* when you're learning math.

2. Most students have more ability to learn math than they realize.

3. Adults have more practical experience than younger students and they can use this experience to review and learn math.

4. One of the most important factors that determines your ability to do math is self-confidence.

5. Staying calm is important when studying math. Being nervous can interfere with your concentration.

6. Even students who have done poorly in math in the past can improve if they have a never-quit attitude.

7. Students who work hard and who *act* as if they have control over their own success, will become successful.

8. If it's been a long time since you studied math and you've forgotten a lot, you can overcome this deficiency by reviewing and getting help with anything you don't understand.

Source: #1–5 adapted from S. Kogelman & J. Warren (1978). *Mind over math.* New York: McGraw-Hill; and # 6–8 from R. M. Smith (1998). *How to be a GREAT math student* (3rd ed.). Pacific Grove, CA: Brooks/Cole.

Overcoming Math Anxiety Discussion Questions

1. Do the members of your group agree with the statement?

2. Does anyone have an experience or example that demonstrates the truth of the statement?

3. How can you apply this information to help change your attitude about math?

4. What do the members of your group already know and do that demonstrate their ability to do math? The following examples require the use of applied math. Can you think of others?

   a. Using and balancing a checkbook
   b. Shopping
   c. Paying taxes
   d. Applying for a student loan
   e. Measuring
   f. Estimating distances
   g. Sewing and shop projects
   h. Building and working around the house

Health Care Occupations

1. Certified Nurse's Assistant

2. Dental Assistant

3. Dental Hygienist

4. Dental Laboratory Technician

5. Diagnostic Medical Sonographer

6. Emergency Medical Technician

7. Health Information Technician

8. Home Health Aide

9. Medical Assistant

10. Insurance Coding Specialist

11. Medical Laboratory Assistant

12. Medical Transcriptionist

13. Mental Health Technician

14. Occupational Therapy Assistant

15. Ophthalmic Technician

16. Phlebotomist

17. Physical Therapist Assistant

18. Practical/Vocational Nurse

19. Radiologic Technician

20. Registered Nurse

21. Respiratory Therapist

22. Surgical Technologist/Technician

Questions for Group Discussion

1. In each of the occupations you discussed, what effect can math accuracy have on patient safety and well-being?

2. What effect can it have on facility efficiency? For example, how would accuracy affect the use of time? Of supplies?

3. What impact could it have on the cost of patient care and other finances of the organization?

4. How can understanding the ways that math will be applied on the job help motivate you to work on developing your math skills?

Number Cards

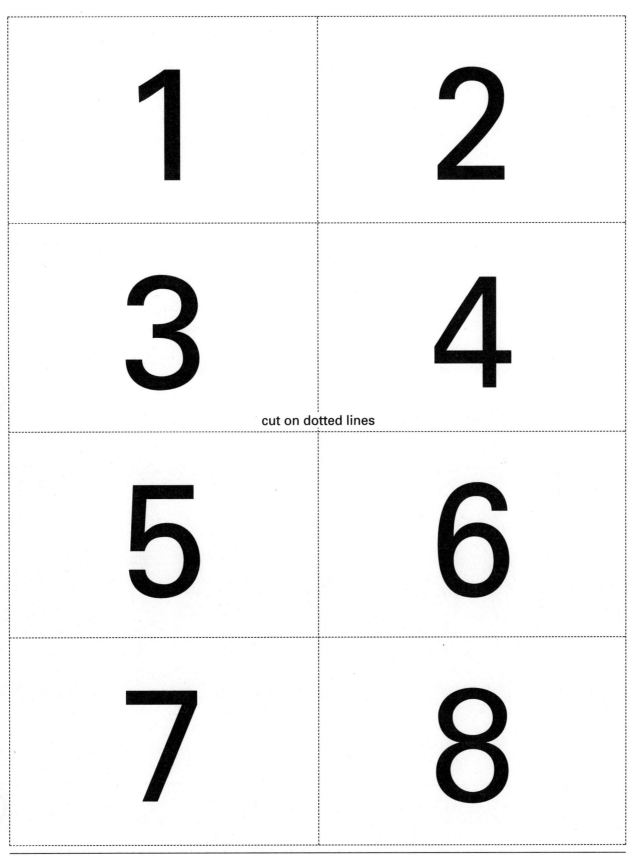

cut on dotted lines

Forming Fractions

1. Arrange the cards to form as many fractions as possible. Write your list below. (The fractions do not have to be in their lowest terms.)

2. Which fraction on your list has

   a. the greatest value?

   b. the least value?

3. Arrange cards to create two examples of improper fractions. Write them below.

4. Arrange cards to create two examples of mixed numbers. Write them below.

5. Create two fractions that are equivalent in value. Write them below.

6. Create three fractions. Now move the cards to create their reciprocals. Write the original fractions and their reciprocals below.

Fraction Flash Cards I

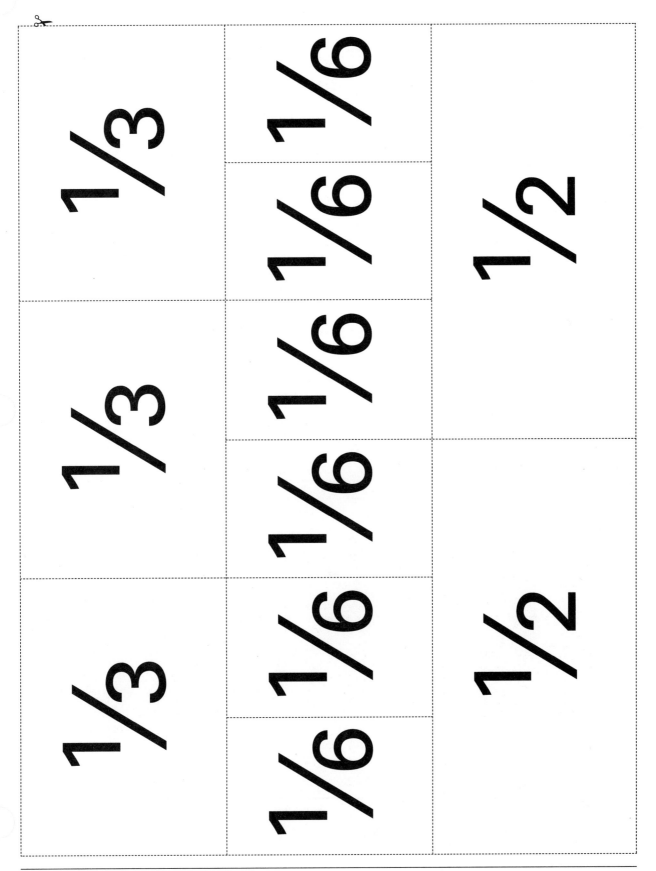

Fraction Flash Cards II

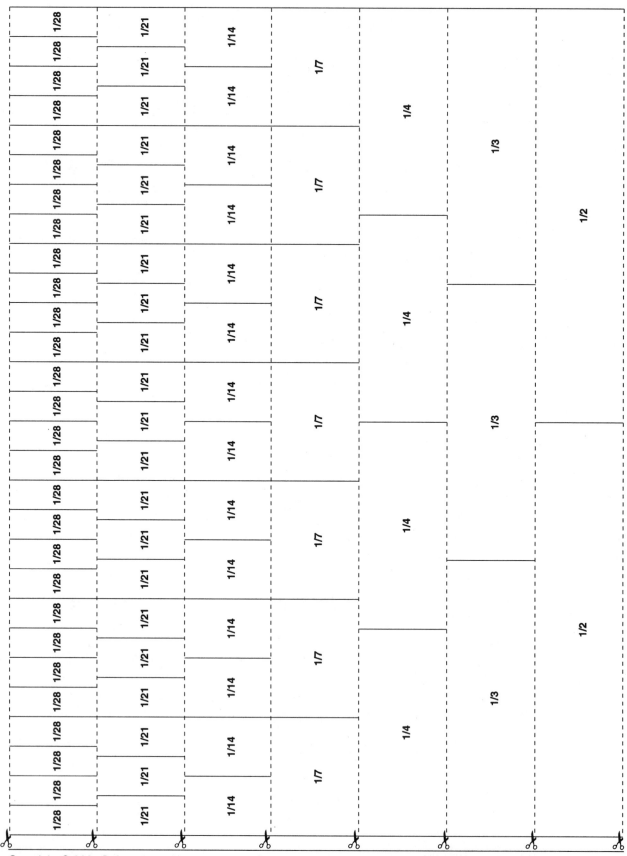

Comparing Fractions

Fraction Facts

- The top number in a fraction is the *numerator*.

- The bottom number in a fraction is the *denominator*.

- Fractions whose denominators cannot be divided evenly by the same number will not have any equivalent forms.

- A fraction is in its lowest terms when the numerator and denominator can no longer be evenly divided by the same number.

Use Handout 5-8 to answer items 1 through 5:

1. In the following pairs, circle the fraction that represents the largest amount;

   ⅙ and ⅓

   ½ and ⅙

2. Fill in the blank in the following sentence:

   The smaller the denominator, the _____ the amount represented by the fraction.

3. Using only the fractions given on the handout, write all the ways that each of the following can be expressed:

   ⅓ =

   ³⁄₆ =

   ⅔ =

   ½ =

   ²⁄₆ =

4. Write "yes" next to the pair(s) of fractions that are equivalent in value. Write "no" next the pair(s) that are not equivalent.

   ⁵⁄₆ and ⅔

   ⅓ and ⁴⁄₆

   ½ and ³⁄₆

5. Circle the fraction in each pair that is expressed in its lowest terms.

   ²⁄₆ and ⅓   ⅔ and ⁴⁄₆   ½ and ³⁄₆

Use Handout 5-9 to answer items 6 through 8:

6. Using only the fractions given on the handout, write all the ways that the following can be expressed:

   ½ =

   ⅓ =

   ¼ =

7. Write "yes" next to the pair(s) of fractions that are equivalent in value. Write "no" next the pair(s) that are not equivalent.

   ⅐ and ²⁄₁₄

   ½ and ²⁄₇

   ⅓ and ³⁄₁₄

   ½ and ¹⁴⁄₂₈

   ¼ and ⁷⁄₂₈

   ⅓ and ⁸⁄₂₈

8. Circle the fraction in each pair that is expressed in its lowest terms.

   ³⁄₂₁ and ⅐

   ⁷⁄₂₈ and ¼

   ½ and ⁷⁄₁₄

STUDENT HANDOUT **5-11**

Using Paper Models to Show Multiplication of Fractions

1. Take a piece of paper and fold it into thirds one way. Then fold it in half the other way. Note that the value of each small square formed by the folds is $\frac{1}{6}$. Refold your paper to demonstrate the following problems:

   a. $\frac{1}{2} \times \frac{1}{3} = \frac{1}{6}$

   b. $\frac{2}{3} \times \frac{1}{2} = \frac{2}{6} = \frac{1}{3}$

2. Use a second sheet of paper and fold it in half three times. Note that the value of each small square formed by the folds is $\frac{1}{6}$. Refold your paper to demonstrate the following problems:

   a. $\frac{1}{4} \times \frac{1}{2} = \frac{1}{8}$

   b. $\frac{3}{4} \times \frac{1}{2} = \frac{3}{8}$

3. Use a third sheet of paper and fold it into fourths one way and thirds the other way. Note that the value of each small square formed by the folds is $\frac{1}{12}$. Refold your paper to demonstrate the following problems:

   a. $\frac{2}{3} \times \frac{3}{4} = \frac{1}{2}$

   b. $\frac{1}{4} \times \frac{1}{3} = \frac{1}{12}$

Decimal Cards

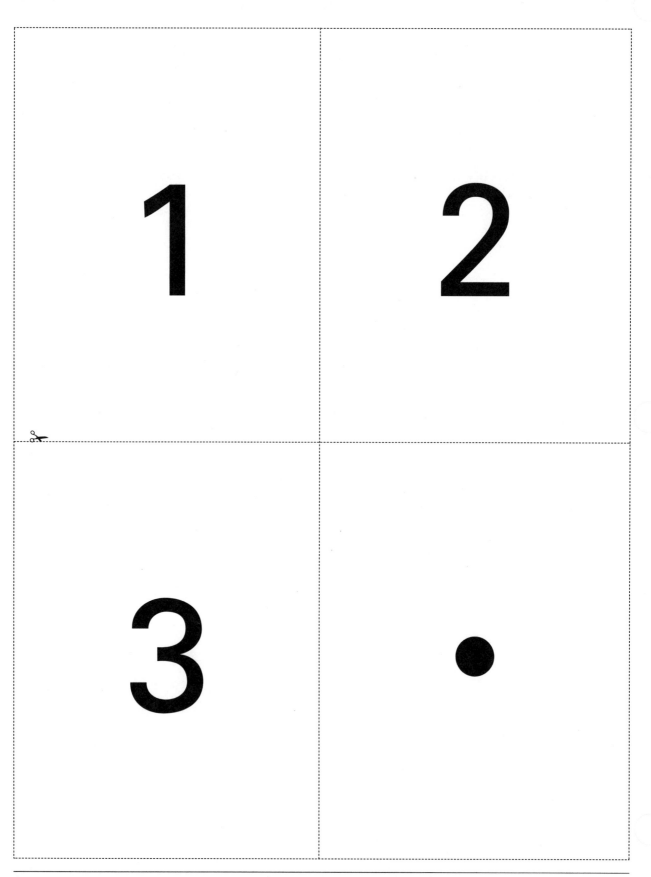

Percentage Grids

#1

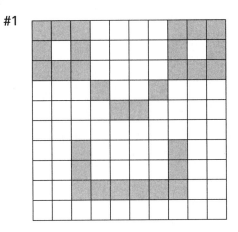

percent:

fraction:

#2

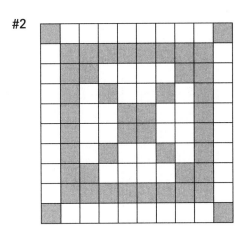

percent:

fraction:

#3

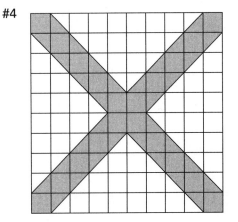

percent:

fraction:

#4

percent:

fraction:

Create Your Own Percentage Grids

#1

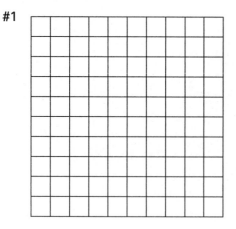

percent:

fraction:

#2

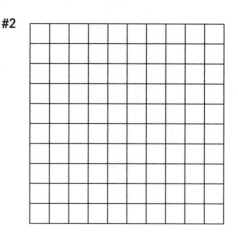

percent:

fraction:

#3

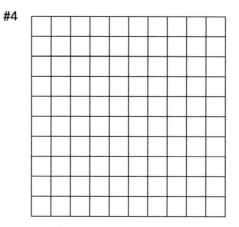

percent:

fraction:

#4

percent:

fraction:

Measuring

MEASUREMENT SIZES

Cubic Centimeters (cc), Milliliters (ml), Teaspoons (tsp), Drops (gtts), and so on

Five, ten, and fifteen milliliters are common sizes of medication orders for liquids such as eye drops and ear drops. They can also be common sizes of dosage administration. It is important that you have an idea of how much 5 ml, 10 ml, and 15 ml really are. The following exercises will help you better understand these measurement sizes. It is important to remember, though, that household measurements are approximate and not as accurate a measure as the metric measurements used in medicine.

Calculate approximately how many drops are in 5 ml. (Note that 1 ml is equal to 1 cc.)

What You Need

- An eyedropper
- Household measuring spoons
- A medicine cup, calibrated test tube, spill-proof medicine spoon, or any small container marked in ml measurements
- A cup of water

What To Do

1. Put at least 8 ounces of water in a cup.
2. Use the eyedropper to transfer water from the cup, one drop at a time, into a container that measures milliliters.
3. Count how many drops it takes to reach 5 ml.
4. Repeat steps 1, 2, and 3 two or three more times.

What is the average number of drops it takes to fill 5ml? _____

Now calculate how many teaspoons are in 5 ml, 10 ml, and 15 ml. You can do this by starting with a small amount of water such as ¼ or ½ teaspoon and pouring it into a small container with metric divisions. Do this until you reach 5 ml.

How many teaspoons does it take to equal 5 ml? _____

How many teaspoons does it take to equal 15 ml? _____

If you have containers that are large enough, calculate how a liter compares to a quart. Is it more or less than one quart? _____

Linear Measurements

Using a tape measure or other measuring device that shows both English and metric units, measure common items in your classroom or home and record both sets of measurements. Measure at least 10 items. Here are some examples:

Student desk _____   Height of a chair seat _____

One square floor tile _____   Height of the light switch _____

Instructor's desk _____   Width of classroom window _____

Length of your shoe _____   Your notebook _____

Your textbook _____   Width of chalk or whiteboard _____

Choose a few more items and estimate their size in the metric system. Now measure and see how close you have come. Here are some examples:

	Estimate	**Reality**
Width of a sidewalk	_____	_____
Height of the bulletin board	_____	_____
Width of the doorway opening	_____	_____

Estimate how tall each member of your group is using the metric system. Measure each member and compare your guess to reality.

	Estimate	**Reality**
Member 1	_____	_____
Member 2	_____	_____
Member 3	_____	_____
Member 4	_____	_____

Measuring Temperature

Using the Celsius and Fahrenheit thermometer, observe the outdoor temperature daily for at least 5 days. Record the temperature in Celsius and Fahrenheit. Don't forget to mark your findings with a C to indicate a Celsius measurement or an F to indicate Fahrenheit measurement. Record your observations here:

Day 1	_____	_____
Day 2	_____	_____
Day 3	_____	_____
Day 4	_____	_____
Day 5	_____	_____

Use a Celsius and Fahrenheit thermometer to take the temperature of everyone in your group. What is a normal Celsius body temperature?

Use your imagination to choose other temperatures to compare. Ideas include measuring the temperature of a glass of ice water, a soft drink, hot tap water, and your soup at lunch. Become familiar with the metric system applied to everyday items. Take enough temperatures so that if someone tells you it is 20°C outside, you will know whether you should bring a jacket or wear shorts that day.

Conversions Please!

Conversion formulas from English to metric measurements

1 pound = 0.4545 kilograms

1 inch = 2.5 centimeters

1 mile = 5,280 yards = 1.6 kilometers

1 yard = 0.914 meters

1 meter = 39.37 inches = 3.28 feet = 1.09 yards

1 ounce = 28.4 grams

1 foot = 0.3048 meters

1. "He demanded a pound of flesh."

2. "A miss is as good as a mile."

3. "Every inch a king."

4. "Five foot two, eyes of blue . . . ."

5. "An ounce of prevention is worth a pound of cure."

6. "First down and 10 yards to go"

7. "Give him an inch and he'll take a mile"

Source: Adapted from T. Pappas (1998). *More joy of mathematics: Exploring mathematics all around you.* San Carlos, CA: Wide World Publishing.

Fun With Numbers

Help with Division*

A number is divisible by the numbers listed in column A if it meets the condition stated in column B.

A	B
2	If it ends with an even number.
3	If the sum of the digits of the number is divisible by 3.
4	If the last two digits of the number are divisible by 4.
5	If the number ends in a 5 or 0.
6	If the number ends in an even number and if the sum of the digits is divisible by 3.
8	If the last three digits of the number represent a number divisible by 8.
9	If the sum of the digits of the number is divisible by 9.
10	If the number ends in 0.

Dividing by 9

You can rearrange the digits in a whole number in any order you like and the sum of the difference between the two numbers will be divisible by 9. For example:

Number	Rearranged	Difference	Divided by 9
25	52	27	3
386	836	450	50
386	683	297	33
9,673	7,369	2,304	256

*Source: Adapted from T. Pappas (1998). *More joy of mathematics: Exploring mathematics all around you.* San Carlos, CA: Wide World Publishing.

Help with Your Checkbook

Here is a tool that can help if you are unable to balance when doing bookkeeping. For example, if your checkbook doesn't balance, follow these steps:

1. Subtract the number you get and the balance you should have reached (shown on your statement).

2. Determine if the answer is divisible by 9.

3. If it is, look for a number that you have transposed (written in the wrong order, such as 29 instead of 92).

Remembering the Factors for 9

Notice that if you add 1 to the number in the tens place, the answer is the result of the number being divided by 9.

$\underline{4}5 \div 9 = \underline{4} + 1 = 5$

$\underline{6}3 \div 9 = \underline{6} + 1 = 7$

$9 \div 9 = 1$	$45 \div 9 = 5$	$72 \div 9 = 8$
$18 \div 9 = 2$	$54 \div 9 = 6$	$81 \div 9 = 9$
$27 \div 9 = 3$	$63 \div 9 = 7$	$90 \div 9 = 10$
$36 \div 9 = 4$		

If the sum of the numbers in a group is divisible by 9, the entire number is evenly divisible by 9:

450	297	2,304
$4 + 5 + 0 = \underline{9}$	$2 + 9 + 7 = \underline{18}$	$2 + 3 + 0 + 4 = \underline{9}$
$\underline{9} \div 9 = 1$	$\underline{18} \div 9 = 2$	$\underline{9} \div 9 = 1$
$450 \div 9 = 50$	$297 \div 9 = 33$	$2,304 \div 9 = 256$

Fun with Numbers Worksheet

Without actually doing the math, determine which of the following numbers is evenly divisible by 2:

28	367	98,064	3	2,584,756

44,449	54,690	258	437	395

Without actually doing the math, determine which of the following numbers is evenly divisible by 3:

2,970	107	375	385

Without actually doing the math, determine which of the following numbers is evenly divisible by 9:

3,204	29	2,304	43,101	5,419

Without actually doing the math, determine which of the following numbers is evenly divisible by 6:

168	1,018	1,008	21,942	3,655

Without actually doing the math, determine which of the following numbers is evenly divisible by 8:

2,045	4,712	456	29,184	1,538

Fraction Flash Cards I

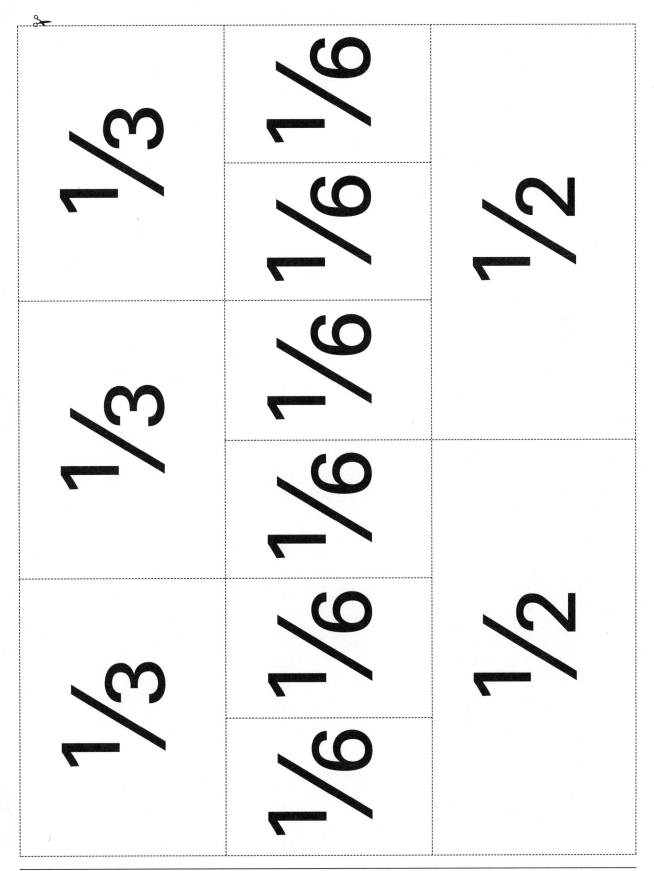

Fraction Flash Cards II

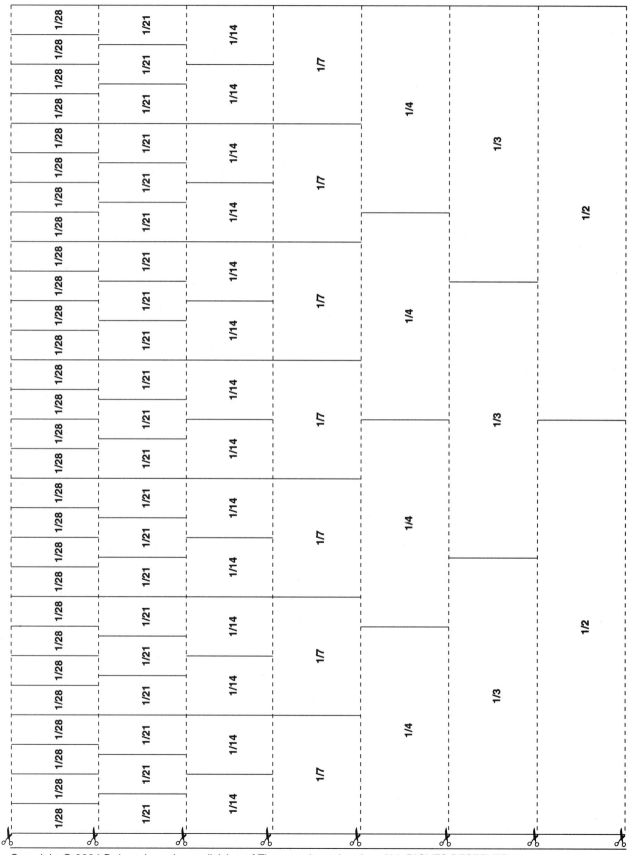

Multiplying Fractions

Operation	Says	
$4 \times 8 = 32$	4 groups *of* 8 = 32	
$9 \times 3 = 27$	9 groups *of* 3 = 27	
$6 \times \frac{1}{2} = 3$	6 groups *of* ½ = 3	
$\frac{1}{2} \times 6 = 3$	½ *of* 6 = 3	
$\frac{1}{2} \times \frac{2}{3} = \frac{1}{3}$	½ *of* ⅔ = ⅓	
$\frac{2}{3} \times \frac{3}{4} = \frac{1}{2}$	⅔ *of* ¾ = ½	

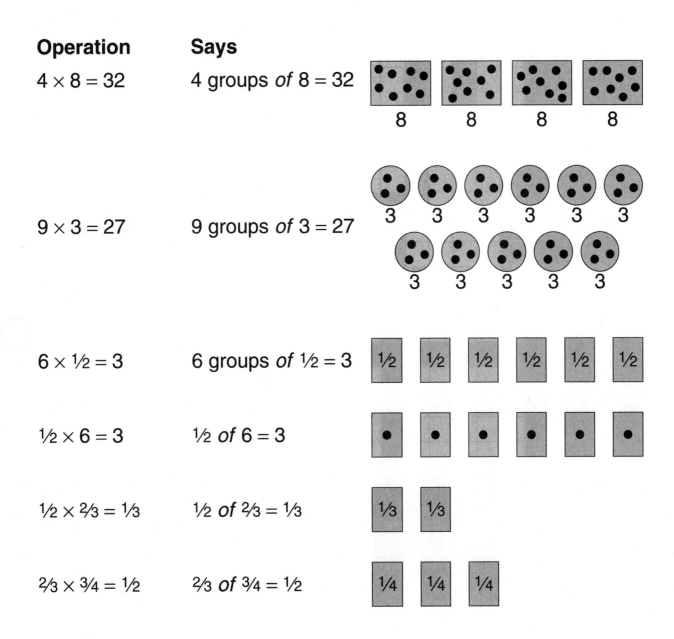

Multiplication Models

1.　(a)　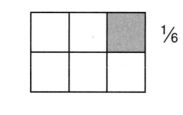 ⅙

$$\frac{1}{2} \times \frac{1}{3} = \frac{1}{6}$$

 　(b)　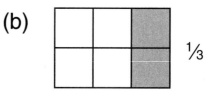 ⅓

$$\frac{2}{3} \times \frac{1}{2} = \frac{2}{6} = \frac{1}{3}$$

2.　(a)　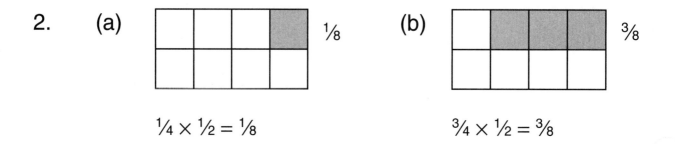 ⅛

$$\frac{1}{4} \times \frac{1}{2} = \frac{1}{8}$$

 　(b)　 ⅜

$$\frac{3}{4} \times \frac{1}{2} = \frac{3}{8}$$

3.　(a)　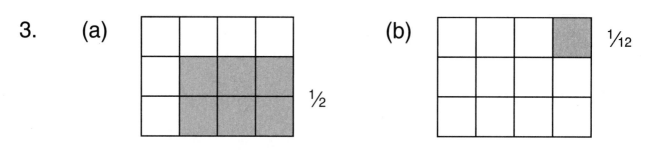 ½

$$\frac{2}{3} \times \frac{3}{4} = \frac{1}{2}$$

 　(b)　 ¹⁄₁₂

$$\frac{1}{4} \times \frac{1}{3} = \frac{1}{12}$$

Dividing with Fractions

Operation	**Say**
$6 \div 3 = 2$	How many 3's are in 6?

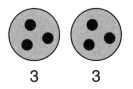

$6 \div \frac{1}{2} = 12$ How many ½'s are in 6?

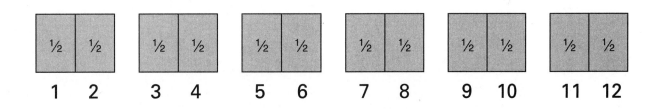

Decimal Point Placement

The following numbers can be formed using the four cards created from Student Handout 5-12:

.1	.12	.123	.13	.132	.2
.21	.213	.23	.231	.3	.31
.312	.32	.321	1	1.2	1.23
1.3	1.32	2	2.1	2.13	2.3
2.31	3	3.1	3.12	3.2	3.21
12	12.3	13	13.2	21	21.3
23	23.1	31	31.2	32	32.1
123	132	213	231	312	321

Source: Adapted from M. Sobel & E. Maletsky (1988). *Teaching mathematics: A sourcebook of aids, activities, and strategies* (2nd ed.). Englewood Cliffs, NJ: Prentice Hall.

Percentage Grids Answers

#1

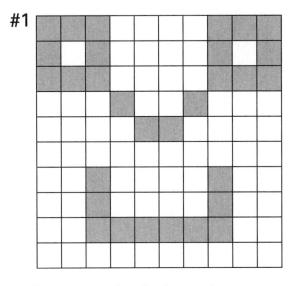

Express shaded portion as
percent: 30%
fraction: $^{30}/_{100} = {}^{3}/_{10}$

#2

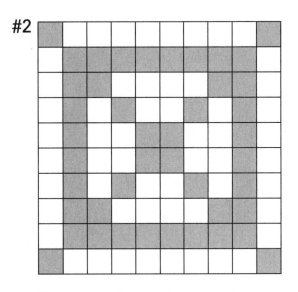

Express shaded portion as
percent: 44%
fraction: $^{44}/_{100} = {}^{22}/_{50}$

#3

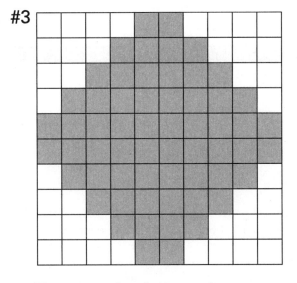

Express shaded portion as
percent: 60%
fraction: $^{60}/_{100} = {}^{3}/_{5}$

#4

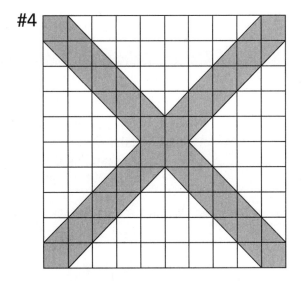

Express shaded portion as
percent: 36%
fraction: $^{36}/_{100} = {}^{18}/_{50}$

CHAPTER **6**

Diversity

INTRODUCTION

In today's world, students will come into contact every day with people who are different from them. These differences can include color, religious beliefs, native language, value systems, sexual orientation, abilities and handicaps, and age. Success in the workplace and in society depends on the ability to understand and accept these differences. Learning about diversity will help students grow and become more open-minded members of society.

Accepting those who are different requires understanding oneself, recognizing what is unique about others, and having empathy. The activities in this chapter are designed to help students learn about themselves and each other. Opportunities are provided to explore differences and discover what makes each of us special. Cultural awareness and sensitivity will help students become more effective members of the health care team.

ACTIVITY 6-1
HOW DO I SEE THE WORLD?

What Students Will Learn*

- Awareness that a variety of factors influence people's perspectives about life and the world.
- Understanding that different perspectives are okay.
- The benefits of understanding the viewpoints of others.

What You Need

- A copy of Student Handout 6-1, How Do I See the World? for each student.

What To Do

1. Distribute Student Handout 6-1 and explain that the worksheets won't be collected.
2. Ask students to write brief answers to the questions. Explain that some of the questions are personal and students may skip them if they are not comfortable answering them.
3. After students have answered the questions, conduct the follow-up discussion.

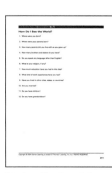
Student Handout **6-1**

---

*Source: Activity adapted from J. Gibbs (1994). *Tribes: A new way of learning together.* Santa Rosa, CA: Center Source Publications.

4. Alternate activity: After students have worked individually to answer the questions, divide the class into groups of up to five students and hand out a copy of the discussion questions for them to discuss in their groups.

Follow-up Discussion

1. How do people's backgrounds give them different perspectives and opinions?
2. What can happen when people believe that everyone else sees the world in the same way they do?
3. How can different perspectives be beneficial in a work situation?
4. How can people learn about the perspectives of others?
5. How can differences in perception lead to conflict?
6. How can conflict due to these differences be resolved?

ACTIVITY 6-2
WHAT IS SPECIAL ABOUT MY CULTURE?

What Students Will Learn

- How different ethnic groups view themselves.
- Something special about each of the cultures represented in the class.
- Something special about their own culture.

What You Will Need

- 3 × 5 card for each student
- White board or chalkboard

What To Do

1. Begin a class discussion by asking students, "What is special about your culture?"
2. Prompt students to consider other unique things about themselves such as family life, age, religion, food preferences, holiday customs, and the like.
3. As the discussion proceeds, write the different ethnicities and what is special about each on the board.
4. Give each student a 3 × 5 card. Ask them to write their name on one side and their ethnicity and one word they believe that describes their ethnic group on the other. (e.g., Italian, passionate). Ask the students to share what they have written and why.

Follow-up Discussion

1. Did you learn anything new about the various cultural backgrounds represented in the class? If so, explain what you learned.
2. What are the advantages of living in a society in which many cultures are represented?
3. Why is it important for the health care worker to be aware of cultural differences?

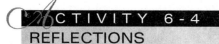

Transparency Master **6-1**

Transparency Master **6-1**
(Continued)

ACTIVITY 6-3
CULTURAL VALUES

What Students Will Learn

- Awareness that each culture has a unique value system.
- Values of other cultures.

What You Will Need

- A copy of Student Handout 6-2, Cultural Values, for each student or Transparency 6-1, Cultural Values.

Student Handout **6-2**

What To Do

1. Start with a class discussion about values. You can have this discussion with or without using Transparency 6-1 or Student Handout 6-2.
2. Discuss ethnocentrism (the belief that one's own cultural group is superior to others) with students. Ask if any have traveled or lived in another country. What differences have they seen? What is the "Ugly American"?

Follow-up Discussion

1. Use the transparency or student handout as a discussion guide.

ACTIVITY 6-4
REFLECTIONS

What Students Will Learn

- We can't know people by their appearance.*

What You Will Need

- A small mirror for each group (class will be divided into groups of three to five students)

What To Do

1. Divide class into groups of three to five students.

*Source: Activity adapted from J. Gibbs (1994). *Tribes: A new way of learning together.* Santa Rosa, CA: Center Source Publications.

2. Working in their groups, students take turns looking into the mirror and stating what they see (hair and eye color, expression on face, and so on).

3. Instruct students to go around the group a second time. This time they make statements about their values, beliefs, or goals.

4. When each student has shared, conduct the follow-up discussion.

Follow-up Discussion

1. Was it difficult to report what you saw in the mirror? If so, why do you think it was difficult?

2. What messages about how you appear to others were reflected in the mirror?

3. What important characteristics about you were not reflected in the mirror?

4. What are your most important characteristics, both those that can and cannot be seen?

5. What can happen if we judge others simply by their appearance?

6. What are some ways to avoid judging people by their appearance?

7. How does not judging people by their appearance apply to your future work in health care?

ACTIVITY 6-5
WHO AM I?

What Students Will Learn

- How we often judge others based on such things as how they look and what they do.

What You Will Need

Student Handout **6-3**

- A willingness to share personal information with your students.
- A copy of Student Handout 6-3, Who Am I?, for each student.

Instructor's Note: The questions on Student Handout 6-3 are about you and you need to be willing to tell the students the correct answers at the end of the exercise. If you are uncomfortable with any of the questions, you can ask students to skip them or retype the handout without them.)

What To Do

1. Distribute Student Handout 6-3.

2. Ask students to write down the answers to the questions, guessing if they do not know.

3. When students have finished answering the questions, tell them the correct answers.

4. Alternate activity: Show students a picture of someone and have them answer the questions about that person. Again, you will need to know the correct answers and share them with the students at the end of the exercise.

Follow-up Discussion

1. How much did you know about me (or the person in the picture)?

2. On what did you base your answers?

3. How much can we know about people from their appearance?

4. How does this exercise apply to your work in health care?

ACTIVITY 6-6
WHO IS THIS PERSON?

What Students Will Learn

- How we have preconceived notions of others based on appearance.

What You Will Need

- An enlarged photograph of someone you know.

What To Do

1. Show the photograph to the class (pass it around if it is too small for everyone to see) and ask students to tell you about the person based on what they see.
2. After the students have given you as much information about the person they can, tell them the facts about the person.

Follow-up Discussion

1. How accurate were your "facts" about the person in the picture?
2. On what did you base your ideas about this person?
3. Why do we associate certain aspects of appearance with certain characteristics?
4. How do you think the health care worker's appearance influences patients' opinions about the care they are receiving?

ACTIVITY 6-7
STEREOTYPES

What Students Will Learn

- An understanding that diversity refers to many kinds of differences among people.
- How to look at people as individuals rather than as members of a group.

What You Will Need

- A copy of Student Handout 6-4, The Many Meanings of Diversity, for each student.

What To Do

1. Distribute Student Handout 6-4.
2. Instruct students to review the list and fill in the chart.
3. When they have completed the handout, conduct the follow-up discussion.

Student Handout **6-4**

Follow-up Discussion

1. How much do you really know about each group?
2. Why do you think stereotypes are developed about people?
3. Who do you know who contradicts the common stereotypes?
4. Can you think of anyone in history who contradicts the stereotype?
5. How can stereotypes interfere with establishing good relationships with other people?
6. How can stereotypes cause problems among co-workers?

7. How can stereotypes affect relationships between health care workers and their patients?
8. What steps can people take to prevent stereotyping others who are different from themselves?

CTIVITY 6-8
WHAT DO WE HAVE IN COMMON?

What Students Will Learn
- How to identify commonalities among people.
- How to use commonalities to establish a base for communication.

What You Will Need
- Transparency 6-2, What Do We Have in Common?

Transparency Master **6-2**

What To Do
1. Have students pair off with someone they don't know well.
2. Once everyone has a partner, give the class 5 minutes to find out what they have in common with their partners. Use Transparency 6-2 as a guide for areas to explore. (Instead of using the transparency with an overhead projector, you can make copies of the transparency master to distribute to each pair for use as a prompt.)

Follow-up Discussion
1. How much did you have in common with your partner?
2. Did you have more or less in common than you expected? Explain.
3. How did you feel about looking for commonalities with someone you didn't know well?
4. Why would establishing commonalities be a good technique when getting to know your co-workers at a new job?
5. How can establishing commonalities be used to create good relationships with patients?

CTIVITY 6-9
THIS IS ME

What Students Will Learn
- How to explore their own backgrounds.
- How to share information about themselves.
- Facts about the backgrounds of their classmates.

What You Will Need
- Materials to make a collage, such as photos, pictures from magazines, colored paper, stickers.
- Students can bring art they have created themselves or small objects they want to use in their projects.
- A new shower curtain liner.

What To Do

1. Ask students to create a picture, shadow box, collage, or other item that represents their background and who they are. Give them a few days to complete the project.
2. Have each student tell the class about his or her project.
3. Display the projects around the room for the remainder of the term.
4. If the projects are on sheets of paper, attach each sheet to the shower curtain liner to make a "diversity quilt." Hang the quilt in your classroom for the remainder of the term.

Follow-up Discussion

1. What did you learn about yourself from this activity?
2. What did you learn about your classmates?

ACTIVITY 6-10
PEER COACHING

What Students Will Learn*

- How people learn at different rates.
- How people vary in their ability to master specific subjects.
- How the experience of helping others learn can be satisfying.

What You Will Need

- No special materials are needed for this activity.

What To Do

1. Choose a topic that has been studied in class with which some of the students are having difficulty. (Topics should be fairly narrow in scope.)
2. Ask for students who think they understand the topic to act as coaches for the students who do not. (Or choose coaches yourself, based on test scores, your observations of the class, and so on.)
3. Divide the class into the number of groups for which you have coaches.
4. Explain that the goal of the coaches is for everyone in their groups to demonstrate understanding of the concept by explaining it, performing a procedure, and so on, as appropriate.
5. Encourage the coaches to use visuals, demonstrations, group interaction, and anything else they can think of to help their group learn.

Follow-up Discussion

1. What did you learn about helping others learn?
2. Were the coaches' explanations helpful in helping you learn? Why or why not?
3. What did you find most helpful? Least helpful?
4. How did the coaches feel about helping their classmates?
5. Did the noncoaches begin to take part in helping others in their group?
6. Did you find it easier to learn when you worked together?
7. How might peer coaching be useful in the workplace?

*Source: Activity adapted from J. Gibbs (1994). *Tribes: A new way of learning together.* Santa Rosa, CA: Center Source Publications.

ACTIVITY 6-11
WHO ARE THE PEOPLE AROUND ME?

Instructor Sheet **6-1**

Student Handout **6-5**

Transparency Master **6-3**

What Students Will Learn

- To explore diversity among the people in their lives.
- How lives can be enriched by seeking to interact with people from a variety of ethnic groups.

What You Will Need

- A clear plastic cup for each student.
- Enough individual containers of red, orange, yellow, green, purple, blue, and white beads so that each student has access to all seven colors of beads
- A copy of Student Handout 6-5, Bead Color Chart, for each student, or Transparency 6-3, Bead Color Chart, to display to the class.
- Instructor Sheet 6-1, Who Are the People Around You?

What To Do

1. Distribute Student Handout 6-5 or use Transparency 6-3 as a bead color guide for the activity.
2. Using Instructor Sheet 6-1, ask the students questions about the people they interact with.
3. Each student is to answer each question by placing one appropriately colored bead in his or her plastic cup.
4. When you have asked all the questions, conduct the follow-up discussion.

Follow-up Discussion

1. How would you describe the composition of your cup?
2. How do you feel about the combination in your cup?
3. Are all the cups the same? Why or why not?
4. Is there value in having a multicolored cup? If yes, what are some of the benefits?
5. Would you like your cup to look different?
6. What are some ways to get your cup to look different?

ACTIVITY 6-12
ANIMAL FARM

What Students Will Learn*

- An understanding that people who are different deserve respect.
- Awareness that differences are not necessarily negative.

What You Will Need

- Four large signs, each with the name of one of these animals: LION, DEER, FOX, DOVE

---

*Source: Activity adapted from J. Gibbs (1994). *Tribes: A new way of learning together.* Santa Rosa, CA: Center Source Publications.

What To Do

1. Before class starts, put up the animal signs in four areas of the classroom, for example, the four corners.
2. Ask students to stand near the sign for the animal that is most like them when they are in the workplace.
3. When all students are standing by a sign, ask them to discuss among themselves why they chose that particular animal.
4. After a few minutes, conduct a whole group discussion using the follow-up questions.

Follow-up Discussion

1. What characteristics did you consider when you chose your animal?
2. With which animal did the largest number of you identify? Why do you think that happened?
3. With which animal did the least number of you identify? Why do you think that happened?
4. Do you think that one animal is better than the others? Why or why not?
5. What does each animal contribute to the world?
6. How can having a variety of individuals in the health care workplace be beneficial?
7. What did you learn about yourself?
8. What did you learn about others?
9. Why do you think it is easier for many people to accept differences in nature—different kinds of plants and animals—than it is among themselves?

ACTIVITY 6-13
CELEBRATING CULTURE

Instructor's Note: This is a long-term activity. Plan ahead and give students at least 4–6 weeks to put things together. Also, this may be an all-school activity that needs to be coordinated with other school staff. Review plans with school administrators.

What Students Will Learn

- Habits and activities of different cultural groups.
- Organizational skills and working with others on a long-term project.

What You Will Need

- A local telephone book.
- An area that can be used for activities. It must be large enough for a small stage with a place for students and staff to gather as an audience.

What To Do

1. Engage the class in planning a culture day.
2. Brainstorm activities that can take place on this day to help students and staff learn about and appreciate other cultures. Activity ideas include:
   - Having a potluck meal with ethnic foods.
   - Door decorating contest (see Activity 6-14).
   - Inviting groups to do folk dancing (hula, belly dancing, Greek, Mexican, and so forth) or to present folk music.

- Inviting a local storyteller, puppeteer, or other performer.
- Exchanging recipes.
- Inviting grandparents or other elders to come talk to students.
- Dressing in native costumes.

3. Choose a date and work with the students to plan a schedule.
4. If more than one activity is planned, divide students into small groups and give each group one activity to work on.
5. Each group should submit a written plan with a schedule for completion.
6. Check in with groups periodically or have them submit progress reports to be sure things are on track.
7. On the appointed day, help students keep things on schedule and have a good time learning more about other cultures.

Follow-up Discussion

1. Conduct a discussion about cultures based on which ones were represented and what activities took place. Encourage students to share what they learned.

ACTIVITY 6-14
DOOR DECORATING

Instructor's Note: Review plans with school administration.

What Students Will Learn

- To celebrate the special and unique characteristics of different cultures.

What You Will Need

- Craft supplies such as tape, glue, colored paper, felt, colored pencils, and ribbon.

What To Do

Instructor's Note: This activity can be done with one class divided into small groups, or it can involve other classes in the school with each class working as its own group. If this is a school activity, have an instructor or advisor work with each class as they plan and decorate their door.

1. Divide students into the number of groups for which there are doors to decorate.
2. Assign a door in the school to each group. Classroom doors work best, but other interior doors work as well.
3. Ask students to decorate their door using a cultural theme. Students can choose to represent one or many cultures on each door. It is best to use fabric or butcher paper as a base on which decorations can be attached. Putting decorations on the hall side of the door will allow other students and staff to enjoy the door and learn a little about other cultures.
4. Give students a week or so to plan what they will do and to gather supplies. Decorating may best be done when classes are not in session.
5. Once the doors are decorated, ask two or three school officials or student body representatives to judge the best door and award a prize, such as a pizza party.

6. Leave doors decorated for a week or two so everyone can enjoy and learn from them.

Follow-up Discussion

1. What cultures are represented?
2. Why did you choose these cultures?
3. Explain any symbolism on your door.
4. Why did you choose the types of decorations you used?
5. What did you learn about other cultures?

ACTIVITY 6-15
LET'S EAT!

What Students Will Learn

- Foods of different cultures.

What You Will Need

- A room in which it is safe to have foods and drinks.
- A 3 × 5 card or recipe card for each student, or Student Handout 6-6, Recipe Card.
- Instructor Sheet 6-2, Pot Luck Sign-Up Sheet.

Instructor Sheet **6-2**

What To Do

1. Choose a day for a potluck.
2. Ask students if anyone has a food allergy. Request that these ingredients, if any, not be used in the dishes or that the contents of the dishes be clearly labeled.
3. Ask students to bring a dish to share that represents their culture.
4. If you wish, use Instructor Sheet 6-2 to be sure you get a nice variety. Otherwise, just pick the day, let students know, and see what happens. In any case, encourage students to bring a variety of dishes including salads, vegetables, and desserts.
5. Remind students the day before so they don't forget to bring their food.
6. Be sure someone (perhaps the school) provides tableware and drinks.
7. Ask students to use Student Handout 6-6 to write down the recipes for their dishes. Collect the recipes and make a cookbook for each class member.

Student Handout **6-6**

Follow-up Discussion

1. What social significance does food have?
2. Were there new dishes you hadn't tried before?
3. What does food tell you about a culture?
4. How might food preferences affect health and patient care?

REFERENCE

Gibbs, J. (1994). *Tribes: A new way of learning together.* Santa Rosa, CA: Center Source Publications.

Who Are the People Around You?

Read these instructions to the students: "As I call out the following phrases, place in your cup the one colored bead that best describes the person or people who complete the phrase for you. If a phrase doesn't apply to you, or you don't know, skip that item and don't put a bead in your cup."

Then recite the following phrases, pausing after each to allow the students a moment to think and respond by dropping beads in their cups:

I am

Most of my co-workers are

My supervisor is

The CEO of my company is (or the Director of my school is)

If I choose to worship, the people I worship with are mostly

My high school classmates were mostly

My teachers were mostly

My children's teachers are mostly

My close friends are mainly

My dentist is

My primary doctor is

My lawyer is

My hairdresser/barber is

My spouse/partner is

People who live in my home are mostly

People who regularly visit my home are mostly

People whose homes I regularly visit are mostly

My neighborhood is predominantly

My closest friend is

The authors of books I read are mostly

Musicians I listen to are mostly

The actors in movies I prefer are mostly

The TV shows I prefer contain actors who are mostly

Artists whose works I prefer are mostly

The writers and publisher of the newspapers and magazines I read are mostly

Pot Luck Sign-Up Sheet

Appetizers

1. _____
2. _____
3. _____

Casseroles

1. _____
2. _____
3. _____

Drinks

1. _____
2. _____
3. _____

Meats/Poultry

1. _____
2. _____
3. _____

Vegetables

1. _____
2. _____
3. _____

Bread

1. _____
2. _____
3. _____

Desserts

1. _____
2. _____
3. _____

Fruits

1. _____
2. _____
3. _____

Salads

1. _____
2. _____
3. _____

Also Needed: paper plates, cups (hot and cold), forks, spoons, knives, serving spoons, sharp knives, tablecloth, ice, creamer, sugar

How Do I See the World?

1. Where were you born?

2. Where were your parents born?

3. How many parents did you live with as you grew up?

4. How many brothers and sisters do you have?

5. Do you speak any language other than English?

6. What is your religion, if any?

7. How much education have you had to this date?

8. What kind of work experiences have you had?

9. Have you lived in other cities, states, or countries?

10. Are you married?

11. Do you have children?

12. Do you have grandchildren?

Cultural Values

1. What are the values of your culture regarding:

Careers for women	Elderly	Money
Children	Environment	Patriotism
City living	Family	Punctuality
Country living	Food	Religion
Dating	Forgiveness	Sex outside of marriage
Discipline	Happiness	Single-parent households
Education	Marriage	Work

2. Do you believe that some values are better than others?

3. Have your family's values changed over the years? In what way?

4. What kinds of values, if any, do we have in common?

5. Do families who come to the United States from other countries find their values changing as they spend more time here?

6. Do you think that there are values that are considered "American"? What are they? Do they differ from other cultural groups?

7. Are the values in the eastern half of the United States different from those in the western half?

8. If you have traveled or lived in another country, what cultural differences have you observed?

9. What is meant by the "Ugly American"?

Who Am I?

Please answer these questions about your instructor:

1. Am I married or single? _____

2. How many children do I have? _____

3. What ages are my children? _____

4. What kind of car do I drive? _____

5. What kind of car would I like to drive? _____

6. What kind of music do I listen to? _____

7. Do I like to read? If so, what kind of books? (for example, mystery, science fiction, biographies) _____

8. Do I live in a house or an apartment? _____

9. If I am married, for how long? _____

10. How old am I? _____

11. Where did I grow up? _____

12. What do I like to do for fun? _____

13. Do I like to play sports?_____

14. Do I like to dance? _____

15. What is my favorite sport to watch on TV? _____

16. What is my favorite color? _____

17. What are my hobbies? _____

18. What kinds of foods do I prefer? _____

19. What is my favorite movie? _____

20. How many brothers and sisters do I have? _____

21. What is my ethnic background? _____

The Many Meanings of Diversity

Characteristic	Positive Stereotypes	Negative Stereotypes
African American		
Asian American		
Caucasian		
Gay/lesbian		
Hispanic		
Native American		
Obese		
Over age 75		
Physically disabled		
Practice religions different from yours		
Recently immigrated to the United States		

Bead Color Chart

African Americans	Red
Asian Americans	Orange
European Americans	Yellow
Hispanic Americans	Green
Middle Eastern Americans	Purple
Native Americans	Blue
Pacific Islanders	White

Recipe Card

NAME

_____

RECIPE NAME

_____

SERVES _____

INGREDIENTS

_____

_____

_____

_____

_____

INSTRUCTIONS

_____

_____

_____

_____

_____

_____

_____

_____

Cultural Values

1. What are the values of your culture regarding:

Careers for Women	Forgiveness
Children	Happiness
City Living	Marriage
Country Living	Money
Dating	Patriotism
Discipline	Punctuality
Education	Religion
Elderly	Sex outside of marriage
Environment	Single-parent
Family	households
Food	Work

2. Do you believe that some values are better than others?

3. Have your family's values changed over the years? In what way?

4. What kind of values, if any, do we have in common?

5. Do families who come to the United States from another country find their values changing as they spend more time here?

6. Do you think that there are values that are considered "American"? What are they? Do they differ from other cultural groups?

7. Are values in the eastern half of the United States different from those in the western half?

8. If you have traveled or lived in another country, what cultural differences have you observed?

9. What is meant by the "Ugly American"?

What Do We Have in Common?

Career goals

Families

Likes

Dislikes

Skills

Hobbies

Work Experience

Values (what's important in life)

Bead Color Chart

African Americans	Red
Asian Americans	Orange
European Americans	Yellow
Hispanic Americans	Green
Middle Eastern Americans	Purple
Native Americans	Blue
Pacific Islanders	White

CHAPTER 7

Empathy

INTRODUCTION

Health care workers who demonstrate empathy can deliver service and care more effectively. Empathizing improves communication because the empathetic listener focuses on the feelings of the speaker. Sympathy, sometimes confused with empathy, focuses on the listener's own feelings of being sorry or sad for the other person. Understanding the difference between sympathy and empathy can be difficult. The exercises in this chapter help students understand the nature of empathy and provide opportunities for them to practice skills that will increase their capacity to experience empathy, demonstrate understanding, reserve judgment, and communicate effectively. When health care workers have empathy with patients, as well as with co-workers, the health care setting is more effective and humane.

ACTIVITY 7-1
UNDERSTANDING PHYSICAL LIMITATIONS

What Students Will Learn

- What it is like to experience the signs and symptoms of various physical conditions.
- To develop empathy with patients and what they are experiencing.

What You Will Need

- Short (3–4 inches) straws that are not very large in diameter. Small cocktail straws work well.
- Nonprescription eyeglasses with clear lenses that have been coated with petroleum jelly.
- Thin cotton gloves like the ones worn by women at night to soften hands.
- Blindfolds for half of your students.
- A wheelchair, crutches, walkers, and canes.
- Earphones or ear muffs.

What To Do

1. Instruct students to use the items on the list to create conditions that simulate physical limitations caused by disease, accident, or aging; for example:
   - Give each student a straw and have them breathe through the straw for 5 minutes (if they can last that long). This activity will simulate what it is like for a premature baby who struggles for air. It also simulates breathing with lung disorders such as asthma, emphysema, and bronchitis.

- Have students put on the glasses coated with petroleum jelly to demonstrate what it is like to have a cataract or other vision disorder.
- Students can wear the gloves and try to perform simple tasks like buttoning a shirt, picking up some coins, writing, and the like. This activity will help them understand what it is like to have an impaired sense of touch.
- Give a short lecture while students are wearing earphones or ear muffs to simulate hearing loss.
- Blindfold half of the students and have the remaining half lead them around campus.
- Have students maneuver around campus using a wheelchair, crutches, walker, or cane. Make an obstacle course and time the students when they go through it in a wheelchair. If possible, have students take the wheelchairs outside to use on the sidewalk and other uneven surfaces. Ask students using assistive devices to open doors by themselves. Have something on the floor for the student to pick up while seated in the chair (be careful they don't fall).

2. Expanded activity: Have students assume the simulated limitations for a day or more. Ask them to note problems encountered and feelings experienced for follow-up discussion in class or individual reporting.

Follow-up Discussion

1. How did it feel to experience a physical limitation?
2. What are ways you might demonstrate empathy for future patients who have physical limitations?
3. What are some ways that you might help patients who have these limitations?

ACTIVITY 7-2
UNDERSTANDING THE EXPERIENCE OF ILLNESS

What Students Will Learn

- An awareness that effective health care workers understand the effects of disease on patients.
- What it is like to experience the signs and symptoms of various diseases and conditions.
- To develop empathy with patients and what they are experiencing.
- To think about how empathy can help them work more effectively with patients.

Student Handout **7-1**

What You Will Need

- Student Handout 7-1, Diseases That Affect the Everyday Lives of Patients, to copy and cut up into cards to distribute to each student.
- A copy of Student Handout 7-2, Understanding the Experience of Illness, for each student.

What To Do

1. Give each student a disease card made from Student Handout 7-1 and a copy of Student Handout 7-2.
2. Ask students to research the disease and consider its possible effects on daily life.

Student Handout **7-2**

3. Ask students to pretend for at least 2 days that they have the condition and be aware of how it would affect everything they do each day. Then they should complete Student Handout 7-2.
4. Conduct discussion of completed handouts.

Follow-up Discussion

1. How would having this disease or condition affect your life? Consider especially self-confidence, relationships with others, work, potential for recreation and doing things you enjoy, and family life.
2. Were you surprised at how much your life would be altered by this condition?
3. How would you want to be treated by health care personnel when being monitored or receiving treatment for this condition?

ACTIVITY 7-3
BE ME

What Students Will Learn

- To consider the problems, feelings, and needs of others.
- To think about and respond more appropriately to the needs of others.

What You Will Need

- A copy of Student Handout 7-3, Be Me, for each student.
- Transparency 7-1, Be Me.

What To Do

1. Divide the class into groups of three to five students.
2. Distribute Student Handout 7-3 and assign each group a scenario to discuss the possible feelings, concerns, and needs of the people in each of the examples.
3. You may have groups discuss all or just one of the examples.
4. Conduct a whole class follow-up discussion in which the groups share their lists for each patient or discuss, in detail, the one patient they were assigned to discuss.
5. Alternate or additional activity: Using Transparency 7-1, conduct a whole class discussion. Solicit responses from students about the possible feelings, concerns, and needs of the people in each of the examples.

Follow-up Discussion

1. Did the exercise help you gain a better understanding of what it would be like to have a serious disease or condition?
2. Why is it important for health care workers to understand the feelings and needs of their patients?

Student Handout **7-3**

Transparency Master **7-1**

ACTIVITY 7-4

WHAT WOULD IT BE LIKE?

What Students Will Learn

- To think about the perspectives of patients who must deal with difficult conditions.
- To develop empathy with patients and what they are experiencing.

What You Will Need

- A copy of Student Handout 7-4, What Would It Be Like . . . ? for each student.

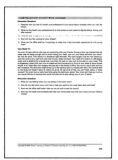

Student Handout **7-4**

What To Do

1. Divide class into groups of three to five students.
2. Distribute Student Handout 7-4 and give the groups several minutes to discuss the questions on the handout.
3. Conduct whole group discussions in which groups share answers to questions in handout.

Follow-up Discussion

1. How is attempting to understand the experiences of others different from feeling sorry for them?
2. What actions can health care workers take to demonstrate empathy for patients?

ACTIVITY 7-5

WALK A MILE IN MY SHOES

What Students Will Learn

- How it feels to be told bad news by your health care provider.

What You Will Need

- Instructor Sheet 7-1, Case Studies of Negative Health Reports.

Instructor Sheet **7-1**

What To Do

1. Read a case study from Instructor Sheet 7-1 to the students and ask them to imagine what the patient is feeling. Ask students to close their eyes, if they wish, and try to put themselves in the place of the patient.
2. Refer to the questions following each case and engage the class in a discussion.
3. Alternate activity: Copy the cases from the instructor sheet to use as student handouts. Students can discuss in groups or answer the questions in writing as an assignment.

Follow-up Discussion

1. What did you learn about patient needs and empathy from the case studies?
2. What other agencies might the families and patients in the cases be referred to for additional help?

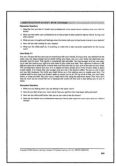

Instructor Sheet **7-1**
(Continued)

ACTIVITY 7-6
EMPATHY ROLE PLAY

What Students Will Learn
- To consider the problems, feelings, and needs of others.
- To respond appropriately to the needs of others.

What You Will Need
- A copy of Student Handout 7-3, Be Me, (same handout used for Activity 7-3), for each student.

Student Handout **7-3**

What To Do
1. Divide the class into groups of three.
2. Distribute Student Handout 7-3.
3. One student in each group plays the part of one of the patients on the list; another plays a health care worker; and the third acts as the observer.
4. The students are to create a situation, such as the patient arriving at the office or clinic, being treated in a hospital; or being visited at home.
5. The student who plays the health care worker asks questions and gives responses in an effort to learn about the needs of the patient.
6. The observers are to note whether the health care worker appears to be listening actively, asking good questions to get useful information, and responding in ways that demonstrate understanding of what the patient is saying.
7. At the completion of each role play, the group members discuss the interaction.
8. Students take turns until they have all played the three roles at least once.

Follow-up Discussion
1. Did the "health care worker" find it difficult to perform the exercise? If so, what made it difficult?
2. Did the "patient" feel that the "health care worker" demonstrated empathy? That is, did he feel listened to? Responded to appropriately?
3. Were the observers helpful in providing insight for the "health care worker?" Why or why not?

ACTIVITY 7-7
VERBAL BARRIERS TO EMPATHY

What Students Will Learn
- An understanding that how we respond verbally to others is an important part of creating empathy.
- Types of commonly used verbal responses that are barriers to empathy.

What You Will Need
- A copy of Student Handout 7-5, Verbal Barriers to Empathy, for each student.
- Student Handout 7-6, Empathy Role Play, to be used by the instructor to make one complete set of statement cards for each group of three students.

Student Handout **7-5**

Student Handout **7-6**

What To Do

1. Distribute Student Handout 7-5 and have students refer to it as you discuss with the class verbal responses that can block true communication and prevent developing empathy for others.
2. After discussing the barriers, divide the class into groups of three.
3. Distribute one complete set of problem cards (created from Student Handout 7-6) to each group.
4. One student reads the problem card; another student, playing the part indicated on the second card ("friend," "co-worker," etc.) provides an empathic response; the third student acts as the observer and listens for responses that might create barriers to empathy.
5. Students take turns with the three roles.
6. After each role play, group members should discuss input from the observer, how they felt as patients, and what difficulties they experienced in responding appropriately.

Follow-up Discussion

1. Was it difficult to avoid responses that might pose barriers to empathy?
2. Did it become easier as you worked through the exercise to respond more empathetically?
3. Why is it important to be empathic when working with patients? With co-workers? With your supervisor?

ACTIVITY 7-8
MY EMPATHY SCORE

What Students Will Learn

- To identify behaviors that demonstrate empathy.
- To review their own behaviors and current level of empathy.
- To differentiate between empowering and enabling behaviors.

What You Will Need

- A copy of Student Handout 7-7, Empathy Inventory, for each student.
- Instructor Sheet 7-2, Suggested Discussion Points for the Empathy Inventory—Student Handout 7-7.

What To Do

1. Distribute a copy of Student Handout 7-7 to each student.

Student Handout **7-7**   Instructor Sheet **7-2**   Instructor Sheet **7-2**
                                                               (Continued)

2. Have students work individually to fill out the inventories. (They may also be completed as a homework assignment.)
3. Explain that there are no right or wrong responses. The purpose of the inventory is to encourage students to explore their current empathy levels.
4. Conduct the follow-up discussion, an essential part of this activity.

Follow-up Discussion

1. Instructor Sheet 7-2 contains suggestions for guiding the discussion of the individual items on the inventory.

ACTIVITY 7-9
HOW DOES IT FEEL?

What Students Will Learn

- Awareness of how it feels to be excluded.*

What You Will Need

Student Handout **7-8**

- Student Handout 7-8, Discussion Topics and Volunteer Tasks, cut into cards for distribution to students. Each group of five to six students receives one set of two cards.

What To Do

1. Explain that the class will be conducting an experiment about group dynamics.
2. Divide the class into groups of five or six students.
3. Ask for a volunteer from each group to go outside the room and wait until you ask them to return.
4. Distribute the topic cards from Student Handout 7-8 to the remaining students in each group. Tell the students they are to discuss the topic.
5. Tell the groups that when the volunteers return to their groups, they are to ignore them, even when they try to enter the conversation or share ideas.
6. While the groups are getting organized for their discussion, go out of the classroom and distribute the cards that correspond with their group cards to the volunteers.
7. Tell the volunteers, while still outside the classroom, that, as indicated on their cards, they are to function as "experts" and make the important contribution written on their cards to the discussion.
8. After the volunteers return, observe the groups and stop the activity after a few minutes.

Follow-up Discussion

1. How did you feel when your group ignored your attempts to contribute to the discussion?
2. How did the group members feel about being asked to ignore a classmate?
3. What can happen to people who work together if one person feels left out of decision-making and other group activities?

---

*Source: Activity adapted from J. Gibbs (1994). *Tribes: A new way of learning together.* Santa Rosa, CA: Center Source Publications.

4. Have you ever had an experience when you were ignored by someone who was supposed to be serving or helping you?
5. Have you had any experiences like this in a health care setting?
6. What can be the result if patients feel they are being ignored?

ACTIVITY 7-10
WE ALL SHARE SIMILAR FEELINGS

What Students Will Learn

- An awareness that many people share the experience of having been ridiculed.
- How being ridiculed can have a negative impact on our lives.

What You Will Need

- Chalkboard or whiteboard for writing down students' answers.

What To Do

1. Ask students for reasons people are ridiculed.
2. Write the reasons on the board. Reasons suggested might include hair, clothes, accent, background, religious beliefs, dialect, where they live, freckles, braces, glasses, and disability.
3. Ask students how many of them have been in situations in which they have been ridiculed for one or more of these reasons.

Follow-up Discussion

1. How did you feel when you were ridiculed?
2. How did you deal with it?
3. Was the ridicule frequent (such as constant teasing as a child)?
4. What long-term effect do you think it has had on you?
5. How can we protect our own children from that kind of behavior?
6. Does telling children that "Sticks and stones may break my bones, but names will never hurt me" help them to cope with being ridiculed?

ACTIVITY 7-11
WHAT ARE THE RULES?

What Students Will Learn

- An understanding that social rules vary among social groups: some are spoken, others are unspoken.
- How it feels when you don't understand the social rules.

What You Will Need

- No special materials are required.

What To Do

1. Divide students into two groups and give each group a physical characteristic to identify with (such as brown eyes/blue eyes).

2. Explain to the groups that Group A represents a unique culture, one that is different from Group B, and that Group A is better than Group B.
3. Send Group B out of the room.
4. Have Group A decide on a set of rules for acceptable behavior in the group. They should create a simple language (such as sign language) that Group B will not recognize, a simple set of values (for example, it is good to smile at all times), and simple set of rules.
5. Invite Group B to return to the classroom and interact with Group A. The goal of Group B members is to make friends with Group A and learn as much as they can about its culture and individual members.
6. Alternate activity: Choose one student from Group B to join Group A and interact with them for 5 minutes. Once the 5 minutes are up, the person from Group B must report back to his or her own group with information regarding Group A's language, rules, values, culture, and the like.

Follow-up Discussion

1. Group B, what did you learn about Group A's language, rules, values, culture?
2. Was it easy or difficult to communicate?
3. How did you work out any differences?
4. Group A, how did you feel when you were told that your group is better than Group B? Group B, how did you feel when you received this information?
5. Group A, did knowing you are superior influence your interactions with your visitors from Group B?
6. Group B, did knowing that Group A is superior influence your interactions with its members?
7. How does this exercise reflect our world today?
8. What have you learned from this activity?
9. What are some of the unspoken rules in your home, school, neighborhood, culture?

ACTIVITY 7-12
ACTIVE LISTENING PRACTICE I

What Students Will Learn

- Active listening is the first step toward developing empathy.
- Active listening is more than just hearing.
- Active listening requires special skills and habits.

What You Will Need

Instructor Sheet **7-3**

- Instructor Sheet 7-3, Illness and Patient Behavior Reading Selection.
- A copy of Student Handout 7-9, Illness and Patient Behavior Questions, for each student.
- Instructor Sheet 7-4, Suggested Answers to Illness and Patient Behavior Questions—Student Handout 7-9.
- Alternatively, one or more short newspaper, journal, or magazine articles on a health care topic related to the subject matter of your class or future careers of students and several basic questions about the content of the article.

Instructor Sheet **7-4**

Student Handout **7-9**

What To Do

1. Tell students you are going to read them an article about a subject that applies to their work in health care. Ask them to listen carefully in order to absorb the information and answer a few questions about the material. (Do not tell them this is specifically a listening exercise.)
2. Read the selection from Instructor Sheet 7-3 or the article you have selected.
3. Distribute Student Handout 7-9 or ask the questions you have prepared.
4. Give students a few minutes to write their answers.
5. When they have finished, give the answers (Instructor Sheet 7-4 or the ones you have prepared) and conduct a follow-up discussion.

Follow-up Discussion

1. Were you surprised at how much or how little you heard and remembered?
2. Why is listening sometimes difficult?
3. What kinds of interference did you experience while you were listening to the selection?
4. What are some ways that listening skills can be improved?
5. Why is it important to learn to listen actively?
6. How is active listening related to empathy?
7. What are some examples in health care that demonstrate the importance of active listening?

ACTIVITY 7-13
ACTIVE LISTENING PRACTICE II

What Students Will Learn

- To use active listening skills in conversation.

What You Will Need

- No special materials are required.

What To Do

1. Review the concept of active listening with students.
2. Divide the students into pairs.
3. Tell them they will take turns speaking and listening.
4. The activity starts with one student in each pair explaining a problem, real or imagined, to his or her partner.
5. The listener is to practice active listening skills as the speaker presents the problem. The goal is to practice active listening, not to solve the problem.
6. After 5 minutes, have students change roles.

Follow-up Discussion

1. Was it hard for you to share when you were presenting your problem?
2. How good a listener were you?
3. Did you find yourself using active listening skills?
4. What interfered with your active listening?
5. Were you tempted to give advice?
6. What are some ways that listening skills can be improved?
7. Why is it important to learn to listen actively?

8. What are some examples in health care that demonstrate the importance of active listening?

REFERENCES

Gibbs, J. (1994). *Tribes: A new way of learning together.* Santa Rosa, CA: Center Source Publications.

Milliken, M. E. (1998). *Understanding human behavior: A guide for health care providers.* (6th ed.). Clifton Park, NY: Delmar Learning.

Case Studies of Negative Health Reports

Case Study # 1

Imagine that you are a person in your early fifties. You have not been feeling well lately. Your symptoms have been odd and you are worried. You can't seem to get enough sleep, and you feel thirsty all the time. You are drinking a lot of water and feel like you are in the bathroom all day. Your weight has been dropping, even though you seem to be eating more than usual. You are weak, sometimes dizzy and nauseous. As you sit waiting for your doctor to come into the exam room to give you the results of your recent physical and blood tests, you think about how much fun you will have tomorrow when you help your grandchild celebrate his first birthday. You look forward to the cake you are making for him and the food that will be there for the family celebration. Your doctor comes into the exam room and interrupts your thoughts. She sits down and tells you that you have become diabetic. For the sake of your health and your life, you must dramatically change your eating habits. This includes avoiding sugar (including your grandchild's birthday cake) and monitoring everything you eat. You will have to learn to prick your finger each day to monitor your blood sugar levels and may have to take a daily insulin injection in the future.

Discussion Questions

1. What are you feeling on the way to the office for the exam?

2. What are your feelings while waiting in the waiting and exam rooms?

3. What about on first hearing the disturbing news?

4. What might happen during the first week or two after this visit?

5. How can the office staff help this patient understand his or her health needs?

6. How difficult would it be for you to make a sudden, drastic, permanent change to your diet?

7. Is anyone in the classroom willing to try a diabetic diet for one week with no cheating? (If someone volunteers, ask him or her to report back to the class after one week. The volunteer might want to keep a food diary that includes notes about how he or she is feeling.)

Case Study # 2

Imagine you are a young, active man in your late twenties. You are just about to have your first physical examination since you were in high school sports. You have chosen a male physician because you think you will be more comfortable, but a very attractive, young female assistant has asked you to disrobe for your exam. You are relieved when she leaves the room. Once you are undressed, you are dismayed when the physician and the female assistant return to the room for your exam. You decide to be adult about it, even though you are very uncomfortable, and it is soon over. The doctor asks you to dress and meet him in his office in a few minutes. You wonder what that is about, but you have been feeling fine, so you aren't too worried. Now you are sitting in front of the doctor's desk. He reviews your file and tells you he has some good news and some bad news. The good news is that your blood pressure, heart rate, and general overall health appear to be normal. The bad news is that the doctor felt a small lump on your right testicle. This could be just a benign lump, or it could be something much more serious. You are asked to make an appointment with a surgeon to have a biopsy. The assistant makes the appointment for you, but the soonest you can get in to see the surgeon is in 3 weeks. You are now free to leave the office.

Discussion Questions

1. Describe how you feel if a health care professional is too casual about modesty when you visit the doctor.

2. What can the health care professional do to help preserve each patient's dignity before, during, and after exams?

3. What are your thoughts and feelings when the doctor tells you he has found a lump in your testicle?

4. How will you feel waiting for your biopsy?

5. What can the office staff do, if anything, to make this a less traumatic experience for this young man?

Case Study # 3

You are a 15-year-old boy who was out swimming with your friends. During a dive, you realized that the water was not deep enough and to avoid hitting your head, you turn your body and slam your shoulder into the sand. This results in a shattered right shoulder. You have surgery and are now wearing a cast that covers your right arm and most of your chest and back. Your right arm is bent at a 90-degree angle and is attached by a dowel that runs from the cast on your arm to the cast on your chest. This arrangement means that your arm is raised and bent across and in front of your chest at about breast height. It is 2 days after your surgery and you are in the doctor's office. You are in a lot of pain and you feel nauseous. You think you might throw up in the waiting room or maybe even faint. The medical staff is very busy and doesn't seem to notice you at all. On top of all of this, you can't feed, bathe, or dress yourself. You even have a really hard time using the bathroom alone! Your mom can't help as much as you would like her to because she works full time and is also taking care of your ill father.

Discussion Questions

1. What are you feeling when you are sitting in the exam room?

2. How do you feel when your mom has to help you perform the most basic daily activities?

3. How can the office staff better help you as you wait to see the doctor?

4. How can the health care professionals help your family best cope with your injury and your father's illness?

Suggested Discussion Points for the Empathy Inventory— Student Handout 7-7

Item # 1

- Being concerned about the welfare of others is important for health care workers.

- It's important to differentiate between giving constructive assistance (empowering others) and enabling destructive behaviors.

- Health care workers should be able to provide patient education about issues that can influence the physical and financial well-being of patients.

Item # 2

- Health care workers must be willing to provide the same level of care to people of all socioeconomic levels.

- As in item 1, it is important to differentiate between empowering and enabling.

- The philosophy of individual worth,* meaning that every human being is entitled to respect, is an important concept for health care workers to understand.

Item # 3

- There is a difference between constructive and destructive criticism.

- Constructive criticism should be delivered using the appropriate tone, at the right time, and in the right place.

- It's more effective to criticize actions, not personalities.

Item # 4

- Students need to distinguish between making decisions for oneself, depending on others, and achieving a balance in decision making.

- Future health care workers need to know that in some work, it may not be appropriate to solicit the opinions of others—or that their opinions will not be solicited by their supervisor in certain situations (for example, in emergencies that require quick action).

- The concepts of inclusion and "buy-in" when our actions affect others are important workplace concepts to understand.

- Patients should have input about their options.

Item # 5

- Understanding the problems of others does not necessarily mean the health care worker has to solve them.

- Understanding problems, however, can make the health care worker's efforts more helpful and effective.

Item # 6

- Relationships among employees affect the delivery of effective patient care.

- Employers report that one of their major problems is lack of good relations among employees.

*M. E. Milliken (1998). *Understanding Human Behavior* (6th ed.). Clifton Park, NY: Delmar Learning.

Item # 7

- Problems don't go away if they are covered up.

- There is an appropriate time, place, and manner for discussing problems experienced with others.

- Keep the discussion on the problem, not the personality.

- Use I-messages, as appropriate, rather than attacking the other person (for example, "I feel frustrated when you interrupt me at staff meetings").

Illness and Patient Behavior Reading Selection

Read the following selection to the class. Tell the students to listen carefully and absorb as much information as possible in order to answer a few questions about the material. Do not introduce this specifically as a "listening exercise."

Illness and Patient Behavior

Illness is always a threat to one's sense of security. Even a minor illness or injury is a threat to physical and emotional well-being. The pattern of life is disrupted. There is discomfort and inconvenience. The threat arouses feelings—perhaps fear, anger, or grief. These feelings are often manifested through the patient's behavior, but are not verbalized. Health care providers must have knowledge about specific illnesses: symptoms, diagnostic procedures, therapeutic techniques. Such knowledge is essential to safe and efficient performance as you provide patient care. Your *effectiveness* as a health care provider, however, depends on your skill in applying knowledge about human behavior to relationships with patients. An effective relationship between a health care provider and a patient promotes the patient's well-being. For one patient, reassurance in large amounts is needed to counteract fear and anxiety. For another patient, you may need to build confidence in the health team in order to gain the patient's cooperation in following the therapeutic plan.

Trying to provide a therapeutic atmosphere that is favorable for each patient is a never-ending challenge. Human variability is so great that no one method will serve for all patients. By applying your knowledge about human behavior and the effects of illness, you can become sensitive to patient behaviors and their possible significance in terms of mental and emotional needs.

Patients not only experience the signs and symptoms of a specific illness, but also various physical effects related to emotional reactions, change in daily routine, and numerous other factors. Examples of such general physical effects are fever, pain, nausea, lack of appetite, urinary problems, and difficulty with elimination. The overall effect may range from extreme sluggishness to extreme restlessness. These general effects may be just as distressing to the patient as the symptoms of a specific illness. *The patient's complaints about general or vague effects should be noted*. These general symptoms may indicate either physical or emotional needs. Since interpretation may be beyond the scope of your role, report such complaints to your team leader or supervisor.

Most people react to illness with some degree of negative emotion. These emotional reactions vary in type and intensity. Some patients are mildly annoyed at being sick; others are quite angry. Some patients are apprehensive; others are almost in a state of panic. Some feel somewhat sorry for themselves; while others react with pronounced self-pity. Some people feel bitter about their misfortune; bitterness is a combination of anger and self-pity.

Some patients readily verbalize their feelings. The patient who says, "Why me?" is probably expressing anger. The patient who says, "It seems as though everything happens to me!" is probably expressing self-pity. Obviously, the words alone do not carry the full message. Be alert for additional evidence about the patient's emotional reaction to illness: facial expression, tone of voice, body posture, choice of words, and emphasis given to certain words.

Negative feelings may also be expressed through disguised behavior. The patient who is very talkative may be covering up fear. The patient who is eager to please may be covering up fear, hostility, or other negative feelings. Such patients are just as much in need of understanding and interest from health care providers as those who verbalize their feelings. Do not make the mistake of thinking that the patient who is pleasant does not have fears and anxieties; for these patients, too, illness is a threat. *Each patient reacts to threat in a very individual way.*

Source: From M. E. Milliken (1998). *Understanding human behavior: A guide for health care providers.* (6th ed.), pp. 246–247. Clifton Park, NY: Delmar Learning.

Suggested Answers to Illness and Patient Behavior Questions—Student Handout 7-9

1. According to the author, how is illness a threat to the patient?

   • Threat to security and well-being.

   • May cause disruption, discomfort, and negative feelings.

2. What must effective health care providers have in addition to good technical knowledge and skills?

   • Ability to apply knowledge of human behavior to relationships with patients.

   • Be able to establish good interpersonal relationships.

   • Be able to listen, communicate, and empathize.

3. Why is it important to observe and note patient complaints that are not specific signs or symptoms of their illness or condition?

   • They reveal emotional state and needs.

   • These may be as distressing for the patient as the illness itself.

4. What are some common patient reactions to illness?

   • Annoyance

   • Fear

   • Anger

   • Self-pity

   • Bitterness

   • Apprehension

   • Panic

5. Why is it a mistake to think that patients who behave pleasantly are okay with their condition?

   • Illness is a threat to every patient

   • Patients react to feelings of threat and negative emotions in different ways

Diseases That Affect the Everyday Lives of Patients

Instructor: Cut along dotted lines to make individual cards.

Herpes zoster (Shingles)	Osteoarthritis	Fibromyalgia
• Chronic, often severe pain	• Swelling joints • Pain (*Note:* About 80% of all Americans are affected by osteoarthritis as they age.)	• Chronic muscle and joint pain • Fatigue • Headache • Feelings of numbness and tingling
Epilepsy	**Cerebral Palsy**	**Parkinson's Disease**
• Occasional seizures that can range in severity	• Spastic paralysis of the limbs • Head rolling • Difficulty with speech and swallowing (*Note:* Caregivers need to be aware that patients ferquently have normal or above normal intelligence.)	• Tremors • Shuffling gait • Muscular rigidity
Alzheimer's Disease	**Carpal Tunnel Syndrom**	**Meniere's Disease**
• Difficulty with short-term memory • Confusion • Anxiety • Poor judgement (*Note:* Advanced symptoms do not come on suddenly; many patients understand the implications when told of their diagnosis.)	• Hand pain • Muscle weakness in the hand • Tingling sensations in the hand	Attacks without warning of: • Dizziness • Nausea • Ringing sensation in ears
Diabetes Mellitus, Type I	**Hemophilia**	**Emphysema**
• Daily insulin injections • Controlled diet • Possibility of hypo- and hyperglycemia	• Prolonged clotting time and abnormal bleeding • Necessity of avoiding trauma, even small cuts	• Difficulty breathing • Extreme fatigue

Understanding the Experience of Illness

Disease or condition: _____

Think about how having this disease or condition would affect your thoughts and daily activities and respond to the following questions.

1. Would there be limitations on what you could do, where you could go, and so on? If so, what are they? How would these limitations affect the quality of your life?

   _____

   _____

   _____

2. Do you think that having this disease or condition would cause you to worry or be anxious? If yes, explain why.

   _____

   _____

   _____

3. Are there activities you enjoy now that you might not be able to do? If so, what are they? How would this change affect the quality of your life?

   _____

   _____

   _____

4. Do you think your self-confidence would be affected by this disease or condition? If so, why?

   _____

   _____

   _____

Be Me

Think about each of the following patients and write down what you think their feelings, concerns, and needs might be.

1. Patient who is very hard of hearing and is having difficulty understanding your questions.

   Feelings: _____

   Concerns: _____

   Needs: _____

2. Patient who is frustrated because of wait for authorization from insurance company for an MRI to determine cause of neck pain.

   Feelings: _____

   Concerns: _____

   Needs: _____

3. Patient who has just been diagnosed with cancer.

   Feelings: _____

   Concerns: _____

   Needs: _____

4. Patient without medical insurance who comes to emergency room with very ill child.

   Feelings: _____

   Concerns: _____

   Needs: _____

5. Patient who is very overweight and seems hesitant to disrobe for exam.

   Feelings: _____

   Concerns: _____

   Needs: _____

6. Patient who appears to be in pain but is having difficulty communicating due to limited English.

   Feelings: _____

   Concerns: _____

   Needs: _____

What Would It Be Like . . . ?

Think about what it would be like to have any of the following conditions:

Amputated limb

Blindness

Chronic pain

Colostomy

Deafness

Disfiguring injury, such as facial scars from burns

Paralysis

Serious learning disability

Group Discussion Questions

1. How do you believe each condition might affect your attitude about life?

2. How do you think each might affect your mood?

3. How would your daily life be different?

4. How would each affect the quality of your life?

5. What would you want from health care workers?

Verbal Barriers to Empathy

Technique	Explanation	Example
Belittling	Statement that tends to make light of the patient's beliefs or fears	*Patient:* "I won't leave this place alive." *H. C. Worker:* "That's ridiculous. You shouldn't even think that way."
Disagreeing	Response indicating that the health care worker believes the patient to be incorrect	*Patient:* "Why am I here? Nothing is being done for me and I'm not getting any better." *H. C. Worker:* "You *are* getting better."
Defending	Statement used to hold off a verbal attack	*Patient:* "I had my light on for fifteen minutes!" *H. C. Worker:* "I am doing the best I can. You are not the only patient I have."
Stereotyped statement	Common statement made without sincerity	*Patient:* "I am really worried about my children. I came to the hospital so quickly and I didn't get to see them. They just won't understand. I wish I could have talked to them." *H. C. Worker:* "I know exactly what you're going through."
Changing the subject	Different subject introduced to prevent talking about a difficult topic	*Patient:* "They are doing a biopsy tomorrow. I hope it isn't cancer." *H. C. Worker:* "Are these your children? You have such a nice looking family."
Reassuring cliché	Reassuring statement that is not sincere	*Patient:* "What will I do if it is malignant?" *H. C. Worker:* "Don't you worry. Everything will be all right."
Giving advice	Statement telling the patient what the health care worker thinks the patient should do	*Patient:* "I broke my arm when I fell off a skateboard." *H. C. Worker:* "At your age, I would suggest you give up skateboards."
Agreeing	Statement showing that the health care worker believes the patient's words are correct; may not respond, however, to the patient's real concern	*Patient:* "I'm afraid the doctor won't discharge me tomorrow." *H. C. Worker:* "I am sure you are correct. I doubt he will let you go home so soon."

Source: Adapted from N. Kalman & C. G. Waughfield (1993). *Mental health concepts* (3rd ed.). Clifton Park, NY: Delmar Learning.

Empathy Role Play

Instructor: Cut along the dotted lines to make cards.

Speaker # 1 I'm really worried I might be pregnant. My mom is going to kill me!	**Listener # 1** Friend
Speaker # 2 My dad was just diagnosed with cancer.	**Listener # 2** Friend
Speaker # 3 I think our supervisor doesn't like me.	**Listener # 3** Co-worker
Speaker # 4 I'm really terrified about seeing the dentist.	**Listener # 4** Dental receptionist
Speaker # 5 I've always been afraid of shots.	**Listener # 5** Medical assistant
Speaker # 6 I just don't feel like I'll ever catch up with my work.	**Listener # 6** Supervisor
Speaker # 7 I'd like to go back to school, but I'm afraid I'm too old.	**Listener # 7** Friend
Speaker # 8 I just can't understand this math. I'm thinking about dropping out of school.	**Listener # 8** Classmate
Speaker # 9 My leg is never going to get better. I might as well give up on these exercises!	**Listener # 9** Physical therapist assistant
Speaker # 10 I just know I'll fail at this diet I'm supposed to follow.	**Listener # 10** Licensed Practical/Vocational Nurse
Speaker # 11 My husband isn't supporting my decision to go back to school.	**Listener # 11** Friend or classmate

Empathy Inventory

For each item, choose the sentence completion that best describes your strongest belief or most typical reaction.

1. When I see people I believe are being taken advantage of, I
   - ☐ feel kind of protective toward them.
   - ☐ want to stop the cause of the problem.
   - ☐ believe they should watch out for themselves.
   - ☐ don't really think about it much one way or the other.

2. When I see people who are financially less fortunate than I, I
   - ☐ often have tender, concerned feelings toward them.
   - ☐ want to do what I can to help them improve their situation.
   - ☐ think that in most cases, it's their own fault.
   - ☐ believe it's the government's responsibility to give them more help.

3. Criticizing the actions of others is
   - ☐ okay if I feel sure that what they've done is wrong.
   - ☐ never okay.
   - ☐ appropriate if I first try to put myself in their place.
   - ☐ justified if I am angry about something they've said or how they've treated me.

4. It's important to listen to other people's opinions
   - ☐ infrequently, if at all.
   - ☐ only when I'm not sure if I'm right about something.
   - ☐ if I think they know more than I do about something.
   - ☐ anytime they will be affected by the results of the outcome.

5. When other people are having problems, I
   - ☐ usually don't feel very much pity for them.
   - ☐ am willing to listen and see if I can understand how they are feeling.
   - ☐ want to help them if I can.

6. I believe that trying to understand my co-workers is
   - ☐ only important if they directly affect my work.
   - ☐ always important.
   - ☐ not really my responsibility.

7. When I'm upset with someone, I usually
   - ☐ let them know right away exactly how I feel.
   - ☐ try to consider both sides of the situation before I say anything.
   - ☐ keep my feelings to myself.

Discussion Topics and Volunteer Tasks

Instructor: Cut long the dotted lines to make cards.

Group # 1 Topic	**Group # 1 Volunteer's Task**
Why are health care costs rising so rapidly?	You are an expert on health care economics. Persuade the members of your group that the growing number of aging Americans is one of the main reasons for rising costs.
Group # 2 Topic	**Group # 2 Volunteer's Task**
What is the first thing a health care worker should do to show empathy for a patient?	Suggest to your group that active listening is the first step in creating empathy with patients.
Group # 3 Topic	**Group # 3 Volunteer's Task**
Why is it important for health care workers to protect patient confidentiality at all times?	You are a legal expert. Explain to your group that the law protects patient confidentiality.
Group # 4 Topic	**Group # 4 Volunteer's Task**
How do the lifestyle habits of individuals affect the health care system?	You are a health care policy expert. Inform your group that habits such as smoking and poor nutrition contribute to conditions such as heart disease, that are costly to treat.
Group # 5 Topic	**Group # 5 Volunteer's Task**
What is causing the projected shortage of registered nurses?	You are a health care employment researcher. Inform your group that many nurses are reaching retirement age and not being replaced by sufficient numbers of nursing graduates.

Illness and Patient Behavior Questions

Write brief answers to the following questions based on what you heard in the selection that was just read.

1. According to the author, how is illness a threat to the patient?

   _____

   _____

2. What must effective health care providers have in addition to good technical knowledge and skills?

   _____

   _____

3. Why is it important to observe and note patient complaints that are not specific signs or symptoms of their illness or condition?

   _____

   _____

4. What are some common patient reactions to illness?

   _____

   _____

5. Why is it a mistake to think that patients who behave pleasantly are okay with their condition?

   _____

   _____

Be Me

1. Patient who is very hard of hearing and is having difficulty understanding your questions.

2. Patient who is frustrated because of wait for authorization from insurance company for an MRI to determine cause of neck pain.

3. Patient who has just been diagnosed with cancer.

4. Patient without medical insurance who comes to emergency room with very ill child.

5. Patient who is very overweight and seems hesitant to disrobe for exam.

6. Patient who appears to be in pain but is having difficulty communicating due to limited English.

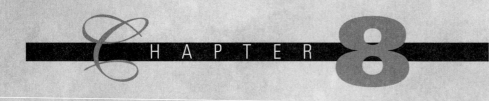

CHAPTER 8

Working as a Team Member

INTRODUCTION

The complexity of modern health care delivery and the challenges faced by health care facilities make the ability to work effectively as a team player more important than ever for today's health care workers. Students should know that outstanding individual performance is no longer sufficient for success in the workplace. They need to understand that achieving team goals, such as providing the best quality service to patients, is more important than achieving personal recognition and gain. The ability to make positive contributions to the work group requires that students respect the contributions of others, take responsibility for their own actions, and be willing to do their part to achieve team goals.

ACTIVITY 8-1
STRENGTHS TARGET

What Students Will Learn*

- Individual team members each bring a unique set of skills to help the team.
- They have skills that will help them make positive contributions to work teams.
- A key to successful teamwork is the variety of skills brought by its members.
- "Synergy," meaning that the combined efforts of two or more people are greater than the sum of their individual efforts, can result when people work together cooperatively.

What You Will Need

- A copy of Student Handout 8-1, Strengths Target, for each student and each team of four to five students.

What To Do

1. Introduce the concept of synergy.
2. Distribute one copy of Student Handout 8-1 to each student.
3. Ask them to spend 5 minutes filling in the target as follows:

Student Handout **8-1**

---

*Source: Activity adapted from an exercise in J. Bormaster & C. Treat (1982). *Building interpersonal relationships through talking, listening, communicating.* Austin, TX: PRO-ED.

- Center circle: their most outstanding individual strengths that they believe will help them contribute to the health care team in the workplace (e.g., enthusiasm).
- Ring around the inner circle: strengths and/or abilities they believe a workplace team possesses by combining the efforts of its members (e.g., variety of health care skills).
- Outer circle: strengths or skills they believe the team might need to seek from others outside the team (e.g., information).

4. When students have completed their lists, divide the class into teams of four or five students each.
5. Give students 10 to 15 minutes to compare and combine their lists into a team list.
6. When they have completed their team lists, have them share them with the class.

Follow-up Discussion

1. Was there great variety in the type of individual strengths brought by each student?
2. What are some ways that combining individual strengths increases the effectiveness of the health care workplace?
3. How do their findings support the concept of synergy?

ACTIVITY 8-2
WHAT ARE MY STRENGTHS?

What Students Will Learn

- Strengths others see in them.
- Strengths they see in others.

What You Will Need

- Enough 3 × 5 cards (or equivalent) for five times the number of students.

What To Do

1. Divide class into groups of three to five students.
2. Each student is to write the name and one strength for each group member on an individual card (one name per card).
3. Allow students to tell their group members what strengths they see in each of them.
4. Each group member gets his or her cards at the end of the exercise. (For example, Mary Gonzalez will get all of the cards the group members have written for her.)
5. This exercise works especially well after students have been together for some time. You may ask students to list any strength, or you may ask them to list strengths that are associated with being a good health care professional.
6. Alternate activity: Tape a 3 × 5 card to each student's back. Give students about 10 minutes to walk around and write a positive trait on each card.

Follow-up Discussion

1. Were you surprised by some of the traits?

2. Did you see a trait of your own that others didn't see?
3. What does this tell us about our perceptions of ourselves?
4. What does this tell us about our perceptions of others?
5. What can we learn about teamwork from this exercise?

ACTIVITY 8-3
BLIND WALK

What Students Will Learn

- How it feels to trust another individual in order to accomplish an assigned task.
- The need for trust in certain situations.

What You Will Need

- Blindfolds for half the number of students in the class.
- An appropriate area, either indoors or out, through which blindfolded students can be safely led by a seeing partner.

What To Do

1. Have the students pair off. They may select their partners or you can have them count off or use some other random method of dividing into pairs.
2. One student in each pair puts on a blindfold and is led on a 5-minute walk by the other. The student leading may use touch and oral instructions.
3. Explain that the seeing partner is responsible for the safety of the blindfolded partner.
4. When the students have all returned, have them switch places.
5. A variation is to have the seeing student describe and have the blindfolded student touch and experience objects on the walk. You can make the exercise more difficult by instructing the partners to not talk during the walks, but rely only on nonverbal communication.

Follow-up Discussion

1. How do you think this exercise relates to trust?
2. How did you feel when you were blindfolded?
3. Did you move freely or did you hesitate?
4. How did you feel about being responsible for someone who couldn't see?
5. Variation: How well did the seeing partners describe the items and provide a meaningful experience for the blindfolded students?
6. Why is it important to develop trust with other members of the workplace health care team?

ACTIVITY 8-4
BLINDFOLD TAG

What Students Will Learn

- How it feels to trust another individual in order to accomplish an assigned task.
- The need for trust in certain situations.

What You Will Need

- Blindfolds for half the number of students in the class.
- An appropriate area, either indoors or out, through which blindfolded students can be safely led by a seeing partner.
- Cones to set an area aside or to set an obstacle course.

What To Do

1. Divide students into pairs.
2. Designate half of the pairs as Team A and half as Team B.
3. Each Team A will compete against a Team B in a game of tag.
4. The team that is "it" tries to avoid being caught by members of the other team. The catch is that one member of the "it" team is blindfolded and must depend on oral directions from the sighted member to avoid being caught.
5. All matched teams can play at the same time if there is sufficient space.
6. Alternate activity: A sighted person is in a wheelchair giving directions to the blindfolded partner who pushes the chair during a game of tag or in a race around cone obstacles.

Follow-up Discussion

1. How did it feel to trust someone else with your safety?
2. How do you earn the trust of others?
3. Were the directions given by your teammates effective?
4. How could they have been improved?

ACTIVITY 8-5
WHEELCHAIR RACE

What Students Will Learn

- Trusting others can aid in accomplishing an assigned task.

What You Will Need

- Blindfolds for $\frac{1}{5}$ of the students.
- Several wheelchairs (or chairs with wheels such as task chairs).
- An open area either indoors or out.
- Two identical obstacle courses (or one course and a stop watch for timing races).

What To Do

1. Divide students into teams of five.
2. Put one student in the chair.
3. Blindfold one student who will push the chair.
4. Other students (including person in chair) each represent a direction: forward, back, left, and right; or north, south, east, and west.
5. Have a race with two groups trying to get through the obstacle courses (or time one group at a time). Blindfolded person pushes and other members of the group give directions according to their assigned representation.

Follow-up Discussion

1. How did it feel to trust someone else with your safety?

2. How do you earn the trust of others?
3. Were the directions given by your teammates effective?
4. How could they have been improved?

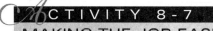

ACTIVITY 8-6
BALLOON GAME

What Students Will Learn
- Working together toward a common goal.

What You Will Need
- An inflated balloon for each team of four students.
- An open area either indoors or out.

What To Do
1. Divide class into teams of four students each. Give each team a balloon and instruct the students per one of the following:
   - Keep the balloon in the air.
   - Hold hands and keep balloon in the air using other parts of their bodies.
   - Use only their feet to move balloon around the circle.
   - Other instructions you create.
2. Call out different instructions every few minutes. All teams should be working at once.

Follow-up Discussion
1. Is this activity easier to accomplish as part of a team or alone?

ACTIVITY 8-7
MAKING THE JOB EASIER

What Students Will Learn
- Working together as a team makes a job easier and more pleasant.

What You Will Need
- Groups of about seven students.
- A clean sheet or large area rug.

What To Do
1. Have one student lie on the sheet or rug with other students arranged around him or her.
2. Using good body mechanics, the standing students will crouch down and attempt to lift the prone student. It will be very easy to do if everyone works together.
3. Students should trade places so everyone gets a turn being lifted.

Follow-up Discussion
1. Why is this activity easier to do as a team?
2. When will this concept be important during your career?

ACTIVITY 8-8
BRAIDING

What Students Will Learn
- Sometimes it takes a team to get the job done.
- The importance of leadership.

What You Will Need
- Enough pieces of rope about 7 feet long each so that each student can have one piece.

What To Do
1. Divide class into groups of three and give each student a rope.
2. Have students tie one end of the three ropes together.
3. Have a student hold the tied ends of the three ropes.
4. The object is to braid the rope. This is done when each member of the team holds one end of the rope and walks back and forth to make a braid.
5. Team members cannot pass the rope, but must continue to hold onto their ends.
6. Make this a race and see which team braids the rope to the end, without mistakes, first.
7. Some students may not know how to braid. This factor will help your students learn about leadership as they try to verbalize to each other what must be done to accomplish the task.

Follow-up Discussion
1. How well did team members cooperate with one another?
2. Did one member of the team take on the role of leader?

ACTIVITY 8-9
VALUES FOR SUCCESSFUL TEAMS

What Students Will Learn
- The values that are important to making a team successful.
- To work together on a project that requires team consensus.

What You Will Need
- A copy of the suggested team values exercise for each student (Student Handout 8-2, Team Values I, or 8-3, Team Values II).
- Two overhead transparency films and pens, or a sheet of butcher paper, marking pen, and masking tape for attaching to the wall, or white- or blackboard space for teams to write lists of five items (for each team of three to five students).

Student Handout **8-2**

What To Do
1. Divide the class into teams of three to five students.
2. Distribute Student Handout 8-2 or 8-3 to each student and the transparency films or butcher paper or assigned space on the board to each team.

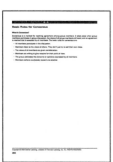

Student Handout **8-3**

3. Instruct the teams to select a recorder to write down their list and a presenter who will share the list with the class and explain why their team selected each item.

4. Give the teams 10 minutes to select the five values they believe to be most important for a team in a health care facility. They are to discuss why they have chosen each value.

5. When they have agreed on their selections, the recorder writes down the lists on the material provided or on the board.

6. The presenters then explain briefly why their teams selected each value.

7. Observe the students as they work in their teams to see evidence of the values under discussion actually being carried out. For example, a team may decide that "respect" is an important value, but not demonstrate it among themselves as they work on compiling their list.

8. Use any examples noted as points to examine during the follow-up discussion.

9. Alternate activity: Using Student Handout 8-3, have teams rank the list of values in order of importance instead of selecting five.

Follow-up Discussion

1. Should the values vary depending on the type of workplace? On the type of team?

2. What did they learn from the process of working together to select or rank the values?

3. Did the teams demonstrate the values they chose as they worked on the assignment?

ACTIVITY 8-10
GETTING CONSENSUS

What Students Will Learn*

- The concept of "consensus."
- To work with others to reach agreements that are accepted by all members of a team.

What You Will Need

- A copy of Student Handout 8-4, Basic Rules for Consensus, for each student.

What To Do

1. Distribute Student Handout 8-4 to each student and briefly discuss the concept of consensus as described on the handout.

2. Divide the class into groups of up to five students.

3. Assign the groups a task such as choosing and ranking in order of importance the ten most important qualities of the health care worker.

4. Before beginning the task, each group should appoint a leader who will facilitate the discussion and encourage everyone to work toward consensus.

5. Allow up to 15 minutes for groups to reach consensus.

Student Handout **8-4**

Source: Activity adapted from V. Payne (2001). *The team-building workshop: A trainer's guide.* New York: AMACOM.

Follow-up Discussion

1. How many groups reached consensus?
2. Did the groups truly decide by consensus? Or did they vote? Or did some people simply give up and go along with the others?
3. Did anyone feel pressured to agree?
4. How did the group handle conflicting views?
5. What attitudes and behaviors helped the groups reach consensus?
6. What attitudes and behaviors made it difficult to reach consensus?
7. What did you learn about consensus decision making?

ACTIVITY 8-11
CONSEQUENCES

What Students Will Learn

- How individual actions affect members of their team and others.
- The importance of keeping commitments.

What You Will Need

- A copy of the same scenario for each student on each team of three to four students (Student Handouts 8-5 through 8-9, scenarios numbered 1 through 5).
- Transparencies 8-1 through 8-5, scenarios numbered 1 through 5, to use in conducting follow-up discussion with entire class.

What To Do

1. Divide class into teams of three or four students.
2. Distribute copies of the scenarios with questions for discussion. (If there are not enough scenarios to go around, you can create a few more or give the same one to more than one group.)

Student Handout **8-5**   Student Handout **8-6**   Student Handout **8-7**   Student Handout **8-8**   Student Handout **8-9**

Transparency Master **8-1**   Transparency Master **8-2**   Transparency Master **8-3**   Transparency Master **8-4**   Transparency Master **8-5**

3. Each group selects a recorder to write down brief answers to the questions and a presenter who will share these answers with the entire class.

4. Allow about 10 minutes for teams to discuss and answer the questions. Then show the overheads for each scenario, have presenters share group answers, and ask the class for additional ideas regarding the possible consequences of each worker's action.

Follow-up Discussion

1. Use the discussion questions at the end of each scenario.

ACTIVITY 8-12
TEAMWORK IN TODAY'S HEALTH CARE WORKPLACE

What Students Will Learn

• Why teamwork is an important component for the success of today's health care delivery system.

What You Will Need

• A copy of Student Handout 8-10, Teamwork in Health Care Today, for each student.

What To Do

1. Divide class into groups of three to five students.

2. Distribute copies of Student Handout 8-10 and give the groups 10 or 15 minutes to discuss the statements and answer the questions.

3. After the allotted time is up, have the class discuss the statement as a group.

Student Handout **8-10**

Follow-up Discussion

1. Use discussion questions on Student Handout 8-10.

ACTIVITY 8-13
DRAWING ON ONE ANOTHER

What Students Will Learn

• Combined efforts of team members produce better results than individual efforts.

Instructor's Note: If labeling drawings of body parts/systems is beyond the current knowledge level of students, develop a task that is challenging but within their scope. Use the same technique described in this activity to demonstrate the combined contributions of team members.

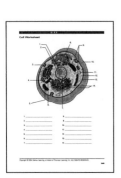

Student Handout **8-11**

What You Will Need

• Seven copies for each group of four students of Student Handouts 8-11, Cell Worksheet; 8-12, Skeleton Worksheet; 8-13, Eye Worksheet; 8-14, Heart Worksheet, and 8-15, Muscles Worksheet, for each student.

• A copy of Student Handouts 8-16, Labeled Cell; 8-17, Labeled Skeleton; 8-18, Labeled Eye; 8-19, Labeled Heart; and 8-20, Labeled Muscles, for each student.

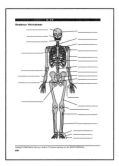
Student Handout **8-12**

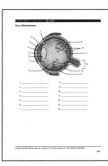
Student Handout **8-13**

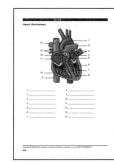
Student Handout **8-14**

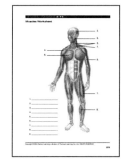
Student Handout **8-15**

What To Do

1. Divide class into groups of four students.
2. Distribute a set of seven copies of one of the handouts to each group. (Groups may have different handouts, but the set of seven given to each group should contain the same handout.)
3. Each student takes one handout from the group's pile. Instruct students to work *individually* and without references to label their drawings. Give them about 5 minutes to complete this part of the activity.
4. Within the groups, students form pairs (two in each group) and have about 5 minutes to label a clean drawing. They may not use references, but can refer to the drawings they labeled individually.
5. The two sets of pairs join and the four students work together for about 3 to 5 minutes, again labeling a clean drawing and using all previously labeled drawings as their only references.
6. When the groups are finished, distribute Student Handouts 8-16 through 8-20 so the students can check their work.
7. Alternate, more difficult, activity: Rather than distributing the drawings for labeling, have students draw and label one of the items. Tell them that the idea is not to draw it perfectly, but to include as many of the components they can in the correct locations. Then have them work in pairs, then groups as in the first activity. Did the drawings improve as more students were brought together to complete the task?

Follow-up Discussion

1. Did the completeness and quality (spelling) of the labeled drawings improve as more students worked on them?

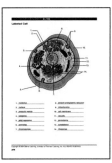
Student Handout **8-16**

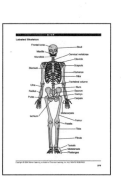
Student Handout **8-17**

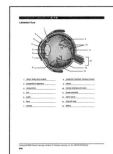
Student Handout **8-18**

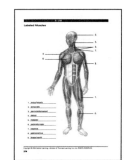
Student Handout **8-19**

Student Handout **8-20**

2. Were there individuals who had the drawings correctly completed on their own?
3. How did they feel about sharing their drawings with the others?
4. Were there individuals who filled in none or only a few of the labels? If so, how did they feel when it came time to share with the others?
5. What did you learn from this activity about working with others to complete a task?

ACTIVITY 8-14
TOGETHER IT WORKS: GROUP TEACHING PROJECT

What Students Will Learn

- Working with others toward a common goal.
- The importance of details.

What You Will Need

- Paper and writing instrument.

What To Do

1. Divide class into groups of three to five students (groups may be larger if you have a very large class).
2. Assign each group a topic or skill that relates to the class content. Emphasize that it is important for them to complete the project in a way that can help the other students in the class learn.
3. Each group is to write a short manual that can be used to teach the chosen topic. The manual should include:
   a. What we are going to teach
   b. Why this information is important to know
   c. Steps to perform the activity to be taught
   d. Instructions
   e. Follow-up
4. The groups then use their manuals to teach the topic or skill to the rest of the class.
5. Alternate activity: Groups exchange manuals and see how well they can follow the directions created by others.

Follow-up Discussion

1. Discuss the quality of the manuals and how the manuals reflected the teamwork efforts of the groups.

REFERENCES

Bormaster, J., & Treat, C. (1982). *Building interpersonal relationships through talking, listening, communicating.* Austin, TX: PRO-ED.

Mitchell, J., & Haroun, L. (2002). *Introduction to health care.* Clifton Park, NY: Delmar Learning.

Payne, V. (2001). *The team-building workshop: A trainer's guide.* New York: AMACOM.

Strengths Target

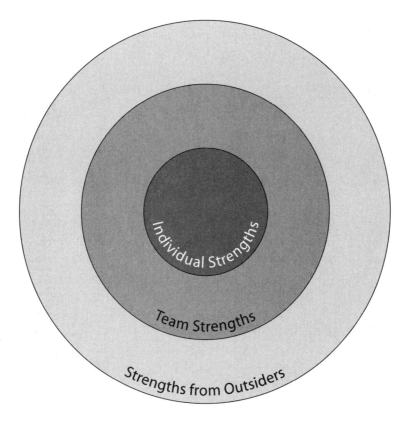

Team Values I

Work as a team to select from the following list the five most important values for a successful team. Fill in the chart with your selections and your reasons for choosing them.

1. Cooperation
2. Courtesy
3. Creativity
4. Dependability
5. Diversity
6. Efficiency
7. Empathy

8. Fairness
9. Honesty
10. Openness
11. Respect
12. Sharing
13. Trust
14. Enthusiasm

Team Choices	Reason Value Is Important
1.	
2.	
3.	
4.	
5.	

Team Values II

Work as a team to rank the following values in order of importance for a successful workplace with the number 1 being the most important.

1. Cooperation
2. Courtesy
3. Creativity
4. Dependability
5. Diversity
6. Efficiency
7. Empathy

8. Fairness
9. Honesty
10. Openness
11. Respect
12. Sharing
13. Trust
14. Enthusiasm

Team Ranking

1. _____
2. _____
3. _____
4. _____
5. _____
6. _____
7. _____

8. _____
9. _____
10. _____
11. _____
12. _____
13. _____
14. _____

Basic Rules for Consensus

What Is Consensus?

Consensus is a method for reaching agreement among group members. It takes place when group members participate in group discussion, the views of all group members are heard, and an agreement is reached that is accepted by all members. The basic rules for consensus are:

- All members participate in the discussion.

- Members listen to the views of others. They don't just try to sell their own ideas.

- The views of all members are given consideration.

- Members are willing to give reasons for their point of view.

- The group addresses the concerns or opinions expressed by all members.

- Members behave courteously toward one another.

Scenario #1

Robert Chin loves his work as a physical therapy assistant. He is a favorite among patients for his cheerful attitude and the encouragement he offers each one. However, Robert dislikes the paperwork aspects of his job and is often careless about the documentation he prepares after each patient session. He writes his chart notes quickly and other health care workers find them difficult, if not impossible, to read.

Discussion Questions

1. What are the potential consequences of Robert's poor-quality documentation?

   (a) For his co-workers?

   (b) For his supervisor?

   (c) For his patients?

   (d) For his career?

2. How do his actions show a lack of consideration for the health care team as a whole?

Source: Scenario adapted from J. Mitchell & L. Haroun (2002). *Introduction to health care.* Clifton Park, NY: Delmar Learning.

Scenario #2

Graciela Lopez is a respiratory therapist in a large hospital. Her schedule is often hectic because there are many patients, some in critical condition. Graciela is a competent therapist and is well-liked by her patients because of her easy-going nature. However, she often fails to return equipment to its storage place or to report, as is hospital policy, when supplies need to be reordered.

Discussion Questions

1. What are the potential consequences of Graciela's failure to return equipment and report low supply levels?

    (a) For her co-workers?

    (b) For the patients?

    (c) For her career?

2. How do her actions show a lack of consideration for the health care team as a whole?

Scenario #3

Sally Jensen works as a medical assistant in a three-physician office in a small community. Sally has both administrative and clinical skills, although she works mainly in the back office assisting Dr. Rashid with patients. Sally has strong skills and performs her work competently, but she arrives for work up to half an hour late at least once a week.

Discussion Questions

1. What are the potential consequences of Sally's consistent tardiness?

   (a) For Dr. Rashid?

   (b) For the patients?

   (c) For her co-workers?

   (d) For her career?

2. How do her actions show a lack of consideration for the health care team as a whole?

Scenario #4

Craig Johnson was recently hired by High-Tech Medical Labs after graduating from a laboratory technician program. He finds the work interesting and especially likes performing the various tests that are part of the daily workload. He was given a facility policy and procedure manual at his new-employee orientation but has not taken the time to read it. He finds it easier to continually ask his co-workers for the location of supplies and equipment and for methods of performing various lab procedures.

Discussion Questions

1. What are the potential consequences of Craig's constant questions?

   (a) For his co-workers?

   (b) For the efficiency of the lab?

   (c) For the patients and facilities being served by the lab?

   (d) For his career?

2. How do his actions show a lack of consideration for the health care team as a whole?

Source: Scenario adapted from J. Mitchell & L. Haroun (2002). *Introduction to health care.* Clifton Park, NY: Delmar Learning.

Scenario #5

John Nguyen is a registered nurse at Valley View Hospital. His work with patients is well-regarded by his supervisor. However, John is frequently late for the weekly meetings held by the director of nursing. These meetings include discussion of the weekly schedule, problems the staff may be experiencing, and any other matters brought up by staff members. In addition to being late, John tends to be inattentive and rarely asks questions or participates in the discussions.

Discussion Questions

1. What are the potential consequences of John's tardiness and lack of participation in meetings?

   (a) For his co-workers?

   (b) For his patients?

   (c) For his career?

2. How do his actions show a lack of consideration for the health care team as a whole?

Teamwork in Health Care Today

1. There is a continuing demand to do things better, faster, and cheaper.

2. Workplace problems require a mix of skills.

3. Good team members receive more benefits than they give.

4. When health care team members work together effectively, patients feel more positive about the care they receive.

5. Quality cannot be improved if people blame each other when things go wrong in the workplace.

6. Health care organizations today are facing serious challenges to their existence.

7. Health care organizations must focus on customer/patient retention and loyalty.

8. New systems and technology require that people work together.

Discussion Questions

1. Does your group agree with the statement?

2. What are some examples of how the statement applies to health care today?

3. How does the statement apply to the future work environment of the members of the group?

Cell Worksheet

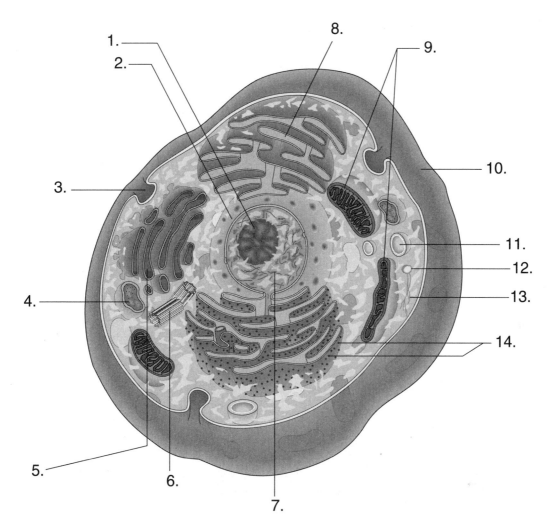

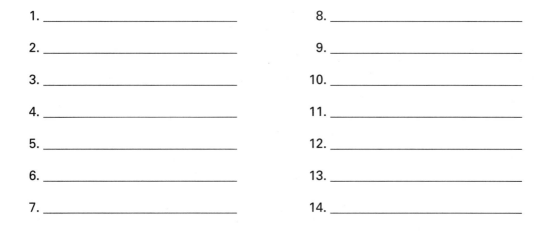

1. _____	8. _____
2. _____	9. _____
3. _____	10. _____
4. _____	11. _____
5. _____	12. _____
6. _____	13. _____
7. _____	14. _____

Skeleton Worksheet

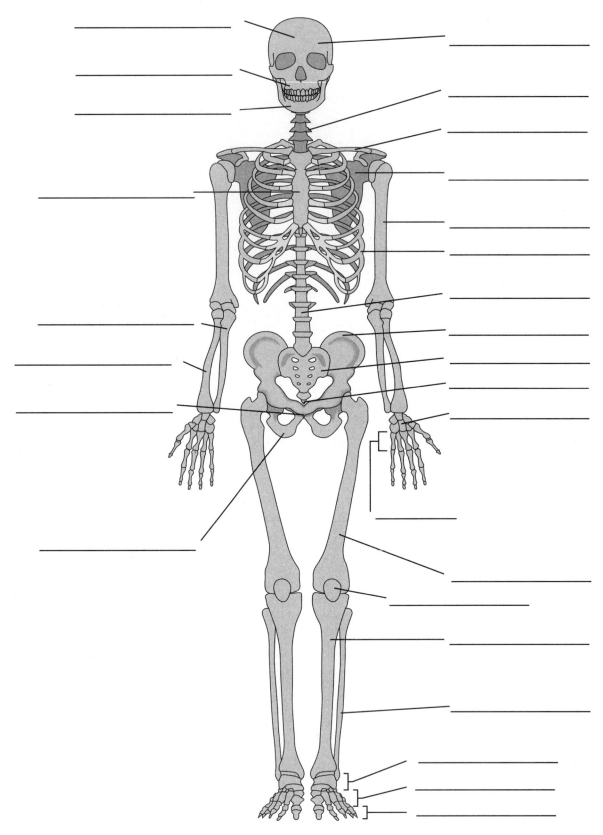

Eye Worksheet

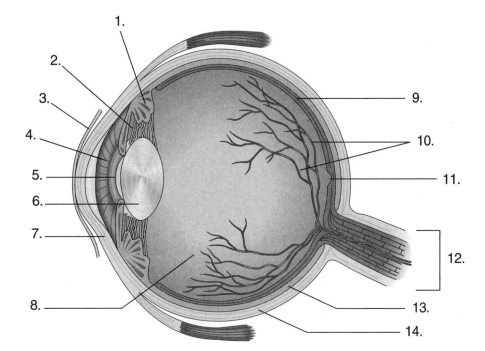

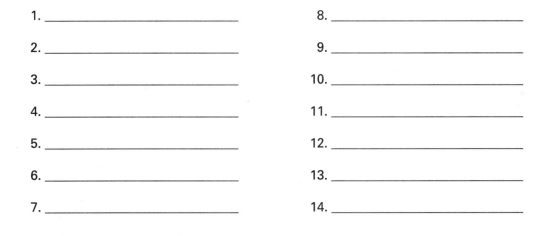

1. _____

2. _____

3. _____

4. _____

5. _____

6. _____

7. _____

8. _____

9. _____

10. _____

11. _____

12. _____

13. _____

14. _____

Heart Worksheet

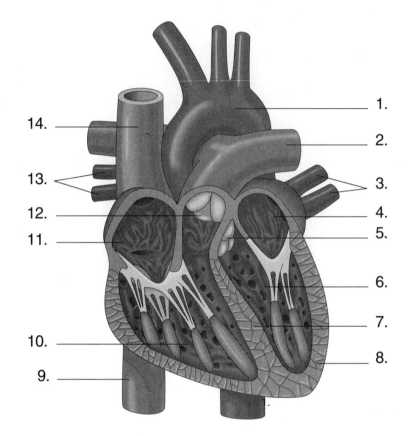

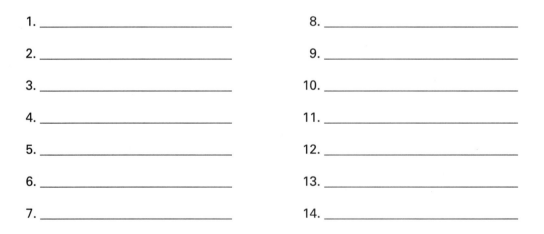

1. _____

2. _____

3. _____

4. _____

5. _____

6. _____

7. _____

8. _____

9. _____

10. _____

11. _____

12. _____

13. _____

14. _____

Muscles Worksheet

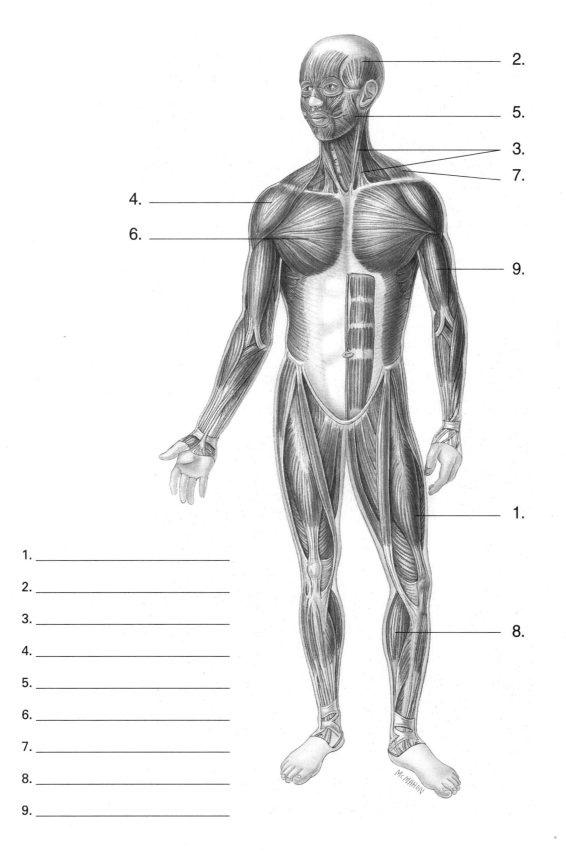

2.

5.

3.

7.

4. _____

6. _____

9.

1.

8.

1. _____

2. _____

3. _____

4. _____

5. _____

6. _____

7. _____

8. _____

9. _____

Labeled Cell

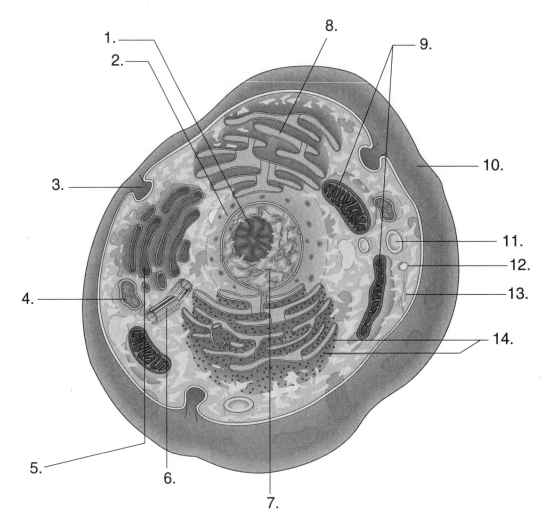

1. nucleolus
2. nucleus
3. pinocytic vesicle
4. lysosome
5. golgi apparatus
6. centrioles
7. chromosomes

8. smooth endoplasmic reticulum
9. mitochondria
10. cell membrane
11. vacuole
12. peroxisome
13. cytoskeleton
14. ribosomes

Labeled Skeleton

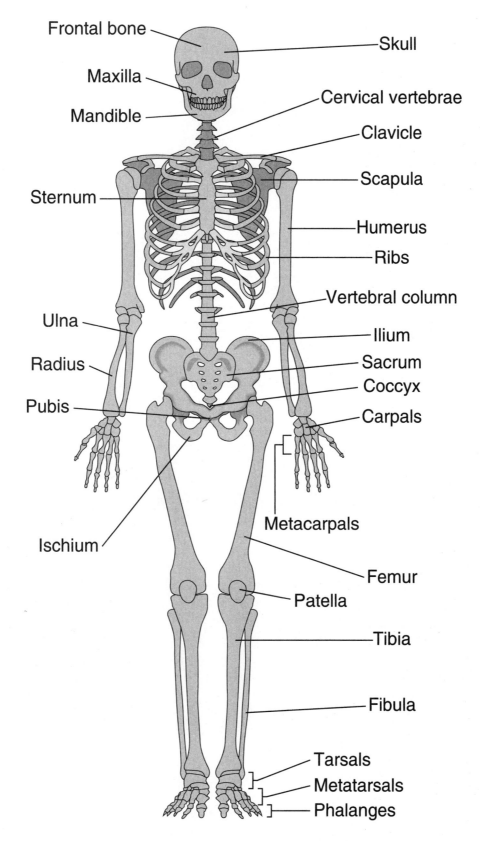

Frontal bone

Skull

Maxilla

Cervical vertebrae

Mandible

Clavicle

Scapula

Sternum

Humerus

Ribs

Vertebral column

Ulna

Ilium

Radius

Sacrum

Coccyx

Pubis

Carpals

Metacarpals

Ischium

Femur

Patella

Tibia

Fibula

Tarsals

Metatarsals

Phalanges

Labeled Eye

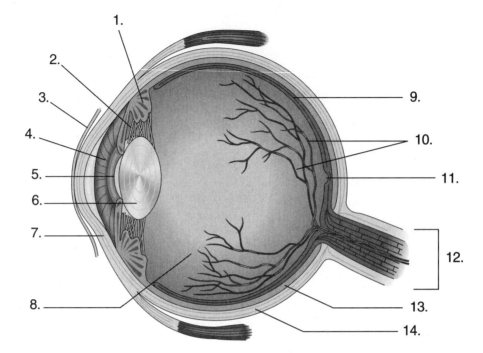

1.
2.
3.
4.
5.
6.
7.
8.
9.
10.
11.
12.
13.
14.

1. ciliary body and muscle

2. suspensory ligament

3. conjunctiva

4. iris

5. pupil

6. lens

7. cornea

8. posterior chamber vitreous humor

9. retina

10. retinal arteries and veins

11. fovea centralis

12. optic nerve

13. choroid coat

14. sclera

Labeled Heart

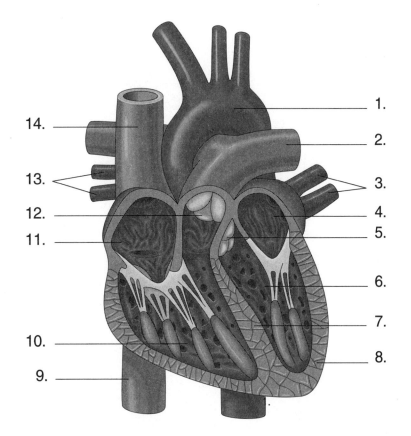

1. __aorta_____

2. __left pulmonary artery_____

3. __left pulmonary veins_____

4. __left atrium_____

5. __aortic semilunar valve_____

6. __left ventricle_____

7. __septum_____

8. __myocardium_____

9. __inferior vena cava_____

10. __right ventricle_____

11. __right atrium_____

12. __pulmonary semilunar valve__

13. __right pulmonary veins_____

14. __superior vena cava_____

Labeled Muscles

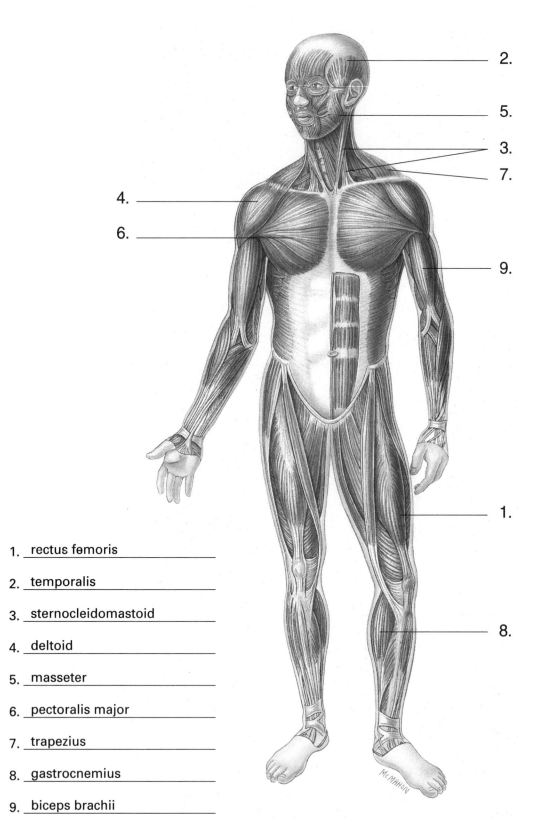

1. rectus femoris
2. temporalis
3. sternocleidomastoid
4. deltoid
5. masseter
6. pectoralis major
7. trapezius
8. gastrocnemius
9. biceps brachii

Scenario #1

Robert Chin loves his work as a physical therapy assistant. He is a favorite among patients for his cheerful attitude and the encouragement he offers each one. However, Robert dislikes the paperwork aspects of his job and is often careless about the documentation he prepares after each patient session. He writes his chart notes quickly and other health care workers find them difficult, if not impossible, to read.

Scenario #2

Graciela Lopez is a respiratory therapist in a large hospital. Her schedule is often hectic with many patients, some of them in critical condition. Graciela is a competent therapist and is well-liked by her patients because of her easy-going nature. However, she often fails to return equipment to its storage place or to report, as is hospital policy, when supplies need to be reordered.

Scenario #3

Sally Jensen works as a medical assistant in a three-physician office in a small community. Sally has both administrative and clinical skills, although she works mainly in the back office assisting Dr. Rashid with patients. Sally has strong skills and performs her work competently, but she arrives for work up to half an hour late at least once a week.

Scenario #4

Craig Johnson was recently hired by High-Tech Medical Labs after graduating from a laboratory technician program. He finds the work interesting and especially likes performing the various tests that are part of the daily workload. He was given a facility policy and procedure manual at his new-employee orientation but has not taken the time to read it. He finds it easier to continually ask his co-workers for the location of supplies and equipment and for methods of performing various lab procedures.

Scenario #5

John Nguyen is a registered nurse at Valley View Hospital. His work with patients is well-regarded by his supervisor. However, John is frequently late for the weekly meetings held by the director of nursing. These meetings include discussion of the weekly schedule, problems the staff may be experiencing, and any other matters brought up by staff members. In addition to being late, John tends to be inattentive and rarely asks questions or participates in the discussions.

CHAPTER 9

Dealing with Conflict

INTRODUCTION

Conflict is a natural part of human interaction. The nature of health care work causes stress and there is potential for conflict both among workers themselves and with the patients they serve. Learning to manage conflict to make it a more constructive experience is a vital skill for interpersonal success. The activities in this chapter will help students explore the nature of conflict and learn ways to manage it so they can deal with it effectively.

ACTIVITY 9-1
WHAT COLOR IS CONFLICT?

What Students Will Learn

- How they feel about conflict.

What You Will Need

- A large quantity of 4-inch by 4-inch construction paper squares in a wide variety of colors. Be sure to have plenty of red, black, brown, and gray.

What To Do

1. You may keep the class as one large group or divide it into groups of five to six students.
2. If working as a whole class, ask each student to select a square of the color (or colors) that he or she thinks represents conflict.
3. Ask students to explain why they chose their colors.
4. If the students worked in groups, have them share with the whole group which colors they chose and why.

Follow-up Discussion

1. Conduct a discussion about the nature of conflict based on the answers given by the students. For example, if they all report conflict as being negative, ask them why they believe this.

ACTIVITY 9-2
I REPRESENT CONFLICT

What Students Will Learn

- How they normally react to conflict.

What You Will Need

- No special materials are required for this activity.

What To Do

1. Place yourself in the middle of the room and say, "Imagine that I represent conflict. Think about how you usually react when you experience a conflict personally or witness a conflict happening nearby. Then stand, in relation to me, somewhere in the room in a way that indicates your first response to conflict or disagreement."
2. Conduct the follow-up discussion while students are still in the locations and positions they have chosen.

Follow-up Discussion

1. Which direction are you facing? Explain why.
2. How far are you from the conflict? Explain why.
3. What conditions might determine your reactions to conflict?
4. If this represents your first reaction, what might your second reaction be, after thinking about the conflict?

ACTIVITY 9-3
PUTTING UP A FIGHT

What Students Will Learn

- What is important to them and what they would be willing to fight for.

What You Will Need

- No special materials are required for this activity.

What To Do

1. Go around the group and have students answer the question: "What is something you have that you would put up a serious fight for—even risk your life for—if someone tried to take it away?" (This can be a material thing, like a gold chain, or something intangible, like a good reputation.)
2. Ask students to explain why this is important to them.

Follow-up Discussion

1. How do we place value on things in our lives?
2. How have your values influenced your decision to work in health care?
3. What would you be willing to give up in order to succeed in school?
4. What would you be willing to give up in order to succeed on the job?
5. What would you not be willing to give up?

ACTIVITY 9-4
CONCENTRATE ON THE POSITIVE

What Students Will Learn

- Giving positive feedback is an important way to establish and maintain good interpersonal relationships.

What You Will Need

- No special materials are required for this activity.

What To Do

1. Divide the class into pairs, one student being "A" and the other "B." It is best if the students in the pairs know each other, at least slightly.
2. Explain to students that the pairs are to take turns giving each other compliments.
3. Allow 1–2 minutes for student "A" to compliment student "B."
4. When you call time, have students reverse roles and allow the same amount of time for "B" to compliment "A."

Follow-up Discussion

1. How did it feel to give compliments?
2. How did it feel to receive compliments?
3. Do you think people are given enough acknowledgment for their skills and good qualities?
4. How can giving deserved recognition improve relationships in the workplace?
5. How can giving recognition help prevent conflict in the workplace?
6. If conflicts do occur, how can the ability to give deserved recognition contribute to conflict resolution?

ACTIVITY 9-5
CONSTRUCTIVE CONFLICT

What Students Will Learn

- Conflict can be constructive.
- Each person's attitude influences whether conflict has positive or negative results.

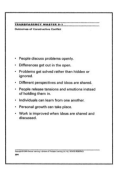

Transparency Master **9-1**

What You Will Need

- Transparency 9-1, Outcomes of Constructive Conflict.

What To Do

1. Introduce the concept that conflict can have positive results. Conflict may be demonstrated by people disagreeing, expressing different opinions, or arguing different points of view. An example of constructive conflict is when a group airs differences and is then able to establish stronger relationships between the members.
2. Divide the class into groups of three to five students.
3. Ask the groups to brainstorm positive outcomes from conflict in the workplace. One group member should record the ideas.

4. Allow about 10 minutes for the brainstorming, then have the groups share their ideas.
5. Transparency 9-1 can be used to suggest ideas and encourage discussion about constructive conflict.

Follow-up Discussion

1. Can you think of constructive experiences you have had with conflict?
2. What have you learned from this activity about how conflict can help you learn new ideas or ways of looking at things?

ACTIVITY 9-6
CONFLICT POSTERS

What Students Will Learn

- To think about ways that conflict can be constructive.
- To work together to create a group project.

What You Will Need

- A copy of Student Handout 9-1, Statements About Conflict—What Do They Mean? for each student
- Supplies for groups to make posters: posterboard, marking pens, glue, old magazines, colored paper, and so on.

What To Do

1. Divide the class into groups of three to five students.
2. Assign each group one of the statements about conflict listed on Student Handout 9-1.
3. The groups are to discuss the meaning of the statement and create a poster that illustrates the meaning.
4. When they finish, ask the groups to present their posters to the class along with their interpretation of the statement. Encourage students to think of examples to support their interpretations.

Follow-up Discussion

1. Do you agree with all statements on the posters? Explain.
2. Why is it sometimes difficult for people to accept differences of opinion?

Student Handout **9-1**

ACTIVITY 9-7
I-MESSAGES

What Students Will Learn

- To share their feelings in conflict situations without assigning blame.

What You Will Need

- Transparency 9-2, I-Messages.
- A copy of Student Handout 9-2, I-Messages, for each student.

Transparency Master **9-2**

Student Handout **9-2**

What To Do

1. Use Transparency 9-2 to initiate a discussion of the use of I-messages to communicate feelings and let other people know how their behavior affects us. An important element of I-messages is to not blame the other person when sharing feelings. Blaming is usually ineffective because it causes defensive reactions. The goal of conflict resolution is to share feelings and work out the problem, not make someone feel wrong.
2. Following the discussion, distribute Student Handout 9-2 and have students work in pairs. Using the situations listed on the handout, ask them to take turns creating I-messages to express their feelings in each situation.

Follow-up Discussion

1. Was it difficult to create I-messages?
2. If so, what made it difficult?
3. How did it feel to receive an I-message?
4. Did the I-message help promote discussion of the conflict? Why or why not?
5. How do you think I-messages could be useful in the workplace?

ACTIVITY 9-8
TRY TO SEE IT MY WAY

What Students Will Learn

- Failing to consider the perspectives of others can result in conflict.

What You Will Need

- A copy of Student Handout 9-3, My Way . . . , for each student.

Student Handout **9-3**

What To Do

1. Divide the class into pairs. Distribute Student Handout 9-3.
2. Ask students to role-play the cases with the goal of reaching a mutually agreeable resolution to the conflict.
3. Encourage them to engage in discussions in which they attempt to understand the other's point of view by asking questions, listening, and so on. They are also to present their own circumstances and needs.

Follow-up Discussion

1. Were you able to reach a mutually agreeable resolution with your partner? If not, why?
2. What worked for you in trying to work out your differences?
3. What is the role of communication in resolving conflict?
4. How can conflict resolution be applied on the job?

ACTIVITY 9-9
CONFLICT ROLE-PLAY

What Students Will Learn

- To use their communication skills to deal with conflict.

Student Handout **9-4**

What You Will Need

- A copy of Student Handout 9-4, Conflict Role-Play, for each student.

What To Do

1. Divide the class into small groups. Distribute Student Handout 9-4.
2. Ask each group to create a skit to demonstrate a conflict that might be encountered in a health care setting, including their ideas about how to best deal with it.
3. Students can create their own conflicts, perhaps from personal experiences, or they can use one of the suggestions on Student Handout 9-4.

Follow-up Discussion

1. Conduct a follow-up discussion on conflict resolution based on what the students present in their skits. Ask students how they might apply what they learned in their future health care employment.

Statements About Conflict—What Do They Mean?

1. It's okay to agree to disagree.

2. Attack the problem, not the person.

3. Conflict can be constructive.

4. Conflict isn't necessarily the problem; it's a symptom that a problem exists.

5. I can be right without you being wrong.

6. Conflict is not necessarily good or bad.

I-Messages

Take turns with your partner creating I-messages for the following workplace situations:

1. You are annoyed with your co-worker for continually failing to return equipment to the proper storage area. Not being able to find equipment results in delays when you want to perform patient treatments.

2. You have a co-worker who loudly disagrees with almost every idea you suggest at department meetings.

3. Your supervisor frequently changes your work schedule without giving you adequate notice so you can properly arrange for childcare.

4. A new co-worker constantly interrupts your work to ask you questions before first checking in the procedure manual.

5. A co-worker has asked you more than once to cover for her by filling in a patient chart for a procedure she forgot to document (you refused each time, but she continues to ask).

6. A co-worker spends much of his time, and yours, complaining about working conditions. He has not discussed his concerns with the supervisor.

7. You have been assigned to work with a co-worker to update the department's procedure manual, but she always has an excuse for not meeting with you to plan the project.

8. Your sister frequently calls you at the office and is hurt when you cut the calls short.

My Way . . .

Role-play the following workplace situations with your partner. Think about the perspective of the person you are playing. Present his or her circumstances and needs. The goal is to reach mutually agreeable resolutions to the conflicts.

Case #1

Dan, the department nursing supervisor, is annoyed about Kari's chronic tardiness. He believes she doesn't really care about her job.

Kari, LVN, thinks that Dan is unsympathetic about her responsibilities at home, which include caring for an invalid husband and several children.

Case #2

Mrs. Mendoza, a patient, is annoyed that she has to wait 45 minutes for her 4:15 appointment with Dr. Hermes.

Kim, Dr. Hermes's medical assistant, is tired of patients complaining about scheduling delays that cannot be avoided when emergencies occur with other patients.

Case #3

Frank Ngyuen, physical therapy client, complains that he is being billed for therapy sessions that he believes should be handled by his insurance company.

May Chen, medical biller, has asked Mr. Ngyuen several times to submit certain information necessary for her to properly submit claims to his insurance company.

Case #4

Sally, radiologic technician, does not want to work on Saturdays for religious reasons.

Kurt, Sally's co-worker in radiology, believes that all staff should be available to cover weekend hours and believes that Sally shouldn't receive special treatment.

Case #5

John is upset because he believes he should have received the promotion just granted to Eliza. He is convinced she was promoted because she is a woman and the facility is seeking to fulfill some kind of "quota" of female supervisors.

Eliza is fed up with people thinking she receives her promotions because she is a woman instead of for her hard work and positive results.

Conflict Role-Play

Use the following suggestions to create a skit to demonstrate an effective way the health care worker might deal with conflict.

Situation #1

Your office has not received payment from Mr. Marulli. You have asked repeatedly for additional insurance information, but Mr. Marulli has not provided the information you need. He has telephoned and is very upset because he just received the past due notice you sent to him.

Situation #2

It is the flu season and the office is very busy. You have overbooked the doctor and now she is late from lunch because she stopped at the hospital to take care of an emergency. It has taken longer than expected and patients are arriving and filling up the waiting room. You have scheduled Ms. Drake at the last minute to have her flu symptoms checked by the doctor. You explained the situation and possible delay to each patient as they arrived, but now Ms. Drake is very upset about the delay. She is standing at the counter being very loud and abusive about having to wait.

Situation #3

Dr. Sanchez is meeting with a patient to discuss a difficult diagnosis and has asked not to be disturbed under any circumstances. Dr. Smith has telephoned and insists on speaking with Dr. Sanchez immediately. Dr. Smith will not tell you what the call is about.

Situation #4

Mrs. Douglas arrived early for her child's appointment with the pediatrician. While she and her son wait in the reception room, Mrs. Douglas's 3-year-old is getting completely out of hand. He is throwing toys, hitting and biting other children, and tearing up the magazines. In addition, he is screaming so loudly that you cannot hear on the telephone to make an appointment for a patient. Mrs. Douglas is ignoring her son's behavior.

Situation #5

A patient the doctor has seen only a couple of times has arrived at the office without an appointment. He insists on being seen immediately, but won't tell you what the problem is. You are completely booked for appointments and the doctor is running about 15 minutes behind. Other patients in the reception room are getting anxious listening to this patient make such a fuss.

Outcomes of Constructive Conflict

- People discuss problems openly.

- Differences get out in the open.

- Problems get solved rather than hidden or ignored.

- Different perspectives and ideas are shared.

- People release tensions and emotions instead of holding them in.

- Individuals can learn from one another.

- Personal growth can take place.

- Work is improved when ideas are shared and discussed.

I-Messages

- Describe feelings of the speaker.

- Don't assign blame.

- Are intended as a first step in resolving conflicts

Example of an I-Message

"It really frustrates me when you arrive late to work and I have to deal with irritated patients."

Example of a Blaming Message:

"You make me really frustrated when you come in late. You have no consideration for others and don't take your responsibilities seriously."

CHAPTER 10

Critical Thinking

INTRODUCTION

Critical thinking is an essential skill for the health care worker. It provides the foundation for the problem-solving and decision-making skills necessary to provide safe, effective health care. Critical thinking has been defined in many ways. A useful definition for health care students is that critical thinking is purposeful thinking that enables students and health care workers to

- Observe carefully.
- Question assumptions.
- Look beyond the obvious.
- Reject stereotypes.
- Distinguish fact from opinion.
- Use logic.
- Examine situations from a variety of perspectives.

The activities in this chapter are designed to help students develop critical thinking skills and recognize that what they see is *not* always what they get!

ACTIVITY 10-1
IT'S AN ILLUSION!

What Students Will Learn

- Perceptions—how we see the world—are influenced by our experiences, beliefs, and what is happening around us.
- We are active participants in the creation of our perceptions.

What You Will Need

- Transparencies 10-1 through 10-10, showing optical illusions.
- Instructor Sheet 10-1, Optical Illusion Hints and Answers.

Instructor Sheet **10-1**

What To Do

1. Show Transparencies 10-1 through 10-10 one at a time to students and ask them to write down the first thing they see for each one.
2. After each illusion has been shown, show each one again and have students report what they saw.
3. If the students have seen only one of the two pictures in each illusion, use the hints listed on Instructor Sheet 10-1 to help them change their perceptions so they can see both pictures.

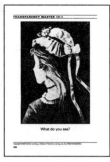

Transparency Master **10-1**

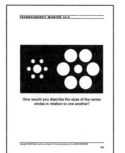

Transparency Master **10-2**

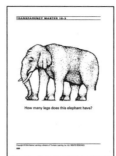

Transparency Master **10-3**

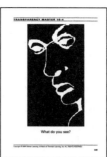

Transparency Master **10-4**

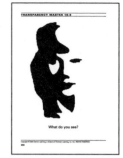

Transparency Master **10-5**

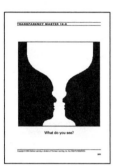

Transparency Master **10-6**

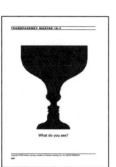

Transparency Master **10-7**

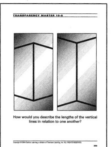

Transparency Master **10-8**

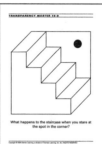

Transparency Master **10-9**

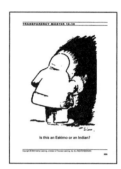

Transparency Master **10-10**

Follow-up Discussion

1. Can you share a situation in which your perception was different than someone else's?

2. How do your perceptions influence your life?

3. Can we change the way we perceive things?

ACTIVITY 10-2

INTERACTIVE STROOP EFFECT EXPERIMENT—OR—YOU OFTEN GET WHAT YOU EXPECT!

What Students Will Learn

- An awareness that beliefs and expectations influence what we see.

What You Will Need

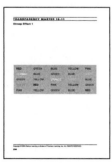

Transparency Master **10-11**

- Transparencies 10-11, Stroop Effect 1, and 10-12, Stroop Effect 2, created as follows:

Word Set #1: (Transparency Master 10-12, Stroop Effect 2): Using colored pens or the computer, print the names of the various colors in the same color ink as the meaning of the word. For example, write the word "red" using red ink.

Word Set #2: (Transparency Master 10-11, Stroop Effect 1): This time, print the same words in ink that is different from the meanings of the words For example, write the word "red" using blue ink.

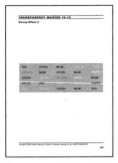

Transparency Master **10-12**

What To Do

1. In this experiment, students are required to say the color of the word, *not* what the word says. For example, for the word, "red" written in blue, they should say "blue."
2. Have a student read Word Set #1 as fast as he or she can.
3. Have another student time how long it takes.
4. Have the same student try again with Word Set #2 and compare the times.
5. Have other students repeat the experiment.

Follow-up Discussion

1. Why was it more difficult to correctly read the examples in the second word set?
2. What does this tell us about perceptions and expectations?
3. What actions have you or others taken that were influenced by expectations rather than facts?

ACTIVITY 10-3
DESCRIBE AN OBJECT I

What Students Will Learn

- We tend to view the world in a general, rather than detailed, way.

What You Will Need

- Actual object or picture of an object for students to draw. Some suggestions: piece of lab equipment, school logo, cell phone, push-button telephone, computer with keyboard.
- Students: a sheet of paper and pen or pencil.

What To Do

1. Show the object or picture to the class for 1–2 minutes. Make sure everyone gets a good look.
2. Remove the object or picture from sight and ask students to draw it including as much detail as possible.
3. Once the object has been drawn, have students compare the details in their own drawing to the actual object or picture.

Follow-up Discussion

1. How close was your drawing to the actual object in terms of details included?
2. Why do you think some details were missing?
3. What does this activity tell us about how we view the world?
4. Why would it be important for health care workers to improve their skills of observation?
5. Can you think of examples in health care when the ability to observe and remember details would be important?

ACTIVITY 10-4
DESCRIBE AN OBJECT II

What Students Will Learn
- Each of us sees differently through our own perceptual lenses.

What You Will Need
- Chalkboard, whiteboard, or flip chart and chalk or felt pen.
- Students: paper and pen or pencil.

What To Do
1. Choose an everyday object that is familiar to all of your students, but different from the one selected for Activity 10-3; for example, a house, church, dog, family, or restaurant.
2. Ask students to each draw the same object in any way they wish. They are not to be concerned with artistic ability.
3. Once the object is drawn, have students compare their drawings to see how each portrayed the object.
4. You can ask four or five students to replicate their drawings on the board or flip chart so everyone can see them.

Instructor's Note: Drawing ability and detail are not the issue; the idea is to see how many ways one common object can be interpreted.

Follow-up Discussion
1. Were you thinking of a particular house/church/dog/family/restaurant from your past when you were drawing?
2. Do you think your past experiences influenced your interpretation? If so, in what way?
3. What can you learn from this activity about making assumptions about what other people say and do?
4. Did you learn anything that might help you in working with patients or clients?

ACTIVITY 10-5
WHAT HAPPENED HERE?

What Students Will Learn
- Each of us sees the world and actions that occur around us in our own way.
- Perceptions can affect beliefs.
- Most of us need to improve our powers of observation.

What You Will Need
- Some people who are not members of the class to act out a scene, or an interesting photograph or painting with at least one person in it.

What To Do
1. Present a scene for students to observe, such as:
   - A brief argument between two people.
   - Someone comes into the room and takes something off the instructor's desk.

- A mock accident such as two people bumping into each other (be very careful with this one so that no one actually gets hurt).

2. After the scene has been enacted, have students write down as many details as they can remember. The actors involved in the scene should not be in the room during this part of the activity.

3. You can prompt the students by asking questions such as the following:
   - What was each person wearing?
   - Hair color?
   - Who started the problem?
   - Who was at fault? Why do you think so?
   - What did the person who entered the room do?
   - Was anything taken? If so, what?
   - What was the argument about?
   - Was anyone acting in an aggressive manner?

4. Have students compare their descriptions.

5. Alternate activity: If you do not want to do a scene, show an interesting drawing on an overhead transparency, a painting, a poster, or a large photograph for about 30 seconds. Then give students a few minutes to write as much as they can remember about what they saw. Encourage them to be as specific as possible. Ask them to share their descriptions about what was taking place along with details about the picture. Ask them to suggest what they think will happen next with the characters in the picture.

Follow-up Discussion

1. Why do you believe your perceptions are different from those of the other students?

2. For the alternate activity: How did you decide what might happen next?

3. When are differences in perceptions highly significant and important to take into consideration? (Examples include: in relationships, in a court of law, when trying to help the police, when a person has a complaint about an organization.)

4. Optional follow-up assignment: Have the students write a paper (about two pages) about a real or imagined incident and show how an observer's perception caused a problem for those involved.

ACTIVITY 10-6
THINKING OUTSIDE THE BOX

What Students Will Learn

- Our assumptions can prevent us from seeing new ways to see and do things.
- The obvious way to do something is not necessarily the only way.

What You Will Need

- A copy of Student Handout 10-1, Puzzles, for each student.
- Blackboard, whiteboard, or flip chart and chalk or felt pen, *or* Transparency 10-13, Puzzles—Solutions for Student Handout 10-1.

What To Do

1. Distribute Student Handout 10-1 and ask students to work on their own to solve the puzzles.

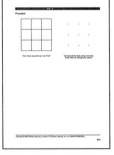

Student Handout **10-1**

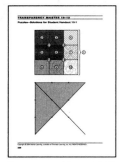

Transparency Master **10-13**

2. If they haven't figured them out after a few minutes, allow them to work in pairs.
3. When the students have either solved the puzzles or given up, show the answers using Transparency 10-13 or recreate them on the board.

Follow-up Discussion

1. How can failing to "see beyond the lines" prevent us from succeeding in school and at work?
2. What happens when people can only see one way of approaching a problem?
3. What did you learn from this activity that you can apply in your own life?
4. What did you learn from this activity that you can use for solving problems on the job as a health care worker?

ACTIVITY 10-7
WHOSE SHOES?

What Students Will Learn

- Assumptions and stereotypes can lead to incorrect conclusions about people.*

What You Will Need

- Several objects of the same type of item such as old shoes, pieces of costume jewelry, or shirts in a variety of styles. The instructor, in advance, creates an "owner" for each item. In some cases, the "owner" will fit the item; for example, a white shirt belonging to a businessman. The idea, however, is to have at least one or more objects with surprise owners to dispel stereotypes about how people dress. Suzanne Chubinski, who developed this exercise using shoes, includes the wonderful example of red-flowered sandals that belonged to an elderly nun. (By the way, she used objects that once belonged to people she knew. You may wish to do this, too.)

What To Do

1. Divide the class into groups of three to five students and distribute one item to each group.
2. Do not reveal the "owners" to the class.
3. Ask students to create a description of the owner of their item, which they then present to the whole class.
4. After each group presents its version of the "owner," you reveal the "real" owner. There should be a few surprises.

Follow-up Discussion

1. How common is it for us to classify people by their appearance and possessions?
2. How might this tendency influence how we deal with our patients or clients?
3. What are some possible negative consequences of making assumptions about people based on their appearance?
4. How can we avoid making these assumptions?
5. What other ways can you think of to get to know who a person "really is"?

---

*Source: Activity exercise adapted from S. Chubinski (1996, November/December). Creative thinking strategies. *Nurse Educator, 21* (6), 23–27.

ACTIVITY 10-8
THE POWER OF STEREOTYPES

What Students Will Learn

- Stereotypes about groups of people influence our perceptions.

What You Will Need

- A whiteboard, chalkboard, or flip chart and chalk or felt pen, or overhead projector.

What To Do

1. Discuss with students the concept of stereotyping: assigning characteristics to an individual because he or she belongs or appears to belong to a certain group. Ask students for examples.
2. Then choose one group of people commonly stereotyped by their gender, ethnicity, hair color, age, dress, choice of music, occupation, and so on.
3. Ask students for common stereotypes about the chosen group. Write these for display.
4. Use the list to discuss how stereotypes influence our perceptions and feelings about things that happen around us.

Follow-up Discussion

1. Why do you think these stereotypes developed?
2. What experiences have you had with false stereotypes?
3. How can stereotyping people interfere with providing all patients or clients with quality health care?

ACTIVITY 10-9
THINGS AREN'T ALWAYS AS THEY SEEM

What Students Will Learn

- Making assumptions about people and situations can lead to unfair or incorrect conclusions.
- Jumping to conclusions can cause unnecessary stress and communication problems.

What You Will Need

- Copies of Student Handouts 10-2 through 10-6, scenarios numbered 1 through 5, for each group of three to five students.
- Instructor Sheet 10-2, the "Real Stories."

Student Handout **10-2**	Student Handout **10-3**	Student Handout **10-4**	Student Handout **10-5**	Student Handout **10-6**

Instructor Sheet **10-2**

What To Do

1. Divide class into groups of three to five students.
2. Give each group a different scenario to discuss. (If the class is large and there are not enough scenarios to go around, you can create a few more or give the same one to more than one group.)
3. Ask each group to come up with as many explanations as possible for the behavior exhibited in the scenario.
4. When the groups have finished creating their lists, use Instructor Sheet 10-2 to give them the "real story" that matches their scenario.

Follow-up Discussion

1. Did your group think of the "real reason" for the behavior of the people in the scenario?
2. How did this activity reveal that "what you see" is *not* always "what you get"?
3. How can we avoid making assumptions about the behavior of others?
4. What implications might learning not to make assumptions have on your future work in health care?

ACTIVITY 10-10
FACTS VERSUS OPINIONS

What Students Will Learn

- To recognize the difference between facts and opinions.*

What You Will Need

- A copy of Student Handout 10-7, Fact or Opinion?, for each student *or* the list prepared as Transparency 10-14, Fact or Opinion?, for the class to view.
- Instructor Sheet 10-3, Fact or Opinion?—Answers (with sources) for Student Handout 10-7.

What To Do

1. For each statement, students discuss whether it is a fact or an opinion and explain why. You might have the class vote on each one.

Student Handout **10-7**

Student Handout **10-7**
(*Continued*)

Transparency Master **10-14**

Instructor Sheet **10-3**

---

*Source: Adapted from M. E. Milliken (1998). *Understanding human behavior: A guide for health care providers*, (6th ed.). Clifton Park, NY: Delmar Learning.

Follow-up Discussion

1. What facts would be needed to support each statement identified as an opinion?
2. For statements that sound like facts, how can they be verified?
3. Were there any facts that were based on "common knowledge"? Ask students to explain.
4. Why is it important to learn to distinguish between facts and opinions?
5. How will distinguishing between facts and opinions be important when working in health care occupations?
6. Point of discussion with students: Do the results of one study make a statement a fact? What would you want to know about a study before deciding how much credibility to give it?

ACTIVITY 10-11
IT'S LOGICAL!

Student Handout **10-8**

What Students Will Learn

- To use logic to determine whether conclusions are true, false, or indeterminable.

What You Will Need

- A copy of Student Handout 10-8, True or False, for each student.

What to Do

1. Discuss with students how reasoning means to draw correct conclusions from statements known as "premises." Conclusions can sound correct—or even be correct—but not be based on the facts given. Or the premises may be false. For example, the facts given may be wrong or a premise may be based on an opinion.
2. Distribute Student Handout 10-8 and ask students to decide which conclusions are most likely true and which are most likely false. Ask them to explain why.

Student Handout **10-8**
(*Continued*)

Follow-up Discussion

1. Were your opinions influenced by strong beliefs you might have?

ACTIVITY 10-12
WHAT'S WRONG WITH THIS LOGIC?

What Students Will Learn

- To recognize statements that have faulty premises or for which conclusions reached don't make sense.

What You Will Need

- A copy of Student Handout 10-9, What's Wrong Here? for each student.
- Instructor Sheet 10-4, Suggested Responses for Student Handout 10-9.

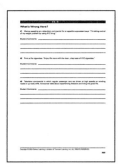

Student Handout **10-9**

Instructor Sheet **10-4**

What To Do

1. Distribute a copy of Student Handout 10-9 to each student.
2. Divide class into groups of three to five students.
3. Each group chooses a recorder and a person to present the group's opinion.
4. Instruct students to discuss in their groups the advertising described on the handouts. Do they notice anything about what the ads are communicating that does not make sense? Allow 5 or 10 minutes.
5. The group's recorder writes down the group's comments.
6. Reconvene the class and have the groups share as a class, discussing what the groups think about the ads.

Follow-up Discussion

1. What other techniques are used in advertising to convince us to buy products?
2. What other examples can you think of that mislead the public about health problems and health care issues?

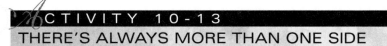

ACTIVITY 10-13
THERE'S ALWAYS MORE THAN ONE SIDE

What Students Will Learn

- Controversial issues have more than one side.
- People bring emotions to discussions about controversial topics.

What You Will Need

- Topics for students to debate. Some ideas include legalization of marijuana for medical use, abortion, health care employees speaking their native languages on the job, dress codes for health care students, smoking in public places (such as restaurants and bars), needle exchange program, and euthanasia. You gather ideas from students by passing out 3 × 5 cards at the beginning of your course and asking students to write down one topic of a controversial nature that they feel strongly about. They do not need to include their names on the cards. Collect the cards and pull one out any time you want to do this activity.

What To Do

1. Divide the class into halves by dividing down the middle of the room or by having students count off in one's and two's and grouping them on either side of the room.
2. Announce the topic to the class and randomly assign one side to argue for and one to argue against.
3. Setting a few ground rules will help keep the debate focused and orderly. Specify that only one student may speak at a time and for a specific period of time such as 1–2 minutes. Each side should have the same amount of time allotted to present its case.

4. Following the presentations, each side should be allotted equal amounts of time to present opposing arguments.

Instructor's Note: The purpose of the debate activity is not to determine a winner and loser, but to illustrate how there is more than one side to any issue and how emotions influence our beliefs and opinions.

Follow-up Discussion

1. Did you observe emotional arguments and responses from your classmates?
2. Were facts used to support arguments? If so, give some examples.
3. What influences our reactions to controversial issues?
4. Do you think it is possible to reach compromises on such issues? If so, how might these be reached?

ACTIVITY 10-14
WHAT'S THE PROBLEM?

What Students Will Learn
- Human behaviors are motivated by many causes.
- It is important not to make assumptions about the behavior of others.

What You Will Need
- A copy of Student Handout 10-10, What's the Problem?, for each student.
- Instructor Sheet 10-5, The Real Problems—Answers for Student Handout 10-10.

What To Do
1. Distribute Student Handout 10-10. Students may read over the scenarios individually before the class discussion. Or, divide the class into small groups with each group assigned to work on one scenario.
2. When they have completed identifying the probable "real" problems, as listed on Instructor Sheet 10-5, discuss how easy it is to fail to recognize underlying problems when we focus only on the behaviors or symptoms of the problem.

Follow-up Discussion
1. How does the inability to identify "real problems" get in the way of finding solutions?
2. How can taking responsibility for a problem be empowering?

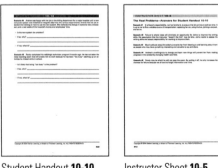

Student Handout **10-10**

Student Handout **10-10**
(*Continued*)

Instructor Sheet **10-5**

REFERENCES

Chubinski, S. (1996, November/December). Creative thinking strategies. *Nurse Educator, 21* (6), 23–27.

Covey, S. (1989). *The 7 habits of highly effective people: Restoring the character ethic.* New York: Simon & Schuster.

Drake, D. (1997). Managed care: A product of market dynamics. *Journal of the American Medical Association, 277,* 311–314.

Milliken, M. E. (1998). *Understanding human behavior: A guide for health care providers* (6th ed.). Clifton Park, NY: Delmar Learning.

Optical Illusion Hints and Answers

Transparency 10-1:   Use the girl's face (jawline) as the old woman's nose.

Transparency 10-2:   The circles are exactly the same. Discuss how things are often viewed in terms of their surroundings.

Transparency 10-3:   Two of the legs have no feet attached. Careful observation is important in health care. A quick glance is not always sufficient to see the real situation.

Transparency 10-4:   The face is almost a profile. The word "liar" begins with a capital L and extends from top left to bottom right.

Transparency 10-5:   The sax player is in black; the woman's face is outlined only on your left side by what also forms the figure of the musician.

Transparencies 10-6 and 10-7:   The stems of the vases make up two identical profiles facing each other.

Transparency 10-8:   The lines are the same length. Again, surroundings make a difference.

Transparency 10-9:   The staircase flips upside down. It takes several seconds of staring at the ball—not the staircase—for this one to work. Discuss how our viewpoint sometimes makes a big difference in what we see in many situations.

Transparency 10-10:   The Eskimo has his back to the viewer. The Indian's profile is directed to the viewer's left.

Corresponds to Student Handouts 10-2 through 10-6

The "Real Stories" Explaining the Behaviors

Scenario #1 Dr. Singh has had a difficult week dealing with various personnel problems. She is not aware that Anita was late for work this morning. Her most pressing problem is to find employees to cover the approaching weekend when the center is open. She plans to ask Anita, who has proven herself to be quite reliable, if she is willing to work overtime. Dr. Singh is worried that if Anita is unable to help out, the center will be understaffed.

Scenario #2 When the patient, Mr. Ferris, comes in, he is rather pushy and annoyed when told he will have to wait 3 weeks for an appointment. Even worse, he looks and sounds a lot like Letisha's abusive stepfather. Although she has left her difficult home situation and created a new life and career for herself, she is still working on dealing with her feelings about being mistreated as a child and teenager. Although she tries to be polite with Mr. Ferris, it is hard to express her usual warmth and friendliness to this man.

Scenario #3 The man's wife, mother of the children, just died in the hospital after a short illness. The children are confused and distraught and the man is grief-stricken and exhausted.

Scenario #4 Ms. Trent left her last job in another state because of criticism that she was too friendly with the staff and allowed her relationships with them to diminish their respect for her as well as her ability to maintain an orderly work environment. She sees this job at Mayflower as a chance to correct her previous mistakes as a manager.

Scenario #5 Mrs. Ling is actually a very kind woman who does not take her wealth for granted. She is, however, terrified of the upcoming surgery because her younger brother died three years ago as a result of a massive infection following a surgical procedure. Finding fault with the hospital is Mrs. Ling's way of trying to cope with her fear.

Fact or Opinion?—Answers (with Sources) for Student Handout 10-7.

1. Opinion.

2. Fact. *Source: Occupational outlook handbook 1998–1999.* U.S. Department of Labor. Published by JIST, Indianapolis, IN. See chart on page 7.

3. Opinion.

4. Opinion.

5. Opinion.

6. Fact. Many sources; for example; D. Drake (1997). Managed care: A product of market dynamics. *Journal of the American Medical Association, 277,* 311–314.

7. Fact, according to the report "The Surgeon General's Call to Action to Prevent and Decrease Overweight and Obesity."

   Available: http://www.seniors.gov/articles/1201/obesity.htm

8. Opinion.

9. Opinion

10. Fact. Many sources.

Suggested Responses to Student Handout 10-9

What's Wrong Here?

#1 Woman speaking on a television commercial for an appetite suppressant says: "*I'm* taking control of my weight problem by using XYZ drug."

Response: Who's really in control, the woman or the drugs? Is relying on drugs an effective way to solve nonmedical problems? What other ways might this woman choose to really "take control" of her life?

#2 Print ads for cigarettes: "Enjoy life more with the clean, crisp taste of XYZ cigarettes."

Response: Since when do cigarette air and breath smell and taste clean? How do cigarettes add to the quality of life, helping us enjoy life more?

#3 Television commercials in which regular passenger cars are driven at high speeds on winding roads or up rocky cliffs. Announcer talks about experiencing freedom and living the good life.

Response: The speeding shown can lead to accidents, and there's nothing free about life in a wheelchair!

The Real Problems—Answers for Student Handout 10-10

Scenario #1 It is Karen's responsibility, not her brother's, to ensure that she arrive at work on time. It is up to her to find a reliable source of transportation: replacing her car, using the bus, joining a carpool, and so on.

Scenario #2 Failure to attend class will eliminate an opportunity for Jaime to improve his writing skills. His assumption that the instructor "doesn't like him" may be false. Jaime needs to assess his writing skills and accept responsibility for working to improve them.

Scenario #3 Myra's attitude about the elderly prevents her from listening to and learning about them as people who may have something interesting and valuable to say and share.

Scenario #4 Andrea's unwillingness to change and learn new things will prevent her from making progress in the constantly changing health care field.

Scenario #5 Randy may be afraid he will not pass the exam. By putting it off, he only increases his chances for failure because we all tend to forget information over time.

Puzzles

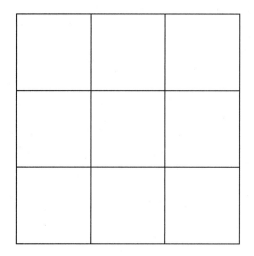

How many squares can you find?

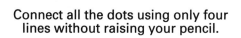

Connect all the dots using only four
lines without raising your pencil.

Scenario #1

Anita recently graduated from a medical assistant program and has been employed in an urgent care center for 4 months. She believes she has been doing a good job, in spite of her lack of experience. Anita arrived for work a few minutes late this morning, although this is only the second time she has done so since she was hired. At about 3 P.M. the director, Dr. Singh, asks Anita to come to her office at 5:00 before she leaves for the day. This is an unusual request. Although Dr. Singh is polite, she is not overly friendly. Anita is nervous and wonders why Dr. Singh would want to see her.

List as many answers as you can.

- Why do you think Dr. Singh asked Anita to report to her office?

_____

_____

_____

_____

- Why is Anita nervous?

_____

_____

_____

_____

Scenario #2

Letisha is the receptionist and administrative assistant for a dentist, Dr. Geary. She enjoys her work and especially likes talking with the patients and helping those who are nervous about visiting the dentist feel less apprehensive. The patients respond well to Letisha and have often mentioned to Dr. Geary how much they appreciate her courteous and reassuring manner. He is very surprised, therefore, when a new patient, Mr. Ferris, calls to complain that Letisha was rude to him and failed to show proper respect when he stopped by the office to make an appointment. Letisha told Mr. Ferris that unless he had an emergency, the next available appointment was 3 weeks away. This was bad enough, Mr. Ferris complains, but the way she said it implied that she could have scheduled him sooner but just didn't want to accommodate him.

List as many answers as you can.

- What might have caused Mr. Ferris to feel this way? Consider possible motivations and actions for both Letisha and Mr. Ferris.

_____

_____

_____

_____

_____

_____

_____

_____

Scenario #3

Kim works in the billing office of a large hospital. Most of her work time is spent preparing bills and filling out paperwork to submit to insurance companies. An organized person, Kim enjoys the relative quiet and orderliness of the office. One day she is eating lunch in the hospital cafeteria with her co-worker, Melissa. The cafeteria is open to the public and a man is there with his two young children who, rather than sitting and eating the sandwiches their father has bought them, run about squealing and bumping into people. The man remains seated at his table and doesn't make a move to stop the children. "Boy," Kim remarks to Melissa, "I can't believe how some people will let their kids get away with murder. Wait till those kids become teenagers. Look out!"

List as many answers as you can.

- What might explain the children's behavior?

_____

_____

_____

_____

- Why might the father be so unresponsive?

_____

_____

_____

_____

Source: Adapted from S. Covey (1989). _The 7 habits of highly effective people: Restoring the character ethic._ New York: Simon & Schuster.

Scenario #4

A new lab supervisor, Ms. Sandra Trent, was hired two months ago to direct daily operations at Mayflower Medical Laboratory. The lab had been without a supervisor for several weeks. During that time, the technicians had worked together as a team keeping the lab running smoothly enough to maintain a steady flow of work. Even so, things were getting a bit disorganized and the staff was tiring of working the overtime hours necessary to complete everything that needed to be done. Therefore, they were pleased when Ms. Trent got right to work restoring order and putting policies and procedures in place. Lately, however, the staff has become dissatisfied with her management style. She insists that everything be done exactly as she directs and constantly checks on the technicians' work. The staff feels offended that they are getting no credit for their ability to keep the lab running on their own. At the same time, Ms. Trent is very businesslike in her manner, almost to the point of being unfriendly.

List as many answers as you can.

- What might account for Ms. Trent's actions and style of management?

_____

_____

_____

_____

Scenario #5

Maria is a nurse who works the evening shift in a major hospital. One of the patients in her area, Mrs. Ling, is scheduled for surgery tomorrow. Mrs. Ling is from a wealthy family and lives in a beautiful home with hired help to cook and clean. She is accustomed to having things "her way." When Maria enters Mrs. Ling's private room to take her vital signs, Mrs. Ling is reluctant to cooperate. She recites a list of complaints to Maria about the hospital, including the lack of responsiveness to her calls to the nursing station, an uncomfortable bed, tasteless food, and so on. Since this hospital usually receives high marks on its evaluation surveys filled out by patients, Maria simply says she is sorry Mrs. Ling is unhappy with the service. She then hurries through her duties so she can leave the room before she has to listen to any more complaints.

List as many answers as you can.

- What might explain Mrs. Ling's complaints about the hospital?

_____

_____

_____

_____

Fact or Opinion?

For each of the following statements, check whether it is most likely a fact or an opinion. Then briefly explain why.

1. Women make better nurses than men.

   ☐ Fact   ☐ Opinion

   Reason: _____

   _____

2. According to the U.S Department of Labor, four of the five fastest growing occupations that require an associate's degree are in health care.

   ☐ Fact   ☐ Opinion

   Reason: _____

   _____

3. The government should take over the costs of providing health care.

   ☐ Fact   ☐ Opinion

   Reason: _____

   _____

4. Sex education should not be allowed in the public schools. Sex education is for adults, not children.

   ☐ Fact   ☐ Opinion

   Reason: _____

   _____

5. Managed care is the best system for providing high quality health care services.

   ☐ Fact   ☐ Opinion

   Reason: _____

   _____

6. Managed care systems were developed to increase efficiency and reduce the growing costs of providing health care.

   ☐ Fact   ☐ Opinion

   Reason: _____

   _____

7. A survey conducted by the RAND research institute found that obese adults are likely to have more chronic health problems than smokers, heavy drinkers, or poor people.

   ☐ Fact   ☐ Opinion

   Reason: _____

   _____

8. People who are obese really don't care that much about their health or appearance.

   ☐ Fact   ☐ Opinion

   Reason: _____

   _____

9. Every health care student is interested in helping the sick.

   ☐ Fact   ☐ Opinion

   Reason: _____

   _____

10. Elderly patients as a group use health care services more frequently than those under the age of 70.

    ☐ Fact   ☐ Opinion

    Reason: _____

    _____

True or False?

#1

Premise: People who smoke have an increased risk of getting lung cancer.

Premise: Mary has smoked two packs of cigarettes a day for 20 years.

Conclusion: Mary will get lung cancer.

This conclusion is: ☐ True ☐ False

Explain why or why not: _____

_____

_____

#2

Premise: People who floss their teeth daily have a decreased risk of gum disease.

Premise: Jim flosses every evening when he brushes his teeth.

Conclusion: Jim has a good chance of staying free of gum disease.

This conclusion is: ☐ True ☐ False

Explain why or why not: _____

_____

_____

#3

Premise: Dental lab technicians need good hand–eye coordination.

Premise: Juan has excellent hand–eye coordination.

Conclusion: Juan should enroll in a dental lab technician program.

This conclusion is: ☐ True ☐ False

Explain why or why not: _____

_____

_____

#4

Premise: Carla has just completed a home health aide program.

Premise: Jobs for home health aides are growing at a much faster rate than for other types of jobs.

Conclusion: It will be easy for Carla to find a job.

This conclusion is: ☐ True   ☐ False

Explain why or why not: _____

_____

_____

#5

Premise: Most infectious diseases that were major killers in the past can now be cured with medication.

Premise: Mohammed contracted an infectious disease while traveling abroad.

Conclusion: Mohammed can be cured if he seeks medical attention immediately.

This conclusion is: ☐ True   ☐ False

Explain why or why not: _____

_____

_____

#6

Premise: Obesity is a risk factor for heart disease.

Premise: An increasing percentage of Americans are obese.

Conclusion: The percentage of Americans who have heart disease is increasing.

This conclusion is: ☐ True   ☐ False

Explain why or why not: _____

_____

_____

What's Wrong Here?

#1 Woman speaking on a television commercial for an appetite suppressant says: "*I'm* taking control of my weight problem by using XYZ drug."

Student Comments: _____

_____

_____

_____

#2 Print ad for cigarettes: "Enjoy life more with the clean, crisp taste of XYZ cigarettes."

Student Comments: _____

_____

_____

_____

#3 Television commercial in which regular passenger cars are driven at high speeds on winding roads or up rocky cliffs. Announcer talks about experiencing freedom and living the good life.

Student Comments: _____

_____

_____

_____

What's the Problem?

Scenario #1   Karen is a respiratory therapist. She is often late for work because her car is old and frequently breaks down. When this happens, she relies on her brother to take her to work. But he doesn't always get her there by 7:30 A.M. when her shift starts. Karen feels that her brother should make more of an effort to help her out.

- Is Karen's brother the problem?

- If so, why? _____

  _____

- If not, what is? _____

  _____

Scenario #2   Jaime is failing his class, "Writing for Health Professionals." He avoids attending class regularly because, as he told his friends, the instructor doesn't like him and it's really a waste of time to go and feel put down.

- Is the instructor the problem?

- If so, why? _____

  _____

- If not, what is? _____

  _____

Scenario #3   Myra works as a CNA in a long-term care facility. Most of the residents are elderly and Myra is bored by their stories about "the old days." She performs her tasks with them as quickly as possible and engages in as little conversation as possible so she can move along and get through the work day.

- Are boring residents the problem?

- If so, why? _____

  _____

- If not, what is? _____

  _____

Scenario #4   Andrea was happy with her job in the billing department for a major hospital until a new computer system was installed to integrate data from the various departments. Andrea has not yet attended the training on how to use the new system. She believes the change in systems was unnecessary and a real waste of the hospital's money and employees' time.

- Is the new system the problem?

- If so, why? _____

  _____

- If not, what is? _____

  _____

Scenario #5   Randy completed his radiologic technician program 5 months ago. He has not taken the state licensing exam that will enable him to work because he has been "too busy" catching up on activities he missed while in school.

- Is it likely that being "too busy" is the problem?

- If so, why? _____

  _____

- If not, what is? _____

  _____

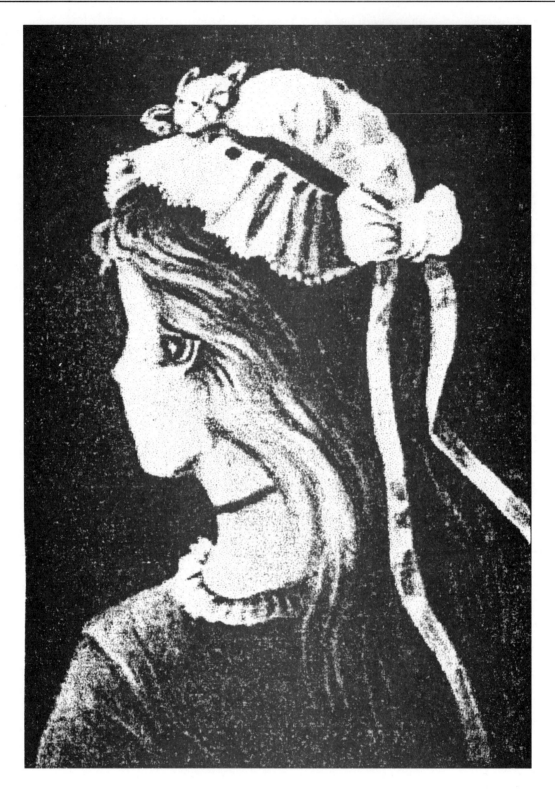

What do you see?

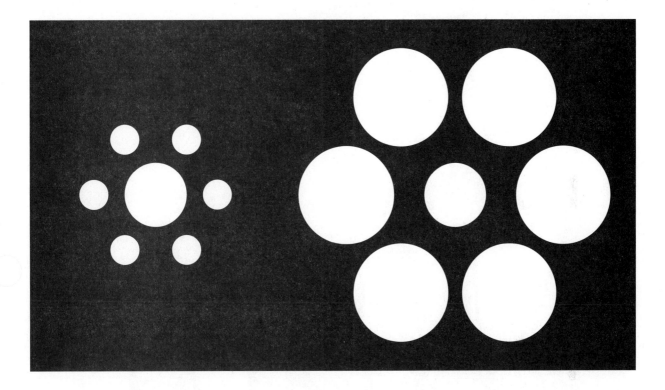

How would you describe the sizes of the center circles in relation to one another?

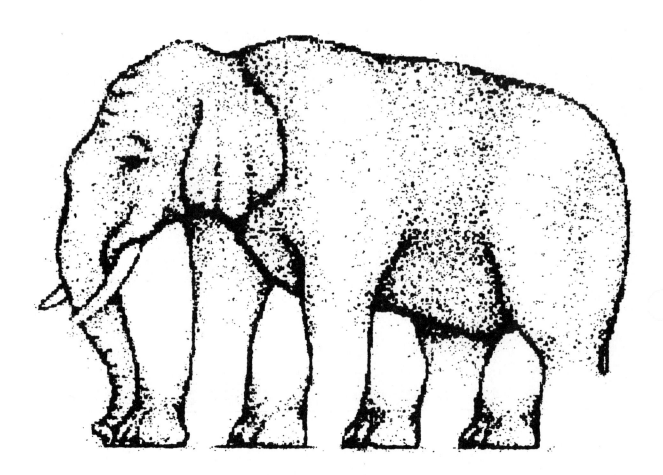

How many legs does this elephant have?

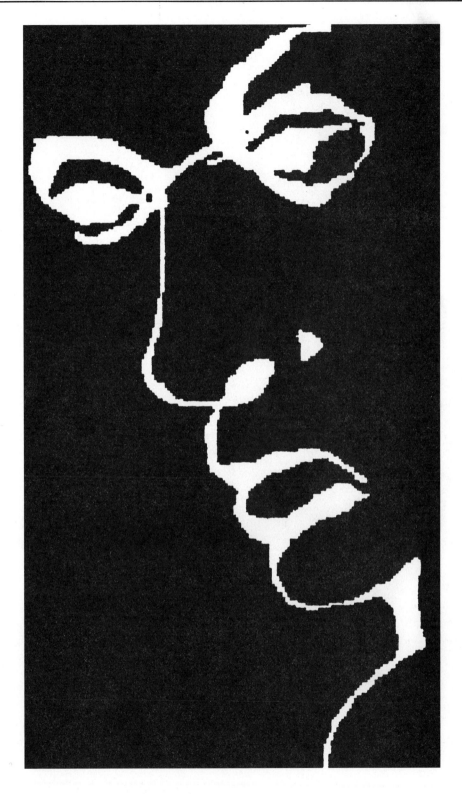

What do you see?

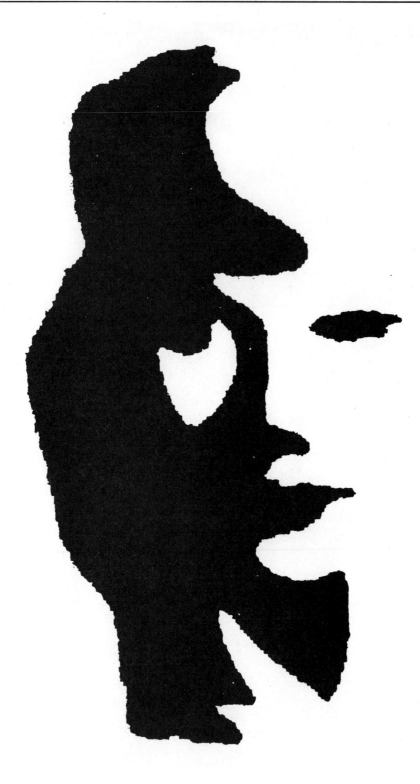

What do you see?

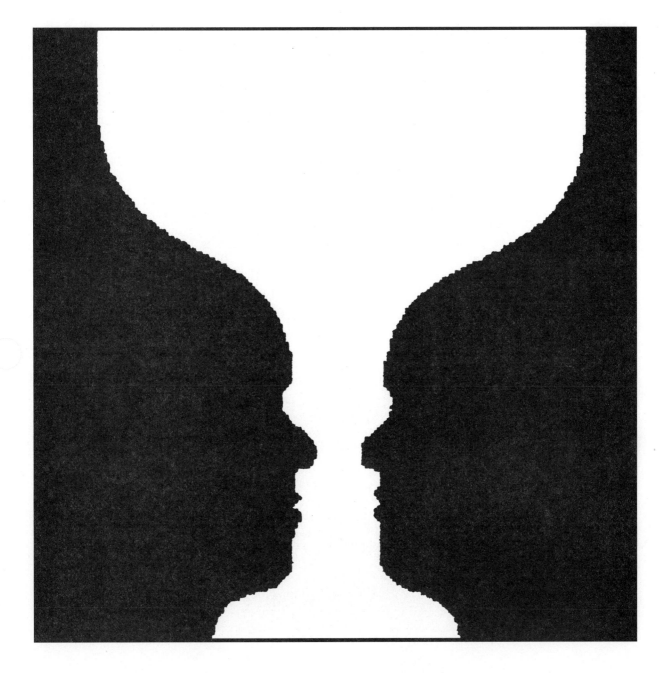

What do you see?

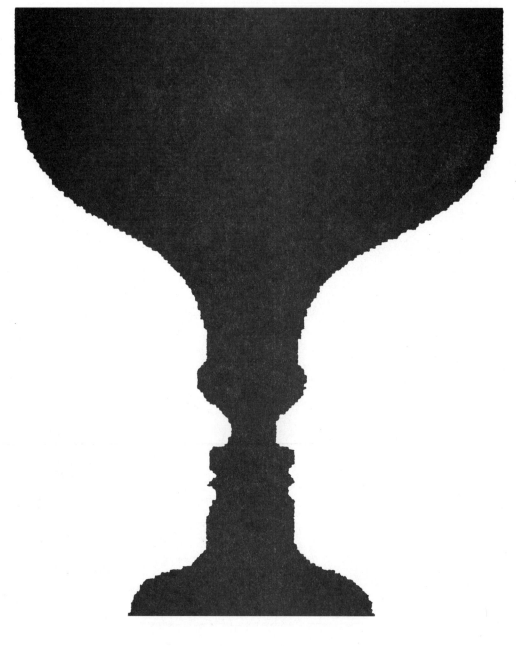

What do you see?

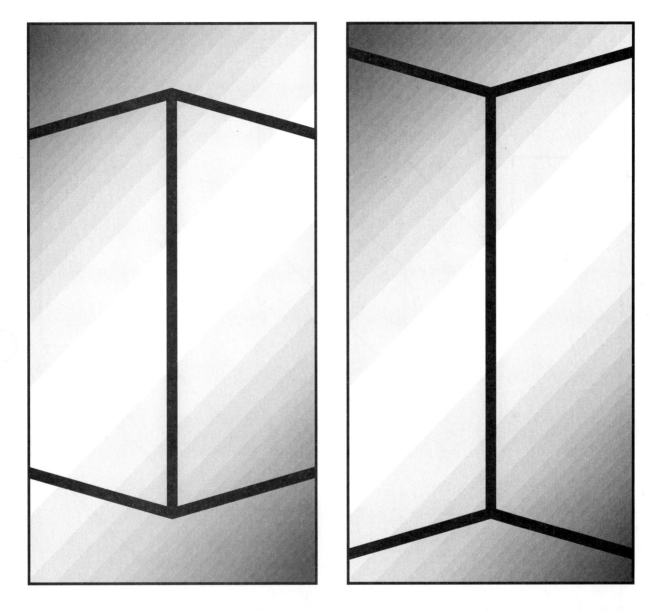

How would you describe the lengths of the vertical lines in relation to one another?

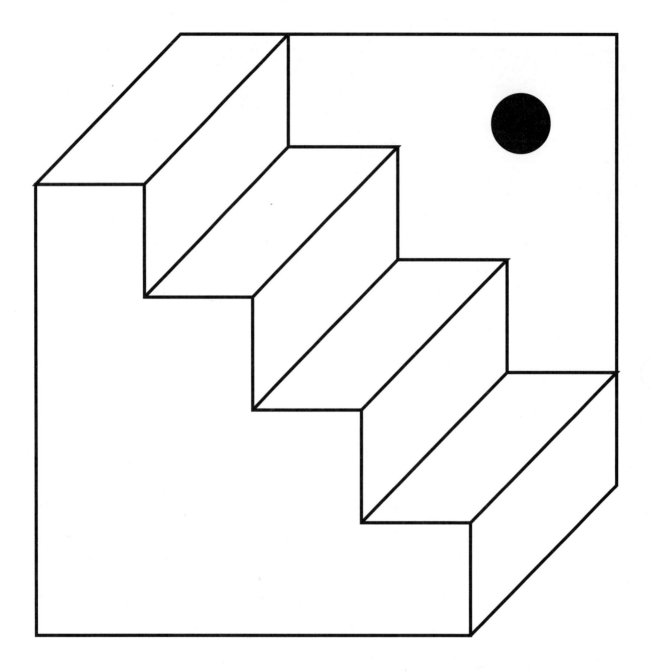

What happens to the staircase when you stare at the spot in the corner?

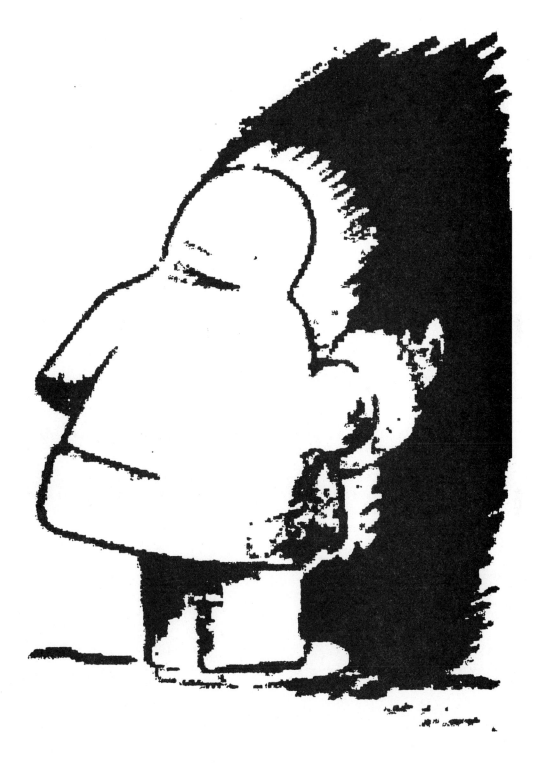

Is this an Eskimo or an Indian?

Stroop Effect 1

RED	GREEN	BLUE	YELLOW	PINK
ORANGE	BLUE	GREEN	BLUE	WHITE
GREEN	YELLOW	ORANGE	WHITE	BLUE
VIOLET	RED	PINK	YELLOW	GREEN
PINK	YELLOW	GREEN	BLUE	RED

Stroop Effect 2

RED	GREEN	BLUE	YELLOW	PINK
ORANGE	BLUE	GREEN	BLUE	WHITE
GREEN	YELLOW	ORANGE	WHITE	BLUE
VIOLET	RED	PINK	YELLOW	GREEN
PINK	YELLOW	GREEN	BLUE	RED

Puzzles—Solutions for Student Handout 10-1

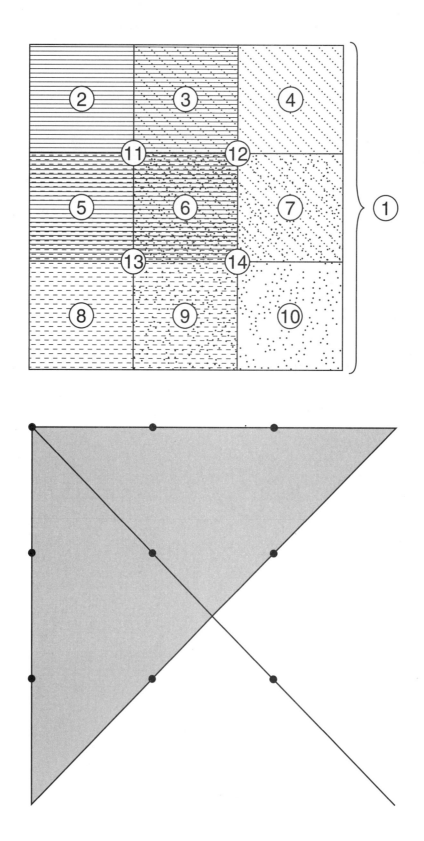

Fact or Opinion?

1. Women make better nurses than men do.

2. According to the U.S Department of Labor, four of the five fastest growing occupations that require an associate's degree are in health care.

3. The government should take over the costs of providing health care.

4. Sex education should not be allowed in the public schools. Sex education is for adults, not children.

5. Managed care is the best system for providing high quality health care services.

6. Managed care systems were developed to increase efficiency and reduce the growing costs of providing health care.

7. A survey conducted by the RAND research institute found that obese adults are likely to have more chronic health problems than smokers, heavy drinkers, or poor people.

8. People who are obese really don't care that much about their health or appearance.

9. Every health care student is interested in helping the sick.

10. Elderly patients as a group use health care services more frequently than those under the age of 70.

CHAPTER 11

Problem Solving and Decision Making

INTRODUCTION

Employers repeatedly tell us that they look for problem-solving and decision-making skills when they hire health care graduates. With its increased demands on health care workers, the current health care environment makes the acquisition of these skills even more critical. This chapter includes activities that range from fun puzzles and games to lessons about applying a useful five-step problem-solving process and using a numerical decision matrix to make important decisions.

ACTIVITY 11-1
HITTING THE JACKPOT

What Students Will Learn

- How to work together to make decisions that benefit all participants.

What You Will Need

- A packet of $25,000 in play money for each group of five students can be used but isn't absolutely necessary.

What To Do

1. Divide class into groups of five students.
2. Distribute a packet of play money to each group, or simply tell each group they have $25,000 to spend.
3. The students must decide as a group how to spend the money. Students should estimate the costs of the items they suggest. Each expenditure should benefit as many of the group members as possible. Encourage students to spend money in ways that will help them as students and as future health care workers, as well as spending for fun.

Follow-up Discussion

1. How easy or difficult was it to decide how to spend the money?
2. Were there wide differences of opinion among the group members? Explain.
3. If so, how did you resolve them?
4. How might the process have been different if you had real money to spend?

ACTIVITY 11-2
CREATIVE COLLABORATION

What Students Will Learn

- How to work together and use their creativity to solve a problem.*

What You Will Need

- A complete set of each of the following six items for each group of four to five students:
    1. Two 3 × 5 cards
    2. Two paper clips
    3. Four toothpicks
    4. One pencil
    5. Two Styrofoam cups
    6. Two medium rubber bands

What To Do

1. Divide the class into groups of four to five students.
2. Give each group a set of the items and tell them they have 12 minutes to work together to invent and build something that would be useful or fun to have in the health care classroom. Encourage them to be creative.
3. At the end of the 12 minutes, ask groups to stop working on the invention and spend 5 minutes preparing a short commercial for their product.
4. Groups present their commercials, explaining the benefits of their inventions, to the class.

Follow-up Discussion

1. How did your group approach the problem of inventing a useful classroom item?
2. How did you decide the best way to proceed with the exercise?
3. Did your group come up with a number of suggestions?
4. How can creativity be applied to solving school and workplace problems?

ACTIVITY 11-3
THINKING OUTSIDE THE BOX

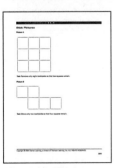

Student Handout **11-1**

What Students Will Learn

- The importance of being creative and "thinking outside the box" when solving problems.†

What You Will Need

- 24 toothpicks for each student.
- A copy of Student Handout 11-1, Stick Pictures, for each student.
- Transparencies 11-1, Solution for Picture A—Student Handout 11-1, 11-2, How to Arrange 11 Toothpicks to Make 9, and 11-3, Solution for Picture B—Student Handout 11-1.

---

*Source: Activity adapted from J. Gibbs (1994). *Tribes: A new way of learning together.* Santa Rosa, CA: Center Source Publications.

†Source: Adapted from "Online Children's Magazine from Amrita Bhavan" at www.dimdima.com.

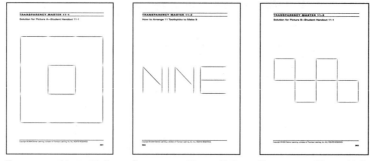

Transparency Master **11-1**   Transparency Master **11-2**   Transparency Master **11-3**

What To Do

1. Distribute Student Handout 11-1 and give each student 24 toothpicks.
2. Have students create picture A that appears on the handout and instruct them to remove only 8 toothpicks so they have two squares remaining.
3. Show the solution using Transparency 11-1.
4. Now ask students to arrange 11 toothpicks to make 9.
5. Show the solution using Transparency 11-2.
6. Finally, ask students to use their toothpicks to create the shape shown in picture B on the handout and instruct them to move only two toothpicks so that four squares remain.
7. Show the solution using Transparency 11-3.

Follow-up Discussion

1. How did you go about trying to solve the puzzles?
2. Was it easier to think about the possible moves or try them out by moving the toothpicks?
3. What is meant by "thinking outside the box"?
4. How might the ability to "think outside the box" be useful on the job?

ACTIVITY 11-4
MORE FUN WITH TOOTHPICKS

What Students Will Learn*

- To solve problems that require strategies.
- To think ahead and predict consequences of actions.

What You Will Need

- 23 toothpicks for each pair of students.

What To Do

1. Have students pair off.
2. Give each pair 23 toothpicks.
3. Instruct students to lay the toothpicks out so they are side by side and tell them to take turns removing one, two, or three toothpicks per turn. The winner is the student whose opponent is stuck with the last toothpick.

*Source: Adapted from "Funky Pages" at www.funkypages.com/navigation.php.

Follow-up Discussion

1. Did you think about and develop a strategy or simply play and hope for the best?
2. If you developed a strategy, what was it?
3. When might thinking and planning ahead be good things to do on the job?

ACTIVITY 11-5
LINE THEM UP

What Students Will Learn

- How to solve problems with others by using nonverbal communication.

What You Will Need

- No special materials are required for this activity.

What To Do

1. Explain to the class that their task is to form a single-file line in the order of their birth dates, from January through December.
2. The rule is that students must form the line without speaking (no lip reading or writing is allowed, either.) Students who share a birthday will stand next to each other in the line.
3. When the line is complete, students call out their birth dates in order, starting with the first person in the line.

Follow-up Discussion:

1. What was the problem that needed to be solved?
2. What skills did you need to use to take the place of speech?
3. How difficult was it to solve the problem without speaking?
4. Were you successful? (Were any students out of order?)

ACTIVITY 11-6
HOW TALL ARE YOU?

What Students Will Learn*

- To use problem-solving skills.
- To work as a team member.

What You Will Need

- A blindfold for each student (or you can ask students to keep their eyes closed during the activity).

What To Do

1. Ask students to stand up and assemble in a space in which they can line up.
2. Distribute the blindfolds and have students put them on (or close their eyes).

Source: Adapted from "Resident Assistant—The Rx for RAs" at www.residentassistant.com.

3. Instruct students to form a straight line by height (tallest to shortest, or shortest to tallest).
4. Students may speak during this exercise, but they may not use their vision.
5. When the line is complete, let students see the results.

Follow-up Discussion

1. What was the problem that needed to be solved?
2. How difficult was it to solve?
3. How could you have solved the problem if, in addition to not being able to see, you could not speak?
4. How important was it to work as part of a team?
5. Was the team successful in solving the problem?

ACTIVITY 11-7
WHAT KIND OF PROBLEM SOLVER ARE YOU?

What Students Will Learn

- The variety of ways that people use to solve problems and make decisions.
- How to identify their preferred method for solving problems and making decisions.

What

- Five   lent.

What

Instructo   one as a class or individually.

1. Ask students to write down five major decisions they have made during the past few years. (An example might be "I decided to return to school to become a medical assistant.") They should write one decision on each card.
2. Ask students to think about the reasons for their decisions and the actions they took when making the decision. They should write these in bullet format under each decision listed on the cards. Examples:
   - Wanted to get ahead
   - Always wanted a job in health care
   - Saw commercial on television
   - Spoke with someone at the school
   - Looked at other schools in the area
   - Made the decision to attend this school
3. Now ask students to discuss the processes they used to make their decisions:
   a. Did they spend a lot of time thinking about what to do or did they make the decisions quickly?
   b. Would they describe their decision making as more guided by their heart (feelings) or head (thoughts)?
   c. Did they gather a lot of information before making a decision or base it on what they already knew?
   d. Did they consult with others or decide for themselves?

Follow-up Discussion

1. Is there one best way to make decisions? Explain your answer.

2. Did the type of decision influence the way you went about making it?
3. Were there similarities among the students in the way they made decisions?
4. What kinds of things influence how we make our decisions? (Examples: level of education of the decision maker, seriousness of decision to be made, length of time person has to make the decision, long-term effects of the decision, etc.)
5. Why is good decision making important for the health care worker?

ACTIVITY 11-8
BRAINSTORMING

What Students Will Learn*

- To use brainstorming to generate new ideas and solve problems.
- To work cooperatively with others in a brainstorming session.

What You Will Need

- A copy of Student Handouts 11-2, Basic Rules for Brainstorming, and 11-3, Problems to Brainstorm, for each student.
- Overhead transparency films and pens, *or* sheets of butcher or flip-chart paper, marking pens, and masking tape for attaching to the wall, *or* white- or blackboard space for teams to write lists (class will be divided into teams of five or six students).

What To Do

1. Distribute Student Handout 11-2 to each student and briefly discuss the purpose and rules of brainstorming.
2. Divide the class into groups of five or six students. Each group selects a person to write down the suggestions and a presenter who will share the suggestions with the whole class at the conclusion of the brainstorming session.
3. Distribute Student Handout 11-3. Assign each group a different problem or have all groups brainstorm the same problem for comparative purposes. Instruct students to brainstorm and list as many ideas as possible during the next 10 or 15 minutes.

Student Handout **11-2**

Student Handout **11-3**

Follow-up Discussion:

1. How many team members came up with ideas?
2. Did the team members expand on ideas suggested by others?
3. Did the groups generate workable solutions that might be effective in solving the problem?
4. How can brainstorming be used by groups to deal with problems in the workplace?

---

*Source: Adapted from T. Justice & T. D. Jamieson (1999). *The facilitator's fieldbook.* New York: AMA-COM.

ACTIVITY 11-9

WHAT'S THE PROBLEM?

What Students Will Learn

- How to clearly identify problems.

What You Will Need

- A copy of Student Handout 11-4, What's the Problem, for each student.
- Instructor Sheet 11-1, The "Real" Problems in the Scenarios—Answers for Student Handout 11-4.

What To Do

1. Distribute Student Handout 11-4 and give the students time to read the scenarios and answer the questions.
2. Conduct a class discussion during which you reveal the "real" problems, referring to Instructor Sheet 11-1. Talk about how easy it is to fail to recognize underlying problems when we focus only on the behaviors or symptoms of the problem.
3. Alternate activity: Divide the class into small groups and assign one scenario to each group for discussion.

Follow-up Discussion:

1. Why is identification of the real problem the first step in problem solving?
2. Why must you be willing to accept responsibility for a problem in order to solve it?
3. What are some other examples you've seen or experienced in which the real problem was not identified?

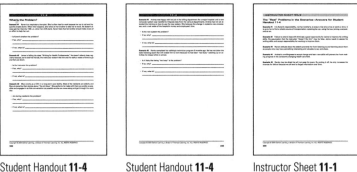

Student Handout **11-4**   Student Handout **11-4**   Instructor Sheet **11-1**
                             (*Continued*)

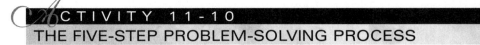

ACTIVITY 11-10

THE FIVE-STEP PROBLEM-SOLVING PROCESS

What Students Will Learn

- The five-step problem-solving process.
- How to apply the five steps to solve a real problem.

What You Will Need

- Transparency 11-4, Five-Step Problem-Solving Process.

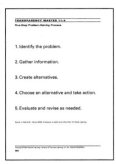

Transparency Master **11-4**

What To Do

1. Choose a problem that affects the class or the school. Look for something the students can take action on to resolve. Or have students discuss and select a problem.
2. Working with the whole class, invite student input and go through the problem-solving process. Use Transparency 11-4 as a guide.
3. Have one student serve as class recorder and list ideas on the board or overhead.
4. As a group, choose a solution.
5. Implement the solution, if appropriate. This can be done as a class, in groups, or by individuals.
6. Follow up to evaluate the effectiveness of the solution and to suggest revisions, if necessary.

Instructor's Note: This activity can be spread over a number of days with students assigned to gather specific kinds of information that they bring to class to share. Or you can complete the activity in one class session, limiting the information gathering to the ideas generated by the group.

Follow-up Discussion

1. How effectively did the problem-solving process work?
2. How can using a process like this one help you find satisfactory solutions to problems?
3. How do you think this process can be applied in the workplace?
4. Do you think this process could be used to deal with personal problems? Explain why or why not.

ACTIVITY 11-11
I'VE GOT A PROBLEM!

Student Handout **11-5**

Student Handout **11-6**

What Students Will Learn

- How to work together to apply the five-step problem-solving process for solving health care problems.

What You Will Need

- Transparency 11-4, Five-Step Problem-Solving Process.
- Problem cards prepared from Student Handout 11-5, Problems for Groups.
- A copy of Student Handout 11-6, I've Got a Problem!, for each student

What To Do

1. Using Transparency 11-4, introduce or review the five-step problem-solving process.
2. Divide class into groups of three to five students.
3. Give each group a problem card prepared from Student Handout 11-5 and give each student a copy of Student Handout 11-6.
4. Allow 15–20 minutes for the groups to work through the first four steps of the process. For step 5, ask them to list potential obstacles for the solution they have chosen and then come up with suggestions about how these obstacles might be avoided or overcome.

Transparency Master **11-4**

5. When the groups have finished, ask a representative from each to read their problem and give a summary of their suggested solution, including how and why they chose it.

Follow-up Discussion

1. How well did this process work for the groups?
2. Do you think using this process makes it easier to come up with good solutions?
3. What did you learn about problem solving from this exercise?

ACTIVITY 11-12
DECISIONS, DECISIONS!

What Students Will Learn

- How to use a decision matrix as a tool for making important decisions.

What You Will Need

- Transparencies 11-5, Decision Matrix, 11-6, Using a Decision Matrix, and 11-7, Sample Decision Matrix.
- A copy of Student Handouts 11-7, Decision Matrix, 11-8, Using a Decision Matrix, and 11-9, Sample Decision Matrix, for each student.

What To Do

1. Use Transparencies 11-5 and 11-6 to introduce decision matrixes. They can be very helpful when making important decisions that have significant consequences such as career choices and major financial commitments. Note that decision matrixes are a bit complex and require students to do a little math.
2. Use the example in Transparency 11-7 to illustrate the use of rankings and ratings. The example involves choosing between staying with a job or moving on to a new one. The results in the example suggest that moving to the new job would be the best choice.
3. Point out that using a decision matrix can be used in the problem-solving process to choose the best alternative.
4. Distribute Students Handouts 11-7, 11-8, and 11-9 and ask students to create a matrix for a real decision they are facing or may face in the future, such as choosing a career or what type of job to seek.

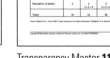

Transparency Master **11-5**

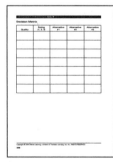

Transparency Master **11-6**   Transparency Master **11-7**   Student Handout **11-7**   Student Handout **11-8**   Student Handout **11-9**

Follow-up Discussion

1. How do you think a decision matrix might help you make important decisions?
2. What variations might work for you?
3. How might a decision matrix be used to help make a group decision in which there are many opinions and ideas about what the decision should be?
4. Will the score always indicate the best choice for you? Why or why not?

REFERENCES

"Funky Pages" at www.funkypages.com/navigation.php.

Gibbs, J. (1994). *Tribes: A new way of learning together.* Santa Rosa, CA: Center Source Publications.

Haroun, L. (2001). *Career development for health professionals.* Philadelphia: W. B. Saunders.

Justice, T., & Jamieson, T. D. (1999). *The facilitator's fieldbook.* New York: AMA-COM.

Mitchell, J., & Haroun, L. (2002). *Introduction to health care.* Clifton Park, NY: Delmar Learning.

"Online Children's Magazine from Amrita Bhavan" at www.dimdima.com.

"Resident Assistant—The Rx for RAs" at www.residentassistant.com.

The "Real" Problems in the Scenarios—Answers for Student Handout 11-4

Scenario #1   It is Karen's responsibility, not her brother's, to ensure that she arrive at work on time. It is up to her to find a reliable source of transportation: replacing her car, using the bus, joining a carpool, and so on.

Scenario #2   Failure to attend class will eliminate a good opportunity for Jaime to improve his writing skills. His assumption that the instructor "doesn't like him" may be false. Jaime needs to assess his writing skills and accept responsibility for working to improve them.

Scenario #3   Myra's attitude about the elderly prevents her from listening to and learning about them as people who may have something interesting and valuable to say and share.

Scenario #4   Andrea's unwillingness to accept change and learn new skills will prevent her from making progress in the constantly changing health care field.

Scenario #5   Randy may be afraid he will not pass the exam. By putting it off, he only increases his chances for failure because we all tend to forget information over time.

Stick Pictures

Picture A

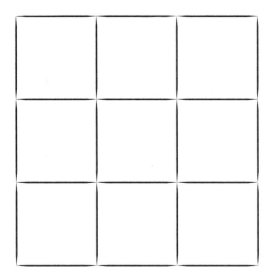

Task: Remove only eight toothpicks so that two squares remain.

Picture B

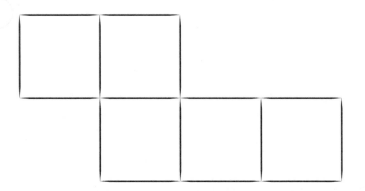

Task: Move only two toothpicks so that four squares remain.

Basic Rules for Brainstorming

What is brainstorming? Brainstorming is a method for generating as many new ideas as possible, especially those that result in solving a problem.

- The goal is to generate a large number of ideas.

- Ideas are not to be evaluated or criticized.

- Wild and silly ideas are welcome.

- It's okay to add to previously suggested ideas or combine ideas into new ones.

- All ideas are recorded exactly as offered.

Problems to Brainstorm

Problem #1   You and your teammates are enrolled in the introductory medical terminology class that is required before you can begin your specialty health care courses. The class is more difficult than you expected and you are all struggling to master the dozens of words that appear on the weekly quizzes.

Brainstorm with your team as many ways as possible to help you study and learn the required medical terms.

Problem #2   Finding a job after graduation from a health care program is an important goal for every member of your team.

Brainstorm with your team as many ways as possible to locate job openings in your community.

Problem #3   Your class wants to raise money for a special field trip to visit a major health care facility in a city 70 miles from your small community.

Brainstorm with your team as many ways as possible to raise the $350.00 necessary to take the trip.

Problem #4   Your graduating class wants to plan special ways to honor classmates who have overcome obstacles and successfully completed their education.

Brainstorm with your team ideas for giving special recognition.

Problem #5   Students at your school sometimes have difficulty attending class due to unreliable transportation.

Brainstorm with your team ways that they can be helped so they don't have to miss class.

What's the Problem?

Scenario #1   Karen is a respiratory therapist. She is often late for work because her car is old and frequently breaks down. When this happens, she relies on her brother to take her to work. He doesn't always get her there by 7:30 A.M. when her shift starts. Karen feels that her brother should make more of an effort to help her out.

- Is Karen's brother the problem?
- If so, why? _____
  _____
- If not, what is? _____
  _____

Scenario #2   Jaime is failing his class "Writing for Health Professionals." He doesn't attend class regularly because, as he told his friends, the instructor doesn't like him and it's really a waste of time to go and feel put down.

- Is the instructor the problem?
- If so, why? _____
  _____
- If not, what is? _____
  _____

Scenario #3   Myra works as a CNA in a long-term care facility. Most of the residents are elderly and Myra is bored by their stories about "the old days." She performs her tasks with them as quickly as possible and engages in as little conversation as possible so she can move along and get through the work day.

- Are boring residents the problem?
- If so, why? _____
  _____
- If not, what is? _____
  _____

Scenario #4 Andrea was happy with her job in the billing department for a major hospital until a new computer system was installed to integrate data from the various departments. Andrea has not yet attended the training on how to use the new system. She believes the change in systems was unnecessary and a real waste of the hospital's money and employees' time.

- Is the new system the problem?

- If so, why? _____

  _____

- If not, what is? _____

  _____

Scenario #5 Randy completed his radiologic technician program 5 months ago. He has not taken the state licensing exam that will enable him to work because he has been "too busy" catching up on activities he missed while in school.

- Is it likely that being "too busy" is the problem?

- If so, why? _____

  _____

- If not, what is? _____

  _____

Problems for Groups

Cut out along the dotted lines to make cards to distribute to groups for discussion.

Problem #1

Enrique needs money for school tuition and expenses.

Problem #2

Kim has two young children who constantly interrupt her when she is studying in the afternoon before attending classes in the evenings.

Problem #3

Lara's spouse is upset about the time she spends in school and studying.

Problem #4

Sam is getting Ds on all his anatomy tests.

Problem #5

Achmed is interested in working in health care but is having a hard time deciding which career to choose.

I've Got a Problem!

> **Five-Step Problem-Solving Process**
>
> 1. Identify the problem.
>
> 2. Gather information.
>
> 3. Create alternatives.
>
> 4. Choose an alternative and take action.
>
> 5. Evaluate and revise as needed.
>
> *Source:* J. Mitchell & L. Haroun (2002). *Introduction to health care.* Clifton Park, NY: Delmar Learning.

Discuss the assigned problem with your group, going through the following steps:

1. State the problem as clearly as possible. Do you think there might be more to the situation than what is stated on the card?

2. What do group members know about ways to resolve the problem? If you had the time, what other information would you want to gather?

3. Think of as many possible solutions as you can. They don't all have to be practical. Sometimes silly ideas lead to good ones that can be used.

4. Which alternative do you think the student having the problem should try first? What are the group's reasons for choosing it?

5. What are possible obstacles to the solution you have chosen? How might the student avoid or overcome these obstacles?

Decision Matrix

Quality	Rating (1, 2, 3)	Alternative #1	Alternative #2	Alternative #3

Using a Decision Matrix

1. List four or five alternative decisions.

2. List the qualities you will use to make the decision.

3. Rate each quality in terms of its importance to you:

   1 = Not very important

   2 = Somewhat important

   3 = Very important

4. Rate each alternative according to how you believe each quality will be met

   1 = Unlikely or unknown

   2 = Probably

   3 = Very likely

5. Multiply the number assigned to each quality by the number assigned to each alternative (multiply the rating number in #3 by the rating number in #4).

6. Add the columns. The alternative with the highest score is most likely to meet your needs.

Sample Decision Matrix

Should I Change Jobs?

Quality	Rating (1, 2, 3)	Current Job	Proposed Job
Specialty	1	1 $1 \times 1 = 1$	2 $1 \times 2 = 2$
Location	2	1 $2 \times 1 = 2$	2 $2 \times 2 = 4$
Salary	3	1 $3 \times 1 = 3$	2 $3 \times 2 = 6$
Training opportunities	2	2 $2 \times 2 = 4$	3 $2 \times 3 = 6$
Possibility of promotion	2	1 $2 \times 1 = 2$	2 $2 \times 2 = 4$
Responsibility	2	1 $2 \times 1 = 2$	2 $2 \times 2 = 4$
Reputation of facility	3	3 $3 \times 3 = 9$	3 $3 \times 3 = 9$
Totals		23	35

Source: Adapted from L. Haroun (2001). *Career development for health professionals.* Philadelphia: W. B. Saunders.

Solution for Picture A—Student Handout 11-1

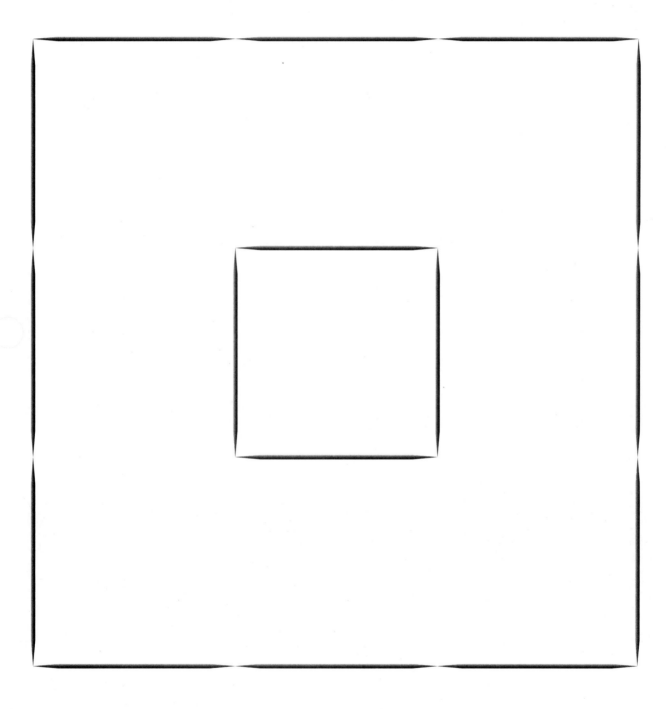

How to Arrange 11 Toothpicks to Make 9

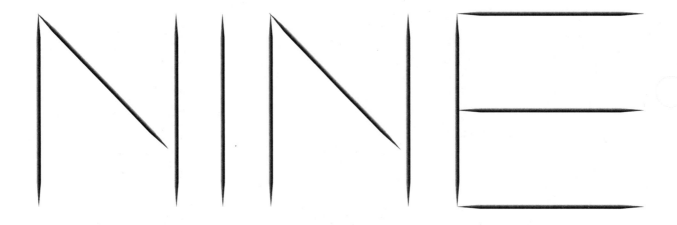

Solution for Picture B—Student Handout 11-1

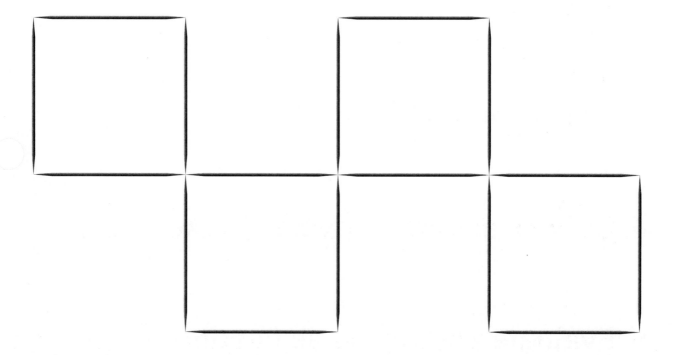

1. Identify the problem.

2. Gather information.

3. Create alternatives.

4. Choose an alternative and take action.

5. Evaluate and revise as needed.

Source: J. Mitchell & L. Haroun (2002). *Introduction to health care.* Clifton Park, NY: Delmar Learning.

Decision Matrix

Quality	Rating (1, 2, 3)	Alternative #1	Alternative #2	Alternative #3

Using a Decision Matrix

1. List four or five alternative decisions.

2. List the qualities you will use to make the decision.

3. Rate each quality in terms of its importance to you:

   1 = Not very important

   2 = Somewhat important

   3 = Very important

4. Rate each alternative according to how you believe each quality will be met:

   1 = Unlikely or unknown

   2 = Probably

   3 = Very likely

5. Multiply the number assigned to each quality by the number assigned to each alternative (multiply the rating number in #3 by the rating number in #4.)

6. Add the columns. The alternative with the highest score is most likely to meet your needs.

Sample Decision Matrix

Should I Change Jobs?

Quality	Rating (1, 2, 3)	Current Job	Proposed Job
Specialty	1	1 $1 \times 1 = 1$	2 $1 \times 2 = 2$
Location	2	1 $2 \times 1 = 2$	2 $2 \times 2 = 4$
Salary	3	1 $3 \times 1 = 3$	2 $3 \times 2 = 6$
Training opportunities	2	2 $2 \times 2 = 4$	3 $2 \times 3 = 6$
Possibility of promotion	2	1 $2 \times 1 = 2$	2 $2 \times 2 = 4$
Responsibility	2	1 $2 \times 1 = 2$	2 $2 \times 2 = 4$
Reputation of facility	3	3 $3 \times 3 = 9$	3 $3 \times 3 = 9$
Totals	15	23	35

Source: Adapted from L. Haroun (2001). *Career development for health professionals*. Philadelphia: W. B. Saunders.

CHAPTER 12

Communication with Patients, Co-workers, and Supervisors

INTRODUCTION

The nature of health care work demands that workers be able to communicate effectively with patients, co-workers, and supervisors on a variety of levels. Many students assume that because they can talk, they can communicate. They are unaware that communication is complex and involves many interrelated skills. This chapter contains activities to practice essential skills that include interpreting nonverbal communication, listening, asking questions, using feedback techniques, and handling special communication situations.

ACTIVITY 12-1
NONVERBAL SIGNALS

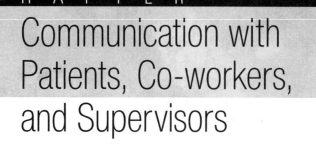

Student Handout **12-1**

What Students Will Learn

- To recognize nonverbal clues that are commonly used in communication.

What You Will Need

- Student Handout 12-1, Nonverbal Clues, cut into cards.

What To Do

1. Divide the class into two teams.
2. Toss a coin to determine the starting team.
3. One person from the starting team draws a card and uses a signal to express what is written on it (for example, holding forefinger perpendicular to lips to indicate "Silence").
4. The members of the same team guess what the signal expresses. Write down how long it takes for them to come up with the correct response.
5. Play alternates between the two teams.
6. The team with the shortest total time wins the game.

Follow-up Discussion

1. What are some other signals we use to communicate nonverbally?
2. Why do we use signals instead of words?
3. How often are they used?
4. Why is it important to understand nonverbal signals?

5. When might nonverbal communication be important in the health care field?

6. What kinds of nonverbal clues might you use in a health care setting?

ACTIVITY 12-2
WHAT IS IT?

What Will Students Learn

- To communicate nonverbally.

What You Will Need

- No special materials are required for this activity.

What To Do

1. Ask students to choose an object to describe nonverbally to the class using gestures and facial expressions. Examples of objects: pencil, key ring, fork, book, paper, pencil sharpener, syringe, vaccutainer, thermometer, stethoscope, blood pressure cuff.

2. Students take turns describing their objects to the class without using words so the other students can guess what the object is.

3. Alternative activity: Divide the class into two or three large groups and make this a contest. Time students as they try to guess the objects. The team that guesses in the least cumulative amount of time wins.

Follow-up Discussion

1. What was most difficult about describing your object?

2. What techniques seemed to work best?

3. When would nonverbal description be helpful in the health care field?

ACTIVITY 12-3
SILENCE!

What Students Will Learn

- To communicate nonverbally when working in a group.

What You Will Need

- A group project for students to complete, for example, cleaning the lab or setting up for a specific lab procedure.

What To Do

1. Divide the class into groups of four or five students.

2. Assign or have groups select a group project.

3. Tell students that there is to be no talking or writing during the 15 minutes they work together to complete the task. All communication by students and instructor must be nonverbal.

Follow-up Discussion

1. How easy or difficult was it to communicate?

2. How did you feel when you tried to communicate?

3. When might you need to use nonverbal communication in health care?

4. What are some ideas you might need to communicate?

5. What are some ways you could communicate with patients nonverbally?

ACTIVITY 12-4
READING BODY LANGUAGE

What Students Will Learn

- How nonverbal communication affects the message they send and receive.

What You Will Need

- A copy of Student Handout 12-2, Body Language for each student.
- Transparency 12-1, Body Language.

Student Handout **12-2**

Transparency Master **12-1**

What To Do

1. Divide the class into groups of two or three students.

2. Give each group one copy of Student Handout 12-2.

3. Use Transparency 12-1 to show students the examples of body language. Ask the student who is holding the handout in each group to choose a category of body language and demonstrate it (without sound) for the other students in the group. Without looking at the handout, the other students guess what the body language indicates. Each student in the group should attempt at least three different categories.

4. Once each member of the group has had a turn, distribute copies of Student Handout 12-2 so that all students have them.

Follow-up Discussion

1. Was it difficult to figure out the message the body language was sending?

2. Do you recall seeing this type of body language in other situations in your life? Explain.

3. How helpful is it to be able to "read" body language?

4. Is it possible to misinterpret body language? Explain.

5. If you are not sure about a person's body language, how can you check on their meaning?

6. Are there cultural differences in body language?

7. Why is reading body language a good skill for the health care worker?

8. How might this skill be applied in the health care setting?

ACTIVITY 12-5
CLOTHING CLUES

What Students Will Learn

- How we communicate through our clothing and appearance.

What You Will Need

- Clothing that students bring.

What To Do

1. At least one day before the activity is scheduled, ask students to bring in at least one item of clothing that they believe represents something about them.
2. Have students share what they've brought and explain what it says about them.
3. Alternate activity: Ask each student to dress in a way that conveys a specific message. Ask classmates to identify the message. Discuss with the class why they were or were not able to identify the message.

Follow-up Discussion

1. What does our clothing communicate about us?
2. Did the class interpret the clothing in the same way as its owner?
3. Why is the way we dress important in the health care workplace?
4. What kind of dress do people expect to see the physician and other health care workers wearing on the job?
5. Why is it important not to judge patients by how they dress?

ACTIVITY 12-6
LISTENING BETWEEN THE LINES

What Students Will Learn

- The importance of listening carefully and thinking about what we hear.

What You Will Need

- Instructor Sheet 12-1, Questions to Read Aloud.

Instructor Sheet **12-1**

What To Do

1. Tell students to listen very carefully to the statements you are going to read aloud.
2. Read the statements and questions to the class, allowing time between each question for the students to write down their answers.
3. Ask them to write the answers on a blank piece of paper. Explain that they need to think about each statement before writing their answer.
4. Once all questions have been asked, ask students to share their answers.
5. Give the correct answers, as needed.

Follow-up Discussion

1. Why is it important to listen carefully when communicating with a doctor, co-worker, or patient?
2. Why is it necessary to think about what you are hearing?
3. What are some ways you can practice and improve your listening skills?

ACTIVITY 12-7
WORDS OF WISDOM

What Students Will Learn

- How our backgrounds and experiences influence how we interpret what we read and hear.

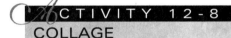

Student Handout **12-3**

What You Will Need

- A copy of Student Handout 12-3, Common Proverbs, for each student.

What To Do

1. Distribute Student Handout 12-3.
2. Ask students to write a short explanation of each proverb on the list.
3. Have students share their answers.
4. Alternate activity: Ask students to write down as many proverbs as they can come up with either individually or as a group. Then have them write an explanation for each.

Follow-up Discussion

1. How different were the interpretations?
2. Were there many proverbs that you had never heard?
3. Did your age influence whether you had heard or knew the proverbs?
4. Did your background and experience influence your interpretation?
5. How might past experiences influence what patients say and hear?
6. How might past experiences influence how the health care worker interprets what a patient says?

ACTIVITY 12-8
COLLAGE

What Students Will Learn

- To explore their own feelings.
- To express themselves orally.

What You Will Need

- Supplies for making collages: old magazines, paper, pens, scissors, glue, etc.
- One piece of posterboard for each student.

What To Do

1. Ask students to create a collage (or other piece of art) that expresses who he or she is. The collage should represent the student's feelings about self and may include the past, present, and/or future. Encourage students to include their goals.
2. Have students present their collages to the class, sharing as much or as little as they are comfortable doing.

Follow-up Discussion

1. How can understanding ourselves help improve our communication with others?
2. How might this understanding help us better understand the needs of patients?

ACTIVITY 12-9
CHECKING FOR UNDERSTANDING

Student Handout **12-4**

Transparency Master **12-2**

Transparency Master **12-3**

What Students Will Learn

- How to use feedback to check for understanding during communication encounters.
- How to ask questions to check for understanding, get clarification, and solicit additional information.

What You Will Need

- Transparencies 12-2, Examples of Paraphrasing, and 12-3, Asking Questions.
- A copy of Student Handout 12-4, Recording Form for Observers, for each student.

What To Do

1. Discuss the use of feedback and, specifically, paraphrasing as communication skills to check your understanding of what you hear. Transparency 12-2 shows examples of paraphrasing the same message.
2. Discuss the use of questions to clarify messages and solicit additional information. Transparency 12-3 lists three types of questions.
3. Distribute Student Handout 12-4.
4. Divide class into groups of three. Students take turns being the "patient" (speaker), "health care worker" (listener), and observer.
5. The patients make up a problem or symptoms that they describe to the health care worker who is to use feedback techniques and questions to learn all he or she can about the patient's needs. The observer writes notes about the encounter on Student Handout 12-4.
6. After each encounter, the observer presents his or her findings and the group briefly discusses the effectiveness of the communication.

Follow-up Discussion

1. How can paraphrasing help you become a better listener?
2. Why is it important to clearly understand the messages we receive from others?
3. How well were you able to paraphrase?
4. How well were you able to use questions?
5. Was it helpful having the observer take notes for follow-up discussion?
6. How do you think these skills will apply in your work in health care?

ACTIVITY 12-10
ASSERTIVE MESSAGES

What Students Will Learn

- How to give assertive messages.
- How to communicate effectively to resolve interpersonal problems.

What You Will Need:

- A copy of Student Handouts 12-5, Giving Assertive Messages, and 12-6, Scenarios for Assertive Message Role-Play, for each student.
- Transparency 12-4, Giving Assertive Messages.

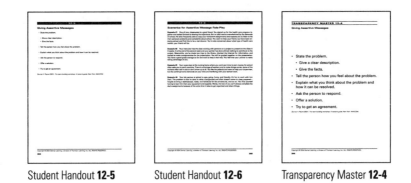

Student Handout **12-5**   Student Handout **12-6**   Transparency Master **12-4**

What To Do

1. Distribute Student Handouts 12-5 and 12-6.
2. Using Transparency 12-4, discuss Student Handout 12-5. Explain the need to be objective when communicating and suggest that students write down their thoughts before beginning encounters they believe may be difficult. This preparation can help them clarify their feelings and organize what they want to say.
3. Give one or two examples so students can see how to deliver these messages.
4. Divide the students into pairs and have them take turns role-playing the scenarios described on Student Handout 12-6.

Follow-up Discussion

1. How would you describe your experiences assuming the roles described in the scenarios?
2. Was it easy or difficult to describe your feelings to the other person? Explain.
3. When you were the receiver of an assertive message, was it stated clearly so that you understood the feelings and concerns of the speaker? Explain what made it clear or unclear.
4. Why is it a good idea to describe the behavior or incident instead of simply saying what you think about the other person?
5. Why should health care students develop skills for bringing problems into the open?
6. What are some examples of giving assertive messages in the health care workplace?

ACTIVITY 12-11
GOSSIP BEGONE

What Students Will Learn

- Effective ways to deal with gossip and negative talk in the workplace.

What You Will Need

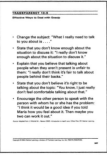

Transparency Master **12-5**

- Transparency 12-5, Effective Ways to Deal with Gossip.
- A copy of Student Handout 12-7, Effective Ways to Deal with Gossip, for each student.
- A copy of Student Handout 12-8, Did You Hear . . .? for each pair of students.

What To Do

1. Discuss the problems caused by gossip, especially in the workplace: lowered morale, breakdown in communications, undermining of patient confidence if they overhear employees' complaints, poor customer service image if patients overhear.

2. Using Student Handout 12-7 and Transparency 12-5, discuss ways to deal with gossip.

3. Distribute Student Handout 12-8 for students to use in pair activity.

4. Have the students pair off and take turns responding to the gossip situations on the handout. Students can also create their own examples of gossip.

Student Handout **12-7**

Follow-up Discussion

1. What are possible consequences of participating in gossip in the workplace?

2. Did you come up with responses for gossip, other than those discussed in class, when doing the exercises?

3. How can spreading gossip hurt the quality of patient care at a facility?

4. How does gossip affect trust between co-workers?

5. What are possible legal consequences of gossiping about a patient?

6. What should you do if you think that something serious you hear might be true? For example, what would you do if someone tells you that another worker is taking illegal drugs while on the job.

Student Handout **12-8**

ACTIVITY 12-12
PATIENTS WITH SPECIAL NEEDS

What Students Will Learn

- Communication techniques for working with patients who have special needs.

What You Will Need

- A copy of Student Handouts 12-9, Communicating with Patients Who Have Special Needs, and 12-10, Observer Notes, for each student.

What To Do

1. Distribute Student Handouts 12-9 and 12-10.

2. Discuss communication techniques that help when working with patients who have special needs.

Student Handout **12-9**

Student Handout **12-9**
(Continued)

Student Handout **12-10**

3. Have students divide into groups of three. Students take turns being the patient (speaker); health care worker (listener); and observer.
4. Assign simple communication encounters that are appropriate for the type of health care program your students are taking.
5. The "patient" assumes a problem or limitation. The "health care worker" uses the suggested techniques, as appropriate, to communicate with the patient. The observer writes notes about the encounter on Student Handout 12-10.
6. After each encounter, the observer presents his or her findings and the group briefly discusses the effectiveness of the communication.

Follow-up Discussion

1. Did you find it easy or difficult to communicate with patients who had special needs? Explain.
2. How might you practice these special communication skills?

ACTIVITY 12-13
WHICH WORD DO I USE?

What Students Will Learn

- The meanings and spelling of easily confused words.

What You Will Need

- A copy of Student Handouts 12-11, Commonly Confused Words, and 12-12, Commonly Confused Words Worksheet, for each student.
- Instructor Sheet 12-2, Answers for Commonly Confused Words Worksheet—Student Handout 12-12.

Instructor Sheet **12-2**

Student Handout **12-11**

What To Do

1. Distribute Student Handout 12-11 and review proper word usage with students. Create examples with the students to show how these words are used. Ask students to think of hints for remembering the meanings. For example, in contractions, the apostrophe takes the place of a word; the word "there" contains its opposite, "here."
2. Distribute Student Handout 12-12 and have students complete the exercise.
3. Correct the worksheets with students using Instructor Sheet 12-2.

Follow-up Discussion

1. Why is it important for health care workers to write accurately?
2. What are possible consequences if health care workers use words incorrectly?

Student Handout **12-12**

REFERENCES

Alexander Graham Bell Association (1996). *Communicating with people who have a hearing loss* [Brochure]. Washington, DC: Author.

Hegner, B., Caldwell, E., & Needham, J. (1999). *Nursing assistant: A nursing process approach* (8th ed.). Clifton Park, NY: Delmar Learning.

Mierenberg, G., & Calero, H. (1973). *How to read a person like a book.* New York: Pocket Books.

Milliken, M. E. (1998). *Understanding human behavior: A guide for health care providers* (6th ed.). Clifton Park, NY: Delmar Learning.

Mitchell, J., & Haroun, L. (2002). *Introduction to health care.* Clifton Park, NY: Delmar Learning.

Payne, V. (2001). *The team-building workshop: A trainer's guide.* New York: AMACOM.

Questions to Read Aloud

Have students write numbers 1 through 12 on a sheet of paper. Read aloud each of the following items and allow a few moments for students to write their answers next to the corresponding number. Answers are in parentheses.

1. Some months have 30 days, some have 31. How many have 28? (All)

2. Does England have a fourth of July? (Yes)

3. I have two coins totaling 55 cents. One is not a nickel. What are the two coins? (A fifty-cent piece and a nickel—one is not a nickel, but the other one is!)

4. If you see three apples and take two apples, how many will you have? (Two)

5. A farmer had sixteen sheep. All but nine died. How many did he have left? (Nine)

6. A doctor gives you three pills. Starting now you are to take one every half hour. How long will they last? (One hour)

7. A woman gave a beggar fifty cents. The woman was the beggar's sister, but the beggar was not the woman's brother. What relation was the beggar? (The woman's sister)

8. Why can't a man living in Winston-Salem, N.C., be buried west of the Mississippi? (He's alive)

9. An archaeologist said he found some coins dated 400 B.C. Do you believe him? (No. People living before Christ was born didn't know he was going to be born, so coins were not dated B.C.)

10. A man built a house with all sides facing the south. A bear came along. What color was it, and why? (White—it was at the North Pole)

11. Do you know how to spell antidisestablishmentarianism? Spell *it*. (I-t)

12. Mississippi. Can you spell *that* without the p's? (T-h-a-t)

Answer Key for the Commonly Confused Words Worksheet—
Student Handout 12-12

1. The reports are ___*all ready*___ to be graded. (already, all ready)

2. Please ___*ensure*___ the work gets done on time. (assure, ensure, insure)

3. We will ___*allot*___ 30 minutes for your break. (a lot, allot)

4. There are ___*a lot*___ of needles in that sharps container. (a lot, allot)

5. Please take this thermometer ___*to*___ examination room C. (to, too, two)

6. There are ___*two*___ extra chairs in this classroom. (to, two, too)

7.. Jose is ___*too*___ tall to fit in that small space. (to, two, too)

8. Martinique got an A. Luis did ___*too*___. (to, two, too)

9. ___*There*___ is the stethoscope I was looking for. (their, they're, there)

10. I drove around until I found ___*their*___ house. (their, they're, there)

11. I'm angry because ___*they're*___ late again. (their, they're, there)

12. Please be sure this is ___*insured*___ against loss. (assured, ensured, insured)

13. Mohammed will ___*assure*___ Jonna that the procedure will not hurt. (assure, ensure, insure)

14. Please pick up ___*your*___ paperwork by noon. (you're, your)

15. ___*You're*___ on ___*your*___ way to a great career. (you're, your)

Nonverbal Clues

Cut along the dotted lines to make cards to distribute to students

Hitchhiking	Good-bye
Yes	No
Maybe	It's good
He's crazy	Stop
Come	Go over there
I want that	Time!
I'm sick	I don't know
It's nice to meet you	Impatient
Victory	We're number one
You're out!	What time is it?

Body Language

Nonverbal messages are often communicated by our posture and body movements. This table contains examples based on typical European and American gestures.

Angry	Defensive
• Body stiff • Skin reddened • Fists clenched • Lips held together tightly • Strong eye contact • Quick, shallow breathing	• Body stiff • Arms crossed in front of the body • Eyes glancing to the side • Minimal eye contact • Looking down • Lips pursed • Fists clenched

Confident	Enthusiastic
• Straight, upright posture • Good eye contact • Fingertips held in the form of a steeple or hands clasped behind the head • Chin tilted up • Slight smile	• Slight or moderate smile • Body held up straight and forward • Hands open and extended • Eyes open and looking alert • Lively, bouncy walk • Peppy voice

Frustrated	Indifferent
• Abrupt gestures made to express frustration, such as taking short breaths, tightly clenching or wringing the hands, and rubbing the back of the neck • Lips closed tightly	• Slouching and glancing around the room • Minimal eye contact • Lips slack • Body pointed toward the door

Nervous	Rejected
• Eyes darting • Lips twitching • Mouth opened slightly • Fingers drumming or fiddling with objects, clothes, or hair • If seated, leaning over slightly in chair • If standing, weight frequently shifted between the feet	• Arms folded • Legs crossed • Body moved away from the other person • Head tilted forward • Eyes squinting • Nose touched or rubbed

Source: Adapted from G. Mierenberg & H. Calero (1973). *How to read a person like a book.* New York: Pocket Books.

Common Proverbs

Write a short explanation of each proverb.

1. A stitch in time saves nine.

_____

_____

2. Variety is the spice of life.

_____

_____

3. A penny saved is a penny earned.

_____

_____

4. Silence is golden.

_____

_____

5. Haste makes waste.

_____

_____

6. Do what I say, not what I do.

_____

_____

7. We do not live by bread alone.

_____

_____

8. Don't count your chickens before they hatch.

_____

_____

9. A bird in the hand is worth two in the bush.

_____

_____

10. You can't know a book by its cover.

_____

_____

Recording Form for Observers

1. What feedback techniques does the "health care worker" use to find out if he or she correctly understands what the "patient" is saying?

   _____

   _____

   _____

   _____

   _____

2. What questions does the "health care worker" ask to clarify or get additional information?

   _____

   _____

   _____

   _____

   _____

3. How does the "health care worker" indicate that he or she understands what the "patient" is saying?

   _____

   _____

   _____

   _____

   _____

4. How does the "health care worker" indicate that he or she does not understand what the "patient" is saying?

   _____

   _____

   _____

   _____

   _____

Source: Adapted from M. E. Milliken (1998). *Understanding human behavior: A guide for health care providers* (6th ed.). Clifton Park, NY: Delmar Learning.

Giving Assertive Messages

- State the problem.

    - Give a clear description.
    - Give the facts.

- Tell the person how you feel about the problem.

- Explain what you think about the problem and how it can be resolved.

- Ask the person to respond.

- Offer a solution.

- Try to get an agreement.

Source: V. Payne (2001). *The team-building workshop: A trainer's guide.* New York: AMACOM.

Scenarios for Assertive Message Role-Play

Scenario #1   One of your classmates is a good friend. You signed up for the health care program together and looked forward to sharing the experience. But he (she) seems overwhelmed by the demands of school. He (she) frequently asks to copy your homework assignments and expects you to listen to his (her) personal problems and complaints about school. You want to help your friend, but have been enjoying school and find this to be a real downer. You're also concerned about what type of health care worker your friend will be.

Scenario #2   Your instructor has the class working with partners on a project to present to the class in 3 weeks. It is the end of the second week and your partner has done almost nothing to contribute to the project. Meanwhile, you've made two trips to the library, checked the Internet for information, and started to make transparencies for the presentation. You will be graded together on the presentation. You have a good grade average so far and want to keep it that way. You feel that your partner is really taking advantage of you.

Scenario #3   Your supervisor at the nursing home where you work part time to earn money for school often asks you to work overtime. There is a shortage of workers and to make things worse, some of the workers often call in sick or don't show up at all. You like the patients and want to help your supervisor, but the continual extra demands on your time are interfering with your school work.

Scenario #4   Your lab partner at school is easy going, funny, and friendly. It's fun to work with him (her). The problem is that he (she) is rather disorganized and often doesn't come to class prepared— forgets to bring a stethoscope, notes, and handouts for lab procedures, and so on. You find yourself having to loan him (her) your equipment and supplies. Worse, the two of you can't always complete the day's assignments because of the extra time it takes to get organized and share things.

Effective Ways to Deal with Gossip

- Change the subject: "What I really need to talk to you about is . . . ."

- State that you don't know enough about the situation to discuss it: "I really don't know enough about the situation to discuss it."

- Explain that you believe that talking about people when they aren't present is unfair to them: "I really don't think it's fair to talk about people behind their backs."

- State that you don't believe it's right to be talking about the topic: "You know, I just really don't feel comfortable talking about that."

- Encourage the other person to speak with the person with whom he or she has the problem: "I think it would be a good idea if you told Maria how you feel about it. Then maybe you two can work it out."

Source: Adapted from J. Mitchell & L. Haroun (2002). *Introduction to health care.* Clifton Park, NY: Delmar Learning.

Did You Hear . . . ?

Take turns presenting and responding to the following examples of workplace gossip.

1. Sam is always telling you about how Daniela doesn't put all the supplies away after finishing patient treatments.

2. Graciela complains that the nursing aides don't get paid enough for all the work they have to do. You are afraid that patients can hear what she's saying.

3. Jose doesn't like his work schedule but there's nothing you can do about it. He hasn't said anything to the supervisor.

4. Nadia places a lot of importance on appearance and how people dress. She often makes unkind remarks about people she thinks look really "awful" and encourages you to join in the criticism.

5. You are new at the workplace and soon learn that a favorite activity of your co-workers is to complain about the supervisor and how supposedly incompetent he is.

6. You are really busy at work when a co-worker who has become a friend wants to discuss what she heard about another co-worker's marital problems.

7. Kim is upset that someone else got the promotion she was hoping for and spends a lot of time complaining about it.

8. The vendor who sells medical supplies to the clinic where you work wants to share a "juicy story" about another clinic in town.

Communicating with Patients Who Have Special Needs

Patients Who Are in Pain, Medicated, Confused, or Disoriented

- Identify yourself and say the patient's name.
- Maintain eye contact.
- Speak slowly and clearly in a low tone of voice.
- Use simple language. Avoid slang and expressions that do not mean exactly what they say.
- Keep each message short and to the point. For example, do not give a series of instructions or ask more than one question at a time.
- Give time to respond.
- Use touch if the patient is comfortable with it.
- Repeat the message as needed, without changing the content or words.
- Review the content with the patient to assess retention of the message.
- When appropriate, give the patient written information that can be referred to later.

Source: From J. Mitchell & L. Haroun (2002). *Introduction to health care.* Clifton Park, NY: Delmar Learning. Originally adapted from Hegner, 1999. B. Hegner, E. Caldwell, & J. Needham (1999). *Nursing assistant: A nursing process approach* (8th ed.). Clifton Park, NY: Delmar Learning.

Patients Who Have Hearing Impairments

- Position yourself close to the receiver and speak face to face.
- Remove or turn off sources of noise.
- Have the light source directed to your face.
- Make sure your mouth is visible to the listener.
- Speak distinctly and do not mumble.
- Speak slowly.
- Do not shout or exaggerate words.
- Maintain a low to moderate pitch of voice.
- Use short sentences.
- Watch for signs of comprehension.
- Do not change the subject without warning.

Source: From J. Mitchell & L. Haroun (2002). *Introduction to health care.* Clifton Park, NY: Delmar Learning. Originally adapted from Alexander Graham Bell Association, 1996. Alexander Graham Bell Association (1996). *Communicating with people who have a hearing loss* [Brochure]. Washington, DC: Author.

Patients Who Have Visual Impairments

- Start all communication by announcing your presence and identifying yourself.

- Before starting a procedure, describe any equipment to be used and its position in relation to the patient.

- As you proceed, explain what will be done and where you will be touching the patient.

- Explain what noises will be heard.

- Give clear and complete directions. For example, say, "Raise your left arm directly in front of you to a forty-five degree angle." *not* "Raise your arm like this."

- Let the patient know when you are leaving the area.

- Give extra verbal information to describe anything that would usually be expressed through facial expressions, gestures, head nods, and other movements.

Source: From J. Mitchell & L. Haroun (2002). *Introduction to health care.* Clifton Park, NY: Delmar Learning. Originally adapted from Hegner, 1999. B. Hegner, E. Caldwell, & J. Needham (1999). *Nursing assistant: A nursing process approach* (8th ed.). Clifton Park, NY: Delmar Learning.

Patients Who Are Angry

- Never respond in anger or argue with the patient.

- Remain calm and courteous.

- Listen attentively to the patient's concerns.

- Offer a sincere apology, if necessary.

- Do not raise your voice.

- Be aware of your body language. Look at the patient.

- Express concern and interest, not annoyance.

- Answer the patient's questions.

Source: From J. Mitchell & L. Haroun (2002). *Introduction to health care.* Clifton Park, NY: Delmar Learning.

Patients Who Speak Little or No English

- A smile is a universal sign of good will.

- Determine if the patient speaks or understands any English.

- Do not raise your voice. It will not help the other person understand.

- Use gestures and pantomime to demonstrate what you need the patient to do.

- Use pictures, if available.

Source: From J. Mitchell & L. Haroun (2002). *Introduction to health care.* Clifton Park, NY: Delmar Learning.

Observer Notes

1. What special techniques does the "health care worker" use to determine what the "patient" needs?

   _____

   _____

   _____

   _____

   _____

2. How does the "health care worker" indicate that he or she understands what the "patient" needs?

   _____

   _____

   _____

   _____

3. How does the "health care worker" indicate that he or she does not understand what the "patient" needs?

   _____

   _____

   _____

4. How does the "health care worker" communicate to the "patient" what he or she should do?

   _____

   _____

   _____

Source: Adapted from M. E. Milliken (1998). *Understanding human behavior: A guide for health care providers* (6th ed.). Clifton Park, NY: Delmar Learning.

Commonly Confused Words

Some words sound the same, but are spelled differently. Other words look similar, but have different meanings.

Words	Meanings
Affect	To influence. "Affect" is a verb.
Effect	To bring about (verb). A result or consequence (noun).
A lot	A large amount of something.
Allot	To set aside something.
Already	Done in the past.
All ready	Complete; completely prepared.
Anyway	In any case.
Any way	Using any method.
Assure	To give someone confidence or reassurance.
Ensure	To be sure or make certain.
Insure	To guard against loss.
Everyday	Ordinary or routine.
Every day	Each day.
Into	Implies entry or change of form.
In to	Prepositional phrase used with a verb.
It's	A contraction for "it is."
Its	Possessive form of "it."
Than	Introduces a phrase of comparison.
Then	At that time; next; therefore.
There	Indicating a place (opposite of "here").
Their	Signifies possession.
They're	A contraction of "they are."
To	In the direction of.
Too	Also; excessively.
Two	The number.
Yours	Possessive.
You're	A contraction of "you are."

Commonly Confused Words Worksheet

Use the correct form of the word in each sentence.

1. The reports are _____ to be graded. (already, all ready)

2. Please _____ the work gets done on time. (assure, ensure, insure)

3. We will _____ 30 minutes for your break. (a lot, allot)

4. There are _____ of needles in that sharps container. (a lot, allot)

5. Please take this thermometer _____ examination room C. (to, too, two)

6. There are _____ extra chairs in this classroom. (to, two, too)

7. Jose is _____ tall to fit in that small space. (to, two, too)

8. Martinique got an A. Luis did _____ . (to, two, too)

9. _____ is the stethoscope I was looking for. (their, they're, there)

10. I drove around until I found _____ house. (their, they're, there)

11. I'm angry because _____ late again. (their, they're, there)

12. Please be sure this is _____ against loss. (assured, ensured, insured)

13. Mohammed will _____ Jonna that the procedure will not hurt. (assure, ensure, in-sure)

14. Please pick up _____ paperwork by noon. (you're, your)

15. _____ on _____ way to a great career. (you're, your)

Body Language

- Angry

- Defensive

- Confident

- Enthusiastic

- Frustrated

- Indifferent

- Nervous

- Rejected

Examples of Paraphrasing

Patient states: "Well, you know, I feel kind of dizzy when I stand up fast.

- "I understood you to say that you only feel dizzy when you stand up quickly."

- "So you feel dizzy when you stand up quickly?"

- "Are you saying you feel dizzy only when you stand up quickly?"

Asking Questions

1. *Closed-ended questions* can be answered with a single word, or phrase, or response of "yes" or "no."

   - "What is your age?"

   - "When did you last see the doctor?"

2. *Open-ended questions* require a more detailed response than simply "yes" or "no."

   - "How did you cut your leg?"

   - "How do you feel just before you get the headaches?"

3. *Probing questions* ask for additional information or clarification.

   - "Can you tell me more about where you feel the most pain?"

   - "What do you mean when you say you feel a little 'strange' after taking the medication?"

Giving Assertive Messages

- State the problem.

  - Give a clear description.

  - Give the facts.

- Tell the person how you feel about the problem.

- Explain what you think about the problem and how it can be resolved.

- Ask the person to respond.

- Offer a solution.

- Try to get an agreement.

Source: V. Payne (2001). *The team-building workshop: A trainer's guide.* New York: AMACOM.

Effective Ways to Deal with Gossip

- Change the subject: "What I really need to talk to you about is . . . ."

- State that you don't know enough about the situation to discuss it: "I really don't know enough about the situation to discuss it."

- Explain that you believe that talking about people when they aren't present is unfair to them: "I really don't think it's fair to talk about people behind their backs."

- State that you don't believe it's right to be talking about the topic: "You know, I just really don't feel comfortable talking about that."

- Encourage the other person to speak with the person with whom he or she has the problem: "I think it would be a good idea if you told Maria how you feel about it. Then maybe you two can work it out."

Source: Adapted from J. Mitchell & L. Haroun (2002). *Introduction to health care.* Clifton Park, NY: Delmar Learning.

Telephone Technique

INTRODUCTION

The telephone is likely to be the first link between patients and health care providers. The quality of the service provided over the telephone has a major impact on patient satisfaction. Today's emphasis on shorter hospital stays means that more patients will be receiving important information by telephone when they have questions about self-care. Developing good telephone technique is required for all health care workers, not simply those whose main job is to answer the telephone.

ACTIVITY 13-1
WHAT'S HELPFUL, WHAT'S NOT

What Students Will Learn
- Why good telephone technique is important.
- The effect of telephone technique on customers/patients.

What You Will Need
- No special materials are required for this activity.

What To Do
1. Divide the class into groups of three to five students.
2. Ask the groups to discuss telephone calls they have made to request information or service. For example, calls to medical facilities, insurance companies, stores, repair shops, and so on. The idea is to share their experiences and level of satisfaction with the calls.
3. Instruct each group to write a list of desirable and undesirable telephone techniques.

Follow-up Discussion
1. What impact can telephone technique have on the success of an organization?
2. Why is good telephone technique important in a health care setting?

ACTIVITY 13-2
GREAT TELEPHONE TECHNIQUE

What Students Will Learn
- Characteristics necessary for great telephone technique.

What You Will Need

- No special materials are required for this activity.

What To Do

1. Ask students for words that describe a person with good telephone technique. They should come up with at least some of the following:

Smiles (the act of smiling is conveyed in the voice)	Friendly attitude	Helpful
	Always positive	Stays focused
Knowledgeable	Picks up quickly	Does not leave on hold long
Takes good messages	Problem solver	
Asks before putting on hold	Identifies self	Clear speaker
	Returns calls when promised	Maintains confidentiality
Uses good grammar		Remains calm at all times
Prioritizes well		

Follow-up Discussion

1. What part does telephone technique play in the delivery of good customer service?

2. What are the most important characteristics of excellent telephone technique in the health care setting?

ACTIVITY 13-3
TELEPHONE TECHNIQUE QUESTIONS

What Students Will Learn

- Skills needed to use the telephone effectively.

What You Will Need

- A soft indoor ball.
- Instructor Sheet 13-1, Questions About Correctly Using the Telephone.

What To Do

1. Have all students stand

2. Toss the ball to a student and ask that student a question from Instructor Sheet 13-1. If the answer is correct, the student remains standing. If the answer is incorrect, the student sits down.

Instructor Sheet **13-1**

Instructor Sheet **13-1**
(Continued)

Instructor Sheet **13-1**
(Continued)

3. Have the student toss the ball to another student.
4. Ask that student a question.
5. Continue until only one student is standing. He or she is the winner

Follow-up Discussion

1. How can students develop good telephone technique for the workplace?

ACTIVITY 13-4
HANDLING ROUTINE CALLS

Student Handout **13-1**

What Students Will Learn

- How to answer routine telephone calls.
- How to write complete telephone messages.

What You Will Need

- A copy of Student Handout 13-1, Routine Telephone Calls, for each student.
- A copy of Student Handout 13-2, Telephone Message Forms, *or* pads of telephone message forms.

What To Do

1. Discuss the basics of telephone etiquette, including properly identifying oneself when answering the telephone.
2. Distribute Student Handouts 13-1 and 13-2 and have the class pair off.
3. Have the pairs sit back-to-back so they cannot see each other.
4. Instruct students to take turns role-playing the situations listed on Student Handout 13-1. When appropriate, they are to prepare a written message.

Student Handout **13-2**

Follow-up Discussion

1. Describe your experiences in role playing the calls: was it easier or more difficult than you expected? Explain.
2. How did the callers feel about the service they received?
3. Did the person taking the call project warmth and interest in the caller?
4. How can future health care workers prepare to be effective on the telephone?

ACTIVITY 13-5
SPECIAL TELEPHONE TECHNIQUES

Student Handout **13-3**

What Students Will Learn

- How to properly transfer calls, put callers on hold, and handle emergency calls.

What You Will Need

- Copies of Student Handouts 13-3, Handling a Variety of Calls, and 13-4, Observer's Notes, for each student.

What To Do

1. Discuss techniques for transferring calls, putting callers on hold, and handling emergency calls.

2. Distribute Student Handouts 13-3 and 13-4.
3. Divide class into groups of three.
4. Students rotate roles so that each has a chance to be the caller, receiver, and observer.
5. The students playing the caller and receiver should sit back-to-back so they cannot see each other. They interact using Student Handout 13-3.
6. The third student listens to the exchange and fills out Student Handout 13-4.

Instructor's Note: The same calls may be repeated by different students or they can vary the details.

Student Handout **13-4**

Follow-up Discussion

1. Did you find it difficult to remember the best way to handle each call?
2. Was it helpful having the observer give you feedback?

ACTIVITY 13-6
HANDLING CHALLENGING CALLS

What Students Will Learn

- How to handle challenging telephone calls.
- How to write complete telephone messages.

Student Handout **13-5**

What You Will Need

- A copy of Student Handout 13-5, Challenging Telephone Calls I, for half of the students.
- A copy of Student Handout 13-6, Challenging Telephone Calls II, for half of the students.
- A copy of Student Handout 13-2, Telephone Message Pages, OR pads of telephone message forms.

Student Handout **13-6**

What To Do

1. Discuss with the class techniques for handling challenging telephone calls.
2. Distribute blank telephone message forms to all the students.
3. Have the class divide into pairs.
4. Give one partner in each pair Student Handout 13-5; give the other partner Student Handout 13-6. The handouts contain information about each of the calls.
5. Ask the pairs to sit back-to-back so they cannot see each other.
6. Instruct students to take turns role-playing the situations described on the handouts.
7. When appropriate, students are to prepare a written message.

Student Handout **13-2**

Follow-up Discussion

1. What was most difficult about dealing with challenging calls?
2. For each case, discuss:
   a. What was most important about handling this call?
   b. What questions should the person receiving the call have asked?
   c. Should this call be charted in the patient's medical or dental record? Explain.

ACTIVITY 13-7
TELEPHONE SCAVENGER HUNT

What Students Will Learn

- How to use the telephone to gather information.

What You Will Need

- A copy of Student Handout 13-7, Telephone Scavenger Hunt: Calls to Make, for each student.

What To Do

1. Distribute Student Handout 13-7 and tell students that they are to conduct a telephone scavenger hunt.
2. Give them a few days to complete this assignment.
3. When the assignment has been completed, conduct a class discussion.

Follow-up Discussion

1. Were they able to easily find what they needed?
2. Did they find it easy or difficult to call and ask for information?
3. How did those receiving the phone calls react? Did they use good customer service skills?

Student Handout **13-7**

ACTIVITY 13-8
VOCAL CLUES

What Students Will Learn

- The influence of vocal clues.
- The importance of not judging people by how they speak.

What You Will Need

- A tape of five or six different voices saying the same few sentences. You may use any sentences you wish. The voices should reflect a variety of accents, ages, and so on.
- A copy of Student Handout 13-8, Vocal Clues, for each student.

What To Do

1. Play your recorded tape in class.
2. Have students answer the questions on Student Handout 13-8.
3. When they have completed answering the questions, have students share their answers with the class.

Follow-up Discussion

1. Were you able to form an impression of the speaker by listening to his or her voice?
2. What vocal clues did you use to answer the questions?
3. Why do students have different answers?
4. What information do we give through our voices?
5. Why should we not judge patients and others who call by their voices?

Student Handout **13-8**

Student Handout **13-8**
(Continued

REFERENCE

Lindh, W., Pooler, M.S., Tamparo, C.D., & Cerrato, J.U. (1998). *Comprehensive medical assisting administrative and clinical competencies.* Clifton Park, NY: Delmar Learning.

Questions About Correctly Using the Telephone

There are many possible correct answers to the following questions. The answers listed here are only suggestions.

1. How can you convey a positive first impression over the telephone?

   - Answer promptly and use a pleasant voice.

   - Use a pleasant voice.

2. What calls are almost always passed directly on to the physician?

   - Family members.

   - Emergencies.

   - Other doctors.

3. What is the best way to put a caller on hold?

   - Find out who is calling, why they are calling, and ask permission.

4. What is an answering service?

   - Usually live operators who will answer calls when no one is available in the office.

5. Is it okay to give patient information over the phone?

   - Only to a referring office *or* if you have a signed patient information release form.

6. What are some important things to remember when answering the phone?

   - Smile. The art of smiling is conveyed in the voice.

   - Enunciate clearly.

   - Sit up straight.

   - Be enthusiastic.

   - Answer as quickly as possible.

7. What kind of information should be written on a message pad?

   - Caller's name.

   - Time of call.

   - Message.

   - Caller's phone number.

   - Date of call.

   - Who the call is for.

   - Nature and urgency of call.

   - Action to be taken: will call back, returned your call, please call back.

   - Your name or initials.

8. True or False: It is always best to wait two or three rings before answering the phone?

   - False.

9. You are a medical assistant in a single doctor's office. What is the best way to answer the telephone?

   • Good morning, Dr. Garcia's office, Jason speaking.

10. What are three types of calls the medical or dental assistant can handle on his or her own?

   • Scheduling appointments or tests.

   • Billing questions.

   • Insurance information.

   • A message about a prescription refill.

   • Routine progress reports from patients.

   • General information about the practice.

   • Salespeople.

11. What are three types of calls that must be handled by the physician or dentist?

   • Request for test results.

   • Emergencies.

   • Medical questions.

   • Other doctors or dentists.

   • Patients who refuse to give you information.

   • Complaints (if there is no office manager).

   • Poor progress report from a patient.

12. When an established patient calls to make an appointment, what information should you write down?

   • Patient's name.

   • Reason for visit.

   • Daytime phone number.

13. What is triage?

   • Evaluation of the urgency of a situation.

14. What are some steps you can take when handling problem calls?

   • Remain calm.

   • Listen carefully.

   • Do not get defensive.

   • Do not take the call tone of the personally.

   • Offer to help.

   • Document the call carefully.

15. Where can you find a list of telephone area codes if you need to make a long distance call?

   • Local telephone directory.

16. What should you have at hand near the telephone?

    • Notepad.

    • Pen or pencil.

    • Clock.

    • Patient chart or insurance information, if appropriate.

17. What should you do if you call and the person answering does not speak fluent English?

    • Speak slowly and clearly.

    • Do not raise your voice.

    • Ask if clarification is needed.

    • Be patient.

18. You call your patient about an uncollected account. The patient is not home, but his wife answers. You know she normally pays all the bills. Can you discuss this account with her?

    • No.

19. What is the advantage of an answering service over a telephone answering machine?

    • A service can make an immediate referral or contact the physician in case of an emergency.

    • A live operator can be reassuring to the patient.

20. What must you be careful of when sending information over a fax machine?

    • Confidentiality.

21. True or False: Cellular signals are not secure and may be heard by others.

    • True.

22. If you are giving a message to the physician about a patient, what should you include?

    • The patient's chart.

23. What should you do when you are transferring a call to someone in your office?

    • Tell the caller the name and extension of the person you are transferring them to.

    • Let the person in the office know who is being transferred to them and why.

24. True or False: Your mood usually comes through when you answer the phone.

    • True.

25. What are some types of calls you might receive in a medical office?

    • Established patients.

    • New patients.

    • Other physicians.

    • Salespeople.

    • Pharmacies.

26. Is the medical assistant permitted to okay a prescription refill over the telephone?

    • Only with the approval of the doctor.

Source: Based on information from W. Lindh, M.S. Pooler, C.D. Tamparo, & J.U. Cerrato (1998). *Comprehensive medical assisting administrative and clinical competencies.* Clifton Park, NY: Delmar Learning.

Routine Telephone Calls

1. You need an appointment for a routine physical exam. You work the afternoon shift and can only make appointments for early in the morning.

2. You have been feeling ill for several days and would like to see the physician as soon as possible.

3. You need a refill for a prescription because you have only one tablet left.

4. You want to know if your insurance company has authorized the diagnostic test the physician recommended.

5. You want to know the results of the tests you had for liver function.

6. You are a physician who wants to refer a patient.

7. You are a drug sales representative who wants to speak with the physician.

8. You are a patient who wants to make an appointment with the physical therapist. You don't know if Medicare has sent the approval yet to the rehabilitation clinic.

9. You are a good friend of the lab technician (who answers the telephone) and want to talk about an urgent personal problem.

10. You are calling from a physician's office and want to schedule a patient for surgery.

Telephone Message Form

Make telephone message forms by copying this page and cutting out individual forms.

PHONE MESSAGE

For _____

M _____

Of _____

Telephone No. _____

○ Telephoned	○ Please Return Call
○ Will Call Again	○ Came In
○ Returned Your Call	○ Important
○ See Me	○ Wants To See You

Message _____

_____

_____

_____

_____

_____

_____

Date _____ Time _____ By _____

Handling a Variety of Calls

Call #1

Caller: You have cut yourself while chopping carrots and are bleeding.

Receiver: You work in a small physician's office. You explain to the caller how to stop the bleeding and then direct her to come to the office.

Call #2

Caller: The director of the laboratory you are calling is a good friend.

Receiver: You transfer the call to the director.

Call #3

Caller: You are calling the dentist to make an appointment.

Receiver: You are on the line with someone else. You put the caller on hold.

Call #4

Caller: Your grandfather collapsed while mowing the lawn.

Receiver: You work for the grandfather's cardiologist. You advise the caller to call 911.

Call #5

Caller: You are a patient who was told to call and speak directly with Dr. Garcia about diagnostic test results.

Receiver: You first try transferring the call, but Dr. Garcia is on another line.

Call #6

Caller: You have called your dentist's office to discuss your bill.

Receiver: While speaking with the patient about her bill, you receive another call and must interrupt the patient and put her on hold.

Observer's Notes

Emergency Calls

Did the receiver . . .

- Speak in a calm, reassuring manner?

  ☐ yes   ☐ no

  Comments _____

- Ask for the caller's name, location, and telephone number at the beginning of the call?

  ☐ yes   ☐ no

  Comments _____

- Ask for details about the condition of the ill/injured person?

  ☐ yes   ☐ no

  Comments _____

- Give clear directions about what the caller should do?

  ☐ yes   ☐ no

  Comments _____

Transferring Calls

Did the receiver . . .

- Explain that he or she would be transferring the call (rather than "one moment"—click!)?

  ☐ yes   ☐ no

  Comments _____

- Ask the caller if he or she would like to leave a message after finding the line was busy?

  ☐ yes   ☐ no

  Comments _____

Putting Callers on Hold

Did the receiver . . .

- Quickly ask the caller if he or she had an emergency before putting on hold?

  ☐ yes   ☐ no

  Comments _____

- Tell the caller he or she would be back shortly?

  ☐ yes   ☐ no

  Comments _____

- Get back to the caller as soon as possible?

  ☐ yes   ☐ no

  Comments _____

Challenging Telephone Calls I

You make the following calls:

1. You are annoyed because you have received several overdue bills from this clinic for bills you believe should have been covered by your insurance company. You wonder if the clinic has submitted the bills properly.

2. You want an appointment with the dentist today (Monday) because you've suffered with a toothache since Friday afternoon.

3. You have the following symptoms: sweating, nausea, and a crushing feeling on your chest. You fear you might be having a heart attack.

You receive the following calls:

1. You are the receptionist in a dental office and you receive a call from a patient who is upset.

2. You work in the ultrasound department as a technologist. You answer the phone and discover it is a sales representative.

3. You are the office manager in a medical clinic and you receive a call from a worried patient.

Challenging Telephone Calls II

You make the following calls:

1. You are very upset because the gold crown the dentist placed on a molar five months ago has fallen off. The crown was quite expensive and this dentist was recommended by a friend.

2. You are a medical equipment sales representative who wants to speak directly with the director of the ultrasound department. You may lose your job if you don't increase your sales.

3. You had a biopsy last week and are calling for the results. You are afraid you have cancer.

You receive the following calls:

1. You are the medical biller for a small medical clinic and you receive a call from a patient who has failed to submit necessary paperwork.

2. You are a dental receptionist and take a call from a patient who wants an appointment as soon as possible.

3. You are the front office medical assistant in a small office. A patient calls who is worried about the symptoms he is experiencing.

Telephone Scavenger Hunt: Calls to Make

1. Find out how much a collection agency charges to collect past due accounts. List the name of the agency and what they charge.

_____

_____

_____

2. Call a local printer and find out the cost of a box of business cards. List the name of the business and the fee.

_____

_____

_____

3. Call three doctors' offices. Tell them you are doing some research for a health care class. Find out what their salary range is for an entry-level medical assistant. List the information here.

_____

_____

_____

4. Call a bank in your community and ask what special services they offer to local businesses. List the information here.

_____

_____

_____

Vocal Clues

Answer the following questions for each recorded voice.

1. What does the person look like?

   A. _____

   B. _____

   C. _____

   D. _____

   E. _____

   F. _____

2. What does he or she do for a living?

   A. _____

   B. _____

   C. _____

   D. _____

   E. _____

   F. _____

3. Where is the person from?

   A. _____

   B. _____

   C. _____

   D. _____

   E. _____

   F. _____

4. How much money does he or she make?

   A. _____

   B. _____

   C. _____

   D. _____

   E. _____

   F. _____

5. How much education does the person have?

   A. _____

   B. _____

   C. _____

   D. _____

   E. _____

   F. _____

6. How old is the person?

   A. _____

   B. _____

   C. _____

   D. _____

   E. _____

   F. _____

CHAPTER 14

Patient Education

INTRODUCTION

The ability to provide good patient education is increasingly important for health care workers. Patients are responsible for more of their own care as procedures that once required hospital stays are now performed on an outpatient basis.

The three leading causes of death in the United States—heart disease, cancer, and stroke—are influenced by lifestyle factors about which patients should be educated. Understanding learning styles and knowing a variety of teaching techniques will increase the value of health care workers at every level.

ACTIVITY 14-1
WHAT'S AVAILABLE ON THE INTERNET?

Student Handout **14-1**

Student Handout **14-2**

What Students Will Learn

- How to locate resources for patients about health care topics.
- How to organize and present information.

What You Will Need

- A copy of Student Handouts 14-1, Health Information Websites, and 14-2, Website Information, for each student.
- Students: Access to the Internet.

What To Do

1. Distribute Student Handouts 14-1 and 14-2 and ask students to select one of the Web sites to explore.
2. Instruct students to fill out Student Handout 14-2 pertaining to the Web site they choose.
3. Ask students to briefly share information about their site with the class.
4. Collect the information forms and make a class resource notebook or copies for each student to take for use on the job.
5. Alternate activity: Students work in pairs rather than individually. You can also have them look for Web sites on other patient education topics, such as HIV and help for patients with visual impairments.

Instructor's Note: Many of the Web sites listed have information for students and health professionals, making them valuable resources for students to use in their classes. Because Web sites change and are updated regularly, answers are not given for this exercise. The information students record on their forms is also subject to individual interpretation and opinions about what is "easy" and so on.

Follow-up Discussion

1. What problems, if any, did you have finding useful information?
2. What suggestions do you have for people looking for health care information on the Internet?

ACTIVITY 14-2
WHAT'S AVAILABLE LOCALLY?

What Students Will Learn

- How to identify local resources for patients.
- How to organize and present information.

What You Will Need

Student Handout **14-3**

- A copy of Student Handout 14-3, Local Resources, for each student.
- Local phone directories.
- Access to the Internet (optional).

What To Do

1. Distribute Student Handout 14-3. Have students work individually or in small groups.
2. Ask students or groups to select an organization to research. Helpful sources for identifying organizations include phone directories (white pages, business section), Chamber of Commerce, hospitals and other health care facilities, local newspaper, neighborhood community centers, and public libraries.
3. Give the class a few days to gather information, using Student Handout 14-3 as a guide. Encourage students to visit organizations, as appropriate, speaking with personnel and collecting brochures and other written information.
4. Have each student or group present its findings to the class in a brief report. Students can also make a bulletin board to display their findings. If appropriate, have them make a resource bulletin board in a central location in the school.
5. Collect the information forms (Student Handout 14-3) and make a class resource notebook or copies for each student to take for use on the job.

Follow-up Discussion

1. Ask students to describe their experiences collecting information.
2. What did you find most helpful as you looked for local resources?

ACTIVITY 14-3
WHAT'S MY LEARNING STYLE?

What Students Will Learn

- The three basic learning styles: visual, auditory, and kinesthetic.
- Their predominant learning style.

Student Handout **14-4**

What You Will Need

- A copy of Student Handout 14-4, Learning Styles Inventory, for each student.

What To Do

1. Discuss learning styles and how we each learn in different ways. When we are teaching others, we often assume that they learn the same way we do and may miss opportunities to present information in the way that is easiest for them to understand.
2. Distribute Student Handout 14-4.
3. Instruct students to circle the items that best describe them. Explain that this is not a test and that they are not expected to circle all the items.
4. Explain that they are to score each checklist by adding all the items they checked and entering the total.

Follow-up Discussion

1. How can understanding your own learning style help you be a better student?
2. How can this understanding help you become more a more effective patient educator?

ACTIVITY 14-4
TAKE ADVANTAGE OF LEARNING STYLES

What Students Will Learn

- How to develop learning and teaching strategies that correspond with the three basic learning styles.

What You Will Need

- No special materials are required for this activity.

What To Do

1. Divide class into groups of 3 to 5 students.
2. Assign a patient education topic to each group (or allow each group to choose a topic), such as the following:
   - Exercise program
   - Basic nutrition
   - Home safety
   - Stress management
   - Immunizations
   - Self-care for specific diseases
   - Prescribed medications
   - Preventive health measures
3. Give groups 10–15 minutes to brainstorm ways to teach patients about their topic. For example, they could show a video or prepare a written handout. Ask them to include methods appropriate for the three learning styles.
4. One member of each group writes down the ideas.
5. At the end of the brainstorming session, ask a representative from each group to present their ideas to the class.
6. Alternate activity: Assign the same topic to three groups and have each group list ideas for one of the three learning styles.

Follow-up Discussion

1. Was it difficult to think of teaching strategies for each of the learning styles? Explain why or why not.
2. When might you apply this information in the health care occupation you have chosen?

ACTIVITY 14-5
GIVING INSTRUCTIONS

What Students Will Learn

- To give clear explanations.

What You Will Need

- No special materials are required for this activity.

What To Do

1. Have the students pair off.
2. Instruct the students to take turns giving each other the directions for driving (or walking, taking public transportation) from the school to their house. They are to give the directions once and include all necessary information. The partners may take notes, then read or say them back for verification.

Follow-up Discussion

1. How clear were your partner's instructions?
2. Why is it sometimes difficult to give clear instructions?
3. What are some ways to make instructions easier for others to understand and follow?
4. Why is it important that patients understand your explanations?
5. What are possible consequences of patients not understanding your instructions?

ACTIVITY 14-6
YOU'RE THE TEACHER

What Students Will Learn

- How to organize and present a lesson.
- How to work with others to complete a project.

What You Will Need

- Copies of Student Handout 14-5, Teaching Plan and 14-6, Patient Education Topics, for each group of three to five students.

What To Do

1. Divide class into groups of three to five students.
2. Distribute copies of Student Handouts 14-5 and 14-6 to each group.

Student Handout **14-5**

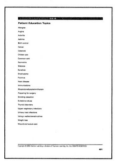

Student Handout **14-5**
(*Continued*)

Student Handout **14-6**

3. Ask each group to pick a topic from Student Handout 14-6.
4. Instruct the groups to prepare a short lesson to present to the class, using Student Handout 14-5 as a guide.
5. One group member acts as the recorder and fills in the plan.
6. The lesson must address the three learning styles and include a short quiz to give the group members feedback about the effectiveness of their teaching. (The "quiz" may ask students to demonstrate knowledge or skill in a way other than a written test.)
7. Alternate activity: Have students complete this activity individually instead of working in groups.

Instructor's Note: You may want to check the written teaching plans before the students present their lessons to the class.

Follow-up Discussion

1. Conduct a discussion about the experience of teaching others and the effectiveness of the lessons presented based on how the students presented their lessons.

ACTIVITY 14-7
CREATE A PAMPHLET

Student Handout **14-6**

Student Handout **14-7**

What Students Will Learn

- Information about common illnesses.
- To communicate in writing.
- How to organize information for effective patient education.

What You Will Need

Instructor's Note: Pamphlets may range from simple hand-lettered projects to more polished products that are created using computers.

- Construction or other type of paper.
- Crayons, colored pencils, scissors, other art materials.
- Computers or typewriters (optional).
- A copy of Student Handouts 14-6, Patient Education Topics, and 14-7, Guidelines for Creating Pamphlets, for each student.

What To Do

1. Distribute Student Handouts 14-6 and 14-7.
2. Ask students to choose a patient education topic, research it, and create an educational pamphlet appropriate for patients.
3. Explain your expectations for the finished product.

Instructor's Note: This activity may be done individually or in small groups.

Follow-up Discussion

1. Why should patients be given written as well as oral instructions?
2. What features make pamphlets most useful for patient education?

ACTIVITY 14-8
GAMES THAT TEACH

What Students Will Learn

- How to teach difficult information to young patients.

What You Will Need

- Posterboard for each group of students.
- Paper supplies for game cards.
- A copy of Student Handout 14-8, Games That Teach, for each student.

Student Handout **14-8**

What To Do

1. Divide the class into groups of four or five students
2. Ask students to design a game to teach children about living with diabetes (or other disease of your/their choice). The game can be a board game, card game, or a physical activity game.
3. Give students a week or two to develop and make their games. You may provide supplies or have students provide their own.
4. Once the games have been developed, have each group present its game to the class.
5. Have groups exchange games and play a game made by another group.
6. Complete the project by having students complete Student Handout 14-8 and turning it in.

Follow-up Discussion

1. How can games be good teaching tools?
2. Were the games the class created effective? Explain why or why not.
3. What were the common features of the most effective games?

ACTIVITY 14-9
LEARNING ABOUT HEART DISEASE

What Students Will Learn

- Facts about the risks that lead to heart disease.

What You Will Need

- White- or chalkboard or flip chart and appropriate writing utensils.
- No special materials are required for this activity.

What To Do

1. Brainstorm with the class risk factors that can lead to heart disease (overweight, high-fat diet, lack of exercise, family history, high cholesterol, smoking, high blood pressure, ethnicity, gender, age, excessive alcohol intake, diabetes, etc). Write these where the class can see them.
2. Ask students to design a questionnaire that will help teach patients about heart disease risk. The questionnaire should include questions, answers, and explanations.
3. Have students share their questionnaires with the class.

Follow-up Discussion

1. Why is a questionnaire a good tool for patient education?
2. How can questionnaires motivate patients to learn more about risk factors?
3. What are some other ways that questionnaires could be used for patient education?

ACTIVITY 14-10
AM I DOING IT RIGHT?

What Students Will Learn

- How to use proper body mechanics when moving patients or other heavy objects.
- How to teach proper body mechanics to caregivers.
- How to teach proper body mechanics to patients using a cane, walker, or crutches.

What You Will Need

- A stationary chair.
- A cane, walker, crutches, and wheelchair.

What To Do

1. Demonstrate to students the proper way to:
   - Help a patient out of a chair.
   - Help a patient into and out of a wheelchair.
   - Push a wheelchair.
   - Walk with a cane, crutches, or a walker.
   - Lift a heavy load, such as a box, off the floor.
2. As a class, develop a list of reminders for proper body mechanics. This list should include items such as the following:
   - Proper stance
   - Bending knees and keeping back straight
   - Squatting rather than bending
   - Pushing or rolling objects rather than lifting, when possible
   - Knowing and respecting own limitations
3. Divide the class into groups of four students.
4. Ask each group to put together and present to the class a skit to demonstrate good body mechanics when caring for someone and when teaching a patient the proper way to walk with a cane, walker, or crutches.

Follow-up Discussion

1. What were the most effective techniques for teaching patients how to perform an activity?
2. Why is it important to learn to explain clearly when teaching health care activities?
3. What did you learn from the skits?

ACTIVITY 14-11
WORD SCRAMBLE

What Students Will Learn

- Which foods raise the blood cholesterol.*

What You Will Need

- Instructor Sheet 14-1, Foods High in Cholesterol.

What To Do

1. Ask students to write down as many foods as they can think of that they believe raise the blood's level of cholesterol.
2. Have students share their lists and correct them as necessary (See Instructor Sheet 14-1 for examples of foods that are high in cholesterol.)
3. Ask students to make a word scramble puzzle by mixing the order of the letters in each word. Have them write these on a clean sheet of paper.
4. Collect the papers and distribute them so that students do not have their own paper. Have them unscramble the words.

Follow-up Discussion

1. How could word puzzles and other games be used in patient education?

Instructor Sheet **14-1**

---

*Source: Activity adapted from G. Ragland (1997). *Instant teaching treasures for patient education.* St. Louis, MO: Mosby.

REFERENCES

Haroun, L. (2001). *Instructor's manual to accompany career development for health professionals.* Philadelphia: W.B. Saunders Company.

Ragland, G. (1997). *Instant teaching treasures for patient education.* St. Louis, MO: Mosby.

Foods High in Cholesterol

One hundred grams of the following foods contain over 100 mg of cholesterol:

Butter

Cheese

Coconut

Cream

Egg Yolks

Fish oil

Lard

Lobster

Organ meats (liver, kidney, heart, brain)

Sardines

Shrimp

Sausage

Tongue (beef)

Whole milk

Health Information Web Sites

Organization	Web Address
National Center for Alcoholism and Drug Dependency	www.ncadd.org
Alcoholics Anonymous World Services	www.alcoholics-anonymous.org
Alexander Graham Bell Association for the Deaf, Inc.	www.agbell.org
Alzheimer's Association	www.alz.org
American Cancer Society, National Center	www.cancer.org
American Diabetes Association	www.diabetes.org
American Foundation for the Blind	www.afb.org
American Heart Association, National Center	www.americanheart.org
American Heart Association, Stroke Connection	www.stroke.org
American Lung Association	www.lungusa.org
American Parkinson's Disease Association	www.apdaparkinson.com
American Red Cross	www.redcross.org
Arthritis Foundation	www.arthritis.org
The Brain Injury Association	www.biausa.org
Cancer Care, Inc.	www.cancercare.org
Epilepsy Foundation of America	www.efa.org
The Glaucoma Foundation	www.glaucoma-foundation.org/info
Multiple Sclerosis Society, National Headquarters	www.nmss.org
Muscular Dystrophy Association, National Headquarters	www.mdausa.org
National Cancer Institute	www.nci.nih.gov
National Kidney Foundation	www.kidney.org
National Osteoporosis Foundation	www.nof.org
Self-Help for Hard of Hearing People	www.shhh.org

Web Site Information

Sponsoring organization:
Web address:
Convenience rating: ___ Very easy to use ___ Okay, not great ___ Confusing, hard to find information
Information is designed for: ___ Patients ___ Their families ___ Health care providers ___ General public
General health topics included:
Special features included:
Interactive features (self-assessments, quizzes, etc.):
Links to other sites:
Other resources available (publications, videos, etc.):

Local Resources

Name of organization:
Address:
Phone number:
Information available:
Services available:
Purpose of organization is to help: ___ Patients ___ Their families ___ Health care providers ___ General public
Comments:

Learning Styles Inventory

Auditory Checklist

☐ I enjoy music activities more than art activities.

☐ If I need to learn something, I would rather have someone explain it to me than read about it.

☐ I tend to talk to myself when I'm performing a task.

☐ I remember things the instructor explains in class better than what I read in my textbook.

☐ I spell better out loud than when writing words out.

☐ Sometimes I don't copy well from the board.

☐ I like jokes that people tell me out loud more than cartoons.

☐ I understand material better if I read it out loud.

☐ Sometimes I don't notice things like a new sign or that a room has been painted unless someone points it out to me.

☐ When I have to go someplace new, I do better with verbal instructions than I do looking at a map.

_____ **Score** (number of checked items)

Visual Checklist

☐ Sometimes I have to ask people to repeat what they have just said.

☐ I sometimes find it difficult to listen to an oral presentation, such as a lecture.

☐ I learn new material better from my textbooks than from listening to the instructor explain it.

☐ I have difficulty understanding instructors or speakers when their backs are turned and I can't see their faces.

☐ It's much easier for me to follow a lecture if the instructor uses overheads or writes on the board.

☐ When I have to go someplace new, I do better with a map or written instructions than if someone explains it to me.

☐ I prefer puzzles done with pencil and paper more than riddles and puzzles that require listening.

☐ It's hard for me to remember things I've been told unless I write them down.

☐ I often draw or doodle on my papers.

☐ I would rather do art than music activities.

_____ **Score** (number of checked items)

Kinesthetic Checklist

☐ When I'm reading or writing, I often say the words quietly to myself.

☐ I often touch things, such as the items for sale in a store when I shop.

☐ Sometimes I count on my fingers.

☐ I prefer games that require the players to move around rather than sit quietly.

☐ I tend to play with things like a pen or pencil while I study.

☐ I find that movements like jiggling my leg or tapping my fingers help me concentrate.

☐ If I have something new to learn, I would rather do a hands-on activity than read or hear about it.

☐ I like to make things with my hands.

☐ I like to move around when I'm listening or learning.

☐ It's easier for me to show someone how to do something rather than explaining it in words or writing down how to do it.

_____ **Score** (number of checked items)

Source: Adapted from L. Haroun (2001). *Instructor's manual to accompany career development for health professionals.* Philadelphia: W.B. Saunders Company.

Teaching Plan

Topic or skill to be taught:

_____

_____

Why this topic or skill is important to know:

_____

_____

What the students or "patients" should know or be able to do as a result of the lesson:

_____

_____

_____

_____

How the skill will be taught:

Visual Presentation/Activity

_____

_____

_____

_____

_____

Auditory Presentation/Activity

_____

_____

_____

_____

_____

Kinesthetic Presentation/Activity

_____

_____

_____

_____

_____

Supplies and/or equipment needed:

_____

_____

_____

_____

_____

_____

Student evaluation: quiz or activity:

_____

_____

_____

_____

_____

_____

Patient Education Topics

Allergies

Angina

Arthritis

Asthma

Birth control

Cancer

Cataracts

Chicken pox

Common cold

Dermatitis

Diabetes

Earaches

Emphysema

Flu/virus

Heart disease

Immunizations

Myopia/presbyopia/amblyopia

Preparing for surgery

Smoking cessation

Substance abuse

Thyroid disorders

Upper respiratory infections

Urinary tract infections

Using a walker/cane/crutches

Weight loss

Wound and suture care

Guidelines for Creating Pamphlets

Use the following questions, as appropriate, to guide the creation of your patient pamphlet:

- What is the topic or disease?

- What are the signs and symptoms?

- How is it diagnosed?

- How is it treated?

- Do I need tests?

- How long does it last?

- How do I catch it?

- When is it likely to occur?

- Is it contagious?

- Is it hereditary?

- What else do I need to know?

- Where can I get more information?

- What can I do to correct the condition?

- What lifestyle changes can I make?

- What are the consequences of this condition?

Games That Teach

Your Group's Game

1. What one new fact about disease did you learn while making your game?

2. How can using a game be helpful for educating young patients?

3. What was the most important medical fact the game taught?

Another Group's Game

1. What did you like best about the other group's game that you played?

2. Did it include all the important information you think needed to be included? If not, what was missing?

3. What did you like least about the game?

4. Is the game appropriate for school-age children?

5. What was the most important medical fact the game taught?

Documentation

INTRODUCTION

Many students report having difficulty with charting once they are on the job. With the increased need for accountability to both the government and third-party payers, all health care workers must understand the importance of complete and accurate documentation. This chapter provides opportunities for reviewing and practicing various types of charting and notation.

ACTIVITY 15-1
DOCU-MATCH

What Students Will Learn

- Terminology and basic concepts of medical records and documentation.

What You Will Need

- Student Handout 15-1, Documentation Terms, for half the students in the class.
- Student Handout 15-2, Definitions and Explanations of Documentation Terms, for the other half of the students.
- Instructor Sheet 15-1, Answer Key for Docu-Match

What To Do

1. Give half the students the cards made from Student Handout 15-1 and the other half the cards made from Student Handout 15-2.
2. If you do not use all the cards, be sure that the ones you do distribute from each handout match each other.
3. Ask students to walk around the classroom and look for the student who has the match for their term/phrase or definition.

Student Handout **15-1**

Student Handout **15-2**

Student Handout **15-2**
(Continued)

Instructor Sheet **15-1**

Instructor Sheet **15-1**
(Continued)

4. Use Instructor Sheet 15-1 to check the matches.
5. When all students are paired up correctly, have them present their terms and definitions to the class.

Instructor's Note: If your class has not studied all the terms included, omit the ones they are not expected to know.

Follow-Up Discussion

1. Why is it important for all health care workers to know the basics of documentation?
2. Are there any terms that need more explanation?

ACTIVITY 15-2
GOOD DOCUMENTATION

What Students Will Learn

- The characteristics of good documentation.

What You Will Need

- Whiteboard, chalkboard, or a flip chart and appropriate writing utensils.
- Transparency 15-1, Characteristics of Good Documentation.

What To Do

1. Ask the class to list as many characteristics of good documentation as they can. Allow 5–10 minutes.
2. Write a compilation of the lists on the board. Use Transparency 15-1 if it contains items the students did not list.
3. Discuss the importance of each of the characteristics and how it contributes to good patient care.
4. Alternate activity: Use Transparency 15-1 to introduce and discuss the characteristics of good documentation. Ask students to compile the lists from recall a day or two after the discussion as a test of recall.

Instructor's Note: This activity can be done in small groups or students can work individually.

Follow-Up Discussion

1. Why is it important for health care documentation to be accurate?
2. How can health care workers ensure that any documentation they write is complete and accurate?

TRANSPARENCY MASTER 15-1
Characteristics of Good Documentation

- Completed as soon as possible after activity being documented.
- Signed by health care worker who performed procedure, spoke with patient, etc.
- Numbers and measurements are written in actual figures rather than described as "small," "many," etc.
- Quotation marks used when reporting patient's statements.
- Dated.
- Legible.
- Clear and concise.
- Spelled correctly.
- Identified with patient's name.
- Written with approved abbreviations.
- Written using correct medical terminology.
- Findings are not duplicated.
- Written in blue or black ink, never in pencil.
- Contains only facts, not opinions or guesses.
- Completed without leaving empty lines.
- Patient's reactions to procedures included.

Transparency Master **15-1**

ACTIVITY 15-3
SUBJECTIVE VERSUS OBJECTIVE INFORMATION

What Students Will Learn

- To distinguish between subjective and objective information.
- To correctly chart subjective and objective information.

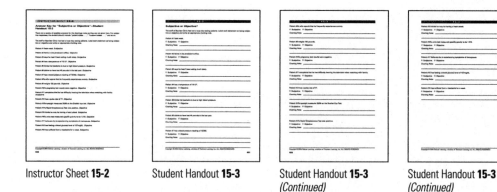

Instructor Sheet **15-2** Student Handout **15-3** Student Handout **15-3** *(Continued)* Student Handout **15-3** *(Continued)*

What You Will Need

- A copy of Student Handout 15-3, Subjective or Objective?, for each student.
- Instructor Sheet 15-2, Answer Key to Subjective or Objective—Student Handout 15-3.

What To Do

1. Divide class into groups of three students.
2. Distribute Handout 15-3 and have group members work together to fill in the handout.
3. Alternate activity: Have students work individually on the handout.
4. Discuss the correct answers as a class.

Instructor's Note: You may omit the charting component of the worksheet if this is too advanced for the students.

Follow-Up Discussion

1. What is the basic difference between subjective and objective information?
2. Were any of the examples difficult to distinguish? Explain.
3. Why is it important in charting to know the difference between subjective and objective information?

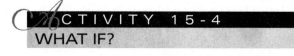

ACTIVITY 15-4
WHAT IF?

What Students Will Learn

- Important concepts and practices related to medical documentation.

What You Will Need

- A copy of Student Handout 15-4, What If? for each student.
- Instructor Sheet 15-3, Suggested Answers to "What If?" Questions—Student Handout 15-4.

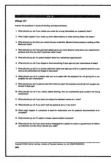

Student Handout **15-4**

What To Do

Version #1: Play as a game in which teams compete to correctly answer the "What If?" questions given by the instructor or a student.

Version #2: Distribute a handout to each student. Students stand up and one starts by asking one of the questions of a classmate. If the classmate answers correctly, he or she remains standing and asks a question of another classmate. Students who cannot answer their questions may ask someone else to answer it, but they must sit down and are out of future play. The student(s) who remains standing at the end of the time limit for play (instructor determines in advance) is the winner.

Version #3: Distribute the handout to students and have them work individually, in pairs, or in groups of three to answer the questions.

Instructor's Note: Explain to students that some of the questions require answers that state the action they should take as the health care worker (question #1 is an example). Other questions require answers that state the consequences of an action already taken (question #2 is an example).

Follow-Up Discussion

1. Conduct a discussion summarizing the importance of accurate documentation in terms of patient safety and well-being, legal and regulatory compliance, and reimbursement.

Instructor Sheet **15-3**

Instructor Sheet **15-3**
(Continued)

ACTIVITY 15-5
HOW DO I CHART IT?

What Students Will Learn

- How to chart objectively and correctly.

What You Will Need

- A copy of Student Handout 15-5, Charting Choices, for each student.
- Instructor Sheet 15-4, Answers to Charting Choices—Student Handout 15-5.

What To Do

1. Discuss the charting practices that are important from a legal standpoint. These include objectivity, avoiding assumptions, avoiding bias, using neutral language, and being complete.
2. Distribute Student Handout 15-5 and ask students to complete the assignment. You may collect this when they are finished or go over it in class using Instructor Sheet 15-5.

Follow-Up Discussion

1. What distinguished the correct from the incorrect choices?
2. How did the answers fulfill the legal requirements for documentation?

Instructor Sheet **15-4**

Student Handout **15-5**

ACTIVITY 15-6
HOW DO I REPORT THIS?

What Students Will Learn
- Diseases that must be reported to local authorities.

What You Will Need
- Whiteboard, chalkboard, or flip chart and appropriate writing utensils.
- Instructor Sheet 15-5, Reportable Diseases and Conditions.

What To Do

1. Ask students to identify health conditions that must be reported to authorities in your area. They may use the Internet or contact local authorities. Assign a completion deadline.
2. On the due date for completion of their research, ask students to share their lists and write their findings on the board. Use Instructor Sheet 15-6 as a guide. (Your students may come up with some different answers because each geographic area is unique and has its own list of conditions that must be reported.)

Follow-Up Discussion

1. What types of diseases must be reported?
2. Why must certain diseases and conditions be reported?
3. How does disease reporting by health care providers help ensure public safety?

Instructor Sheet **15-5**

ACTIVITY 15-7
DRUG-RELATED ABBREVIATIONS

What Students Will Learn
- Common abbreviations used for drugs.

What You Will Need
- A copy of Student Handouts 15-6, Common Drug-Related Abbreviations, and 15-7, Common Drug-Related Abbreviations Worksheet, for each student.
- Instructor Sheet 15-6, Answers for Common Drug-Related Abbreviations Worksheet—Student Handout 15-7.

Student Handout **15-6**

Student Handout **15-7**

Student Handout **15-7**
(Continued)

Instructor Sheet **15-6**

What To Do

1. Distribute Student Handout 15-6.
2. Review drug-related abbreviations as the students refer to their handout.
3. Distribute Student Handout 15-7. Have students complete the worksheet in class or as a homework assignment.

Follow-Up Discussion

1. Why is it essential that health care workers use the correct drug-related abbreviations?
2. What are the potential consequences of using these abbreviations incorrectly?

ACTIVITY 15-8
PRESCRIPTIONS, PLEASE

What Students Will Learn

- The format used for medical prescriptions.

What You Will Need

- Enough used prescription bottles so that each student will have at least one.

What To Do

1. Use a felt-tip marker to black out patient names on the bottles.
2. Distribute the prescription bottles so that each student has at least one.
3. Have each student go to the board and write the prescription as it would have been written when the original script was generated. Ask students to read the prescription aloud.
4. Make any corrections necessary.
5. Continue until each member of the class has had at least one turn.

Follow-Up Discussion

1. What part do pharmaceutical products play in modern medical treatments?
2. Why is it important for health care workers to have a basic knowledge of drug prescriptions?

REFERENCE

Mitchell, J., & Haroun, L. (2002). *Introduction to health care.* Clifton Park, NY: Delmar Learning.

Answer Key for Docu-Match

Word or Phrase	Definition or Explanation
Assessment	A step in charting that records the health care professional's impression of what is wrong with the patient.
What must be done before releasing medical records	A consent authorizing their release must be signed by the patient.
Charting	The recording of information about and observations of patients.
Charting by exception	Only findings that are abnormal for the patient in question are charted.
Chief complaint	The patient's statement of the main reason he or she is seeking medical care.
Corrections on medical documentation	Write these as close as possible to the incorrect information, write "error," and date and initial.
Demographics	Patient data such as address and telephone number.
Documentation	The notes, reports, and various types of information included in medical records.
Errors made when charting	These cannot be erased; instead draw a single line through them.
Flow sheets	Preprinted forms, graphs, checklists, etc. for recording patient data.
Focus charting	A format for charting in which the progress note is divided into three columns: 1st = date/time; 2nd = focus (problem); 3rd = patient care notes.
Golden rule of documentation	If it isn't documented, it wasn't done.
Medical history	Data collected about a patient that includes health, personal, family, and social information.
Medical record	The collection of all documents that are filed together and form a complete health history of a particular patient.
Narrative charting	Writing detailed notes on the chart about all aspects of a patient's care.
Objective information	Direct observations made by the health care professional, including test results and other measurements.
Patients' requests for medical records	Patients must request in writing and include their signature.
PIE	A format for charting in which the letters stand for problem, implementation, evaluation.
Possible consequences of incomplete documentation	Improper or inconsistent patient care; noncompliance with regulations; denial of reimbursement from insurance companies or Medicare.
Problem-oriented medical records	A method of organizing the medical record in which the patient's health problems are assigned numbers that are used for reference throughout the record.

Word or Phrase	Definition or Explanation
Progress note	A written statement about a patient's care.
Sign	Indications of disease or dysfunction that can be observed or measured.
SOAP	A format for charting in which the letters stand for subjective, objective, assessment, plan.
SOAPIE	A format for charting in which the letters stand for subjective, objective, assessment, plan, interventions, evaluations.
Source-oriented medical records	Grouping medical records by category, such as insurance information, progress notes, and lab reports.
Subjective information	Statements made by the patient about his or her condition that cannot be directly observed by the health care professional.
Symptom	Indications of disease or dysfunction that are sensed by the patient.
When charting must be done	Immediately following a procedure, *never* before.
When medical records can be destroyed	Never. Even records for inactive patients must be kept in a safe place.
Why documentation can be used in court	Medical records are legal documents.

Source for some of the definitions: J. Mitchell & L. Haroun (2002). *Introduction to health care.* Clifton Park, NY: Delmar Learning.

Answer Key for "Subjective or Objective"—Student Handout 15-3

There are a variety of possible answers for the chartings notes so they are not given here. For subjective responses, the student should include "patient states . . . ," "husband states . . . ," and so on.

The staff at Bayview Clinic has had a busy day seeing patients. Label each statement as being subjective or objective and write an appropriate charting note.

Patient #1 feels weak. *Subjective*

Patient #2 faints in the physician's office. *Objective*

Patient #3 says he hasn't been eating much lately. *Subjective*

Patient #4 has a temperature of 101.5°. *Objective*

Patient #5 thinks his headache is due to high blood pressure. *Subjective*

Patient #6 claims to have lost 40 pounds in the last year. *Subjective*

Patient #7 has a blood pressure reading of 137/82. *Objective*

Patient #8's wife reports that he frequently experiences anxiety. *Subjective*

Patient #9 weighs 192 pounds. *Objective*

Patient #10's pregnancy test results were negative. *Objective*

Patient #11 complains that he has difficulty hearing the television when watching with family. *Subjective*

Patient #12 has a pulse rate of 77. *Objective*

Patient #13's eyesight measures 20/30 on the Snellen eye test. *Objective*

Patient #14's Rapid Streptococcus Test was positive. *Objective*

Patient #15 thinks he may be having a heart attack. *Subjective*

Patient #16's urine test measured specific gravity to be 1.010. *Objective*

Patient #17 believes she is experiencing symptoms of menopause. *Subjective*

Patient #18 has fasting a blood glucose level of 127mg/dL. *Objective*

Patient #19 has suffered from a headache for a week. *Subjective*

Suggested Answers to "What If?" Questions—Student Handout 15-4

1. What should you do if you realize you wrote the wrong information on a patient's chart?

    Draw a line through the incorrect information, write in the correct information, write "error" (or abbreviation approved by facility), and date and sign the notation.

2. What might happen if you made up some abbreviations to make charting faster and easier?

    It could cause confusion among other health care providers making notes on the charts. It could also cause problems with regulators, insurance companies, and Medicare.

3. What should you do if you realized you had written Mrs. Moreno's blood pressure reading on Mrs. Mariano's chart?

    On Mrs. Mariano's chart: correct the error by drawing a line through the information, writing "error" (or approved abbreviation), and dating and signing the notation. Enter the correct information on Mrs. Moreno's chart. Include the date of the reading and the date of the entry and sign or initial.

4. What should you do if you got interrupted just as you were about to write down your patient's temperature and now you can't remember what it was?

    Retake the temperature and record immediately. Be sure to note the time the recorded temperature was taken and entered.

5. What should you do if a patient doesn't show for a scheduled appointment?

    Write this fact in the patient's chart.

6. What should you do if you forgot to chart something 2 days ago and just remembered it today?

    Record it now. Enter both the date the information was gathered and today's date.

7. What should you do if a co-worker calls from home and asks you to fill in a patient's chart for a procedure she performed and forgot to document?

    Refuse the request. It is illegal to document and sign for someone else.

8. What should you do if a patient tells you he is upset with the physician for not giving him a prescription for pain medication?

    The patient's statement should be written on his chart as directly as possible. Example: Patient states, "I'm really mad at the doctor because he wouldn't refill this prescription."

9. What should you do if a patient calls from home to report his progress recovering from surgery performed 3 days ago?

    Record on his chart what the patient says. Example: Patient states, "I'm feeling better, but I have to change my dressing every couple of hours."

10. What should you do if you realize, before charting, that you accidentally gave a patient the wrong medication?

    Notify the physician or supervisor immediately! Record the information, including time and amount given, on the chart.

11. What should you do if you leave an empty line between entries on a chart?

    Draw a line through the space so it won't be used, causing the notes to be out of chronological order.

12. What should you do if you can't read the previous entry in the chart?

    Report this to your supervisor.

13. What might happen if a physician is sued for malpractice and the patient's documentation is incomplete?

    Incomplete documentation can negatively affect the outcome of a malpractice lawsuit.

14. What should you do if a patient refuses recommended treatment?

    Patients have the right to refuse treatment. Note details on the chart: date, time, what treatment was refused, statements made by patient, your initials. (And report to the physician or supervisor.)

15. What should you do if you leave several messages for a patient to make an appointment for follow-up treatment, but she never returns your calls?

    Note the dates and times of your calls on the patient's chart, along with your initials.

Answers to Charting Choices—Student Handout 15-5

For each pair, check the box next to the chart note that is most appropriate for the patient's chart.

1. You walk into the hospital room and find the patient's IV has been pulled out.

   ☐ The patient pulled out her IV.

   ☐ *The IV was hanging free and no longer in patient's arm.*

2. You walk into an exam room and find the patient lying on the floor.

   ☐ The patient fell off the exam table and is now lying on the floor.

   ☐ *The patient was found on the floor of the examination room.*

3. The patient complains of feeling hot and feverish.

   ☐ The patient appears to have a high fever.

   ☐ *The patient's temperature is 104.5°.*

4. As you enter the patient's room you hear moaning sounds.

   ☐ *Patient states pain level is 7 on a scale of 0–10.*

   ☐ Patient appears to be in pain.

5. You observe the patient as he enters the urgent care clinic.

   ☐ Patient appears to be drunk.

   ☐ *Patient entered the clinic with an unsteady gait. There is an odor of alcohol, muscle tone was lax, and patient was unable to sit upright in a chair when asked to do so.*

6. The doctor has ordered Levoxyl be taken once each day.

   ☐ Levoxyl 1 tab q.o.d.

   ☐ *Levoxyl 1 tab q.d.*

7. You examine a patient's mouth after she complains that the tip of her tongue hurts.

   ☐ *The patient has a spot that is red and about ½ centimeter in diameter on the tip of her tongue.*

   ☐ The patient has a spot that is red and rather large on the tip of her tongue.

8. The patient calls the physician's office requesting an appointment for what he thinks is the flu.

   ☐ *Patient reports vomiting three times since 8 A.M.*

   ☐ Patient reports he has the flu.

Reportable Diseases and Conditions

AIDS

Amebiasis

Animal bites

Anthrax

Arbovirus

Botulism (foodborne, infant)

Brucellosis

Campylobacteriosis

Chancroid

Chlamydial infections

Cholera

Diphtheria

Encephalitis

Food poisoning

Gastroenteritis

Giardiasis

Gonococcal infections

Gonorrhea

Group A beta-hemolytic
streptococcal infections
(including scarlet fever)

Haemophilus influenza Type B

Hepatitis A, B, C

Hepatitis unspecified

Histoplasmosis

Kawasaki disease

Lead poisoning

Legionnaires' disease (Legionella)

Leprosy

Leptospirosis

Lyme disease

Lymphogranuloma venereum

Malaria

Measles

Meningitis

Meningococcal disease

Mumps

Neonatal hypothyroidism

Pertussis

Phenylketonuria

Plague

Poliomyelitis

Psittacosis (ornithosis)

Rabies

Reye's syndrome

Rickettsial disease

Rubella

Salmonellosis

Shigellosis

Syphilis

Tetanus

Toxic shock syndrome

Toxoplasmosis

Tuberculosis

Tularemia

Typhoid and paratyphoid fever

Yellow fever

Answers for Common Drug-Related Abbreviations Worksheet—Student Handout 15-7

1. Take one Toradol 10 mg tablet every 6 hours for inflammation. Dispense 20.

2. Take one Provera 5 mg tablet by mouth daily. Dispense 30.

3. Take one Dyazide 37.5/25 capsule by mouth each day. Dispense 30.

4. Take one Lortab 7.5/500 tablet by mouth every 4–6 hours as needed for pain. Dispense 30.

5. Take one Levoxyl .088 mg tablet by mouth daily. Dispense 30.

6. Take one Motrin 800 mg tablet by mouth 3 times daily with food. Dispense 90.

7. Take one Amoxicillin 500 mg capsule by mouth 3 times daily for 10 days. Dispense 30.

8. Take one Valium 25 mg capsule every 4 hours by mouth as needed for pain. Dispense 20.

9. Place one drop Timoptic .25% in both eyes twice daily. Dispense 10 cc.

Documentation Terms

Cut along the dotted lines to make cards.

ASSESSMENT	WHAT MUST BE DONE BEFORE RELEASING MEDICAL RECORDS
CHARTING	CHARTING BY EXCEPTION
CHIEF COMPLAINT	CORRECTIONS ON MEDICAL DOCUMENTATION
DEMOGRAPHICS	DOCUMENTATION
ERRORS MADE WHEN CHARTING	FLOW SHEETS
FOCUS CHARTING	GOLDEN RULE OF DOCUMENTATION
MEDICAL HISTORY	MEDICAL RECORD
NARRATIVE CHARTING	OBJECTIVE INFORMATION
PATIENTS' REQUESTS FOR MEDICAL RECORDS	PIE
POSSIBLE CONSEQUENCES OF INCOMPLETE DOCUMENTATION	PROBLEM-ORIENTED MEDICAL RECORDS
PROGRESS NOTE	SIGN
SOAP	SOAPIE
SOURCE-ORIENTED MEDICAL RECORDS	SUBJECTIVE INFORMATION
SYMPTOM	WHEN CHARTING MUST BE DONE
WHEN MEDICAL RECORDS CAN BE DESTROYED	WHY DOCUMENTATION CAN BE USED IN COURT

Definitions and Explanations of Documentation Terms

Cut along the lines to make cards

The notes, reports, and various types of information included in medical records.	Never. Even records for inactive patients must be kept in a safe place.
The recording of information about and observations of patients.	A format for charting in which the letters stand for subjective, objective, assessment, plan, interventions, evaluations.
The collection of all documents that are filed together and form a complete health history of a particular patient.	A format for charting in which the letters stand for: problem, implementation, evaluation.
A written statement about a patient's care.	A format for charting in which progress note is divided into three columns: 1st = date/time; 2nd = focus (problem); 3rd = patient care notes.
A format for charting in which the letters stand for subjective, objective, assessment, plan.	A consent authorizing their release must be signed by the patient.
The patient's statement of the main reason he or she is seeking medical care.	These cannot be erased; instead draw a single line through them.
Direct observations made by the health care professional including test results and other measurements.	Patients must request in writing and include their signature.
Statements made by the patient about his or her condition that cannot be directly observed by the health care professional.	Data collected about a patient that includes health, personal, family, and social information.
Indications of disease or dysfunction that can be observed or measured.	Write these as close as possible to the incorrect information, write "error," and date and initial.
Indications of disease or dysfunction that are sensed by the patient.	Preprinted forms, graphs, checklists, etc. for recording patient data.

Only findings that are abnormal for the patient in question are charted.	Immediately following a procedure, *never* before.
Grouping medical records by category, such as insurance information, progress notes, and lab reports.	A step in charting that records the health care professional's impression of what is wrong with the patient.
A method of organizing the medical record in which the patient's health problems are assigned numbers that are used for reference throughout the record.	Improper or inconsistent patient care; noncompliance with regulations; denial of reimbursement from insurance companies or Medicare.
Patient data such as address and telephone number.	Medical records are legal documents.
Writing detailed notes on the chart about all aspects of a patient's care.	If it isn't documented, it wasn't done.

Subjective or Objective?

The staff at Bayview Clinic has had a busy day seeing patients. Label each statement as being subjective or objective and write an appropriate charting note.

Patient #1 feels weak.

☐ Subjective   ☐ Objective

Charting Note: _____

_____

Patient #2 faints in the physician's office.

☐ Subjective   ☐ Objective

Charting Note: _____

_____

Patient #3 says he hasn't been eating much lately.

☐ Subjective   ☐ Objective

Charting Note: _____

_____

Patient #4 has a temperature of 101.5°.

☐ Subjective   ☐ Objective

Charting Note: _____

_____

Patient #5 thinks his headache is due to high blood pressure.

☐ Subjective   ☐ Objective

Charting Note: _____

_____

Patient #6 claims to have lost 40 pounds in the last year.

☐ Subjective   ☐ Objective

Charting Note: _____

_____

Patient #7 has a blood pressure reading of 137/82.

☐ Subjective   ☐ Objective

Charting Note: _____

_____

Patient #8's wife reports that he frequently experiences anxiety.

☐ Subjective   ☐ Objective

Charting Note: _____

_____

Patient #9 weighs 192 pounds.

☐ Subjective   ☐ Objective

Charting Note: _____

_____

Patient #10's pregnancy test results were negative.

☐ Subjective   ☐ Objective

Charting Note: _____

_____

Patient #11 complains that he has difficulty hearing the television when watching with family.

☐ Subjective   ☐ Objective

Charting Note: _____

_____

Patient #12 has a pulse rate of 77.

☐ Subjective   ☐ Objective

Charting Note: _____

_____

Patient #13's eyesight measures 20/30 on the Snellen Eye Test.

☐ Subjective   ☐ Objective

Charting Note: _____

_____

Patient #14's Rapid Streptococcus Test was positive.

☐ Subjective   ☐ Objective

Charting Note: _____

_____

Patient #15 thinks he may be having a heart attack.

☐ Subjective   ☐ Objective

Charting Note: _____

_____

Patient #16's urine test measured specific gravity to be 1.010.

☐ Subjective   ☐ Objective

Charting Note: _____

_____

Patient #17 believes she is experiencing symptoms of menopause.

☐ Subjective   ☐ Objective

Charting Note: _____

_____

Patient #18 has fasting a blood glucose level of 127mg/dL.

☐ Subjective   ☐ Objective

Charting Note: _____

_____

Patient #19 has suffered from a headache for a week.

☐ Subjective   ☐ Objective

Charting Note: _____

_____

What If?

Answer the questions in terms of charting and documentation.

1. What should you do if you realize you wrote the wrong information on a patient's chart?

2. What might happen if you made up some abbreviations to make charting faster and easier?

3. What should you do when you notice that you wrote Mrs. Moreno's blood pressure reading on Mrs. Mariano's chart?

4. What should you do if you got interrupted just as you were about to write down your patient's temperature and now you can't remember what it was?

5. What should you do if a patient doesn't show for a scheduled appointment?

6. What should you do if you forgot to chart something 2 days ago and just remembered it today?

7. What should you do if a co-worker calls from home and asks you to fill in a patient's chart for a procedure she performed and forgot to document?

8. What should you do if a patient tells you he is upset with the physician for not giving him a prescription for pain medication?

9. What should you do if a patient calls from home to report his progress recovering from surgery performed 3 days ago?

10. What should you do if you realize, before charting, that you accidentally give a patient the wrong medication?

11. What should you do if you leave an empty line between entries on a chart?

12. What should you do if you can't read the previous entry in the chart?

13. What might happen if a physician is sued for malpractice and the patient's documentation is incomplete?

14. What should you do if a patient refuses recommended treatment?

15. What should you do if you leave several messages for a patient to make an appointment for follow-up treatment, but she never returns your calls?

Charting Choices

For each pair, check the box next to the chart note that is most appropriate for the patient's chart.

1. You walk into the hospital room and find the patient's IV has been pulled out.
   - ☐ The patient pulled out her IV.
   - ☐ The IV was hanging free and no longer in patient's arm.

2. You walk into an exam room and find the patient lying on the floor.
   - ☐ The patient fell off the exam table and is now lying on the floor.
   - ☐ The patient was found on the floor of the examination room.

3. The patient complains of feeling hot and feverish.
   - ☐ The patient appears to have a high fever.
   - ☐ The patient's temperature is 104.5°

4. As you enter the patient's room you hear moaning sounds.
   - ☐ Patient states pain level is 7 on a scale of 0–10.
   - ☐ Patient appears to be in pain.

5. You observe the patient as he enters the urgent care clinic.
   - ☐ Patient appears to be drunk.
   - ☐ Patient entered the clinic with an unsteady gait. There is an odor of alcohol, muscle tone was lax, and patient was unable to sit upright in a chair when asked to do so.

6. The doctor has ordered Levoxyl be taken once each day.
   - ☐ Levoxyl 1 tab q.o.d.
   - ☐ Levoxyl 1 tab q.d.

7. You examine a patient's mouth after she complains that the tip of her tongue hurts.
   - ☐ The patient has a spot that is red and about ½ centimeter in diameter on the tip of her tongue.
   - ☐ The patient has a spot that is red and rather large on the tip of her tongue.

8. The patient calls the physician's office requesting an appointment for what he thinks is the flu.
   - ☐ Patient reports vomiting three times since 8 A.M.
   - ☐ Patient reports he has the flu.

Common Drug-Related Abbreviations

ABBREVIATION	MEANING	ABBREVIATION	MEANING
A.D.	right ear	I.V.	intravenous
a.m.	morning	kg	kilogram
amt.	amount	lb	pound
A.S.	left ear	m	meter
ASA	aspirin	mg	milligram
A.U.	both ears	M.R. × 1	may repeat once
bid	twice each day	Noct.	night
c	with	N.P.O.	nothing by mouth
caps	capsules	O.D.	right eye
cc	cubic centimeters	O.S.	left eye
d	day	OTC	over-the-counter
/d	per day	O.U.	both eyes
disp	dispense	oz	ounce
DS	double strength	p.c.	after meals
g, gm, GM	gram	p.m.	evening
gt, gtt	drop	P.O.	by mouth
h, hr	hour	prn	as needed
h.s.	hours of sleep (bedtime)	q2h	every 2 hours
I.M.	intramuscular	q4h	every 4 hours
in.	inch	qd	every day
qh	every hour	supp	suppository
qid	4 times a day	susp	suspension
q.n.	every night	t, tsp	teaspoon
qod	every other day	T, Tbs, tbsp	tablespoon
QS	sufficient quantity	tab	tablet
Rx	prescription	tid	three times each day
S.C., SQ	subcutaneous	w/o, s̄	without
Sig	write on label	Ṫ	one
sol., soln	solution	⫶ĪĪ̇I	three
stat	immediately	ÏV̈	four

Common Drug-Related Abbreviations Worksheet

Use Student Handout 15-6 to translate the following orders using medical terminology. The first one has been done for you.

1. Toradol 10 mg

   T̄ tab q6h for inflammation #20

   Answer: Take one Toradol 10 mg tablet every 6 hours for inflammation. Dispense 20.

2. Provera 5 mg #30

   T̄ tab P.O. qd

   _____

   _____

3. Dyazide 37.5/25 #30

   T̄ cap P.O. qd

   _____

   _____

4. Lortab 7.5/500 #30

   T̄ tab P.O. q4–6h prn pain

   _____

   _____

5. Levoxyl 0.088 mg #30

   T̄ tab P.O. qd

   _____

   _____

6. Motrin 800 mg #90

   T̄ tab P.O. tid c food

   _____

   _____

7. Amoxicillin 500 mg #30

   T̄ cap P.O. tid × 10 days

   _____

   _____

8. Valium 25 mg #20

   $\dot{T}$ cap P.O. q4h prn pain

   _____

   _____

9. Timoptic .25% Ophthalmic Sol 10 cc

   $\dot{T}$gtt OU bid

   _____

   _____

Characteristics of Good Documentation

- Completed as soon as possible after activity being documented.

- Signed by health care worker who performed procedure, spoke with patient, etc.

- Numbers and measurements are written in actual figures rather than described as "small," "many," etc.

- Quotation marks used when reporting patient's statements.

- Dated.

- Legible.

- Clear and concise.

- Spelled correctly.

- Identified with patient's name.

- Written with approved abbreviations.

- Written using correct medical terminology.

- Findings are not duplicated.

- Written in blue or black ink, never in pencil.

- Contains only facts, not opinions or guesses.

- Completed without leaving empty lines.

- Patient's reactions to procedures included.

CHAPTER 16

Attitude and Personal Motivation

INTRODUCTION

Employers state over and over again that a positive attitude and good motivation are the most important attributes for success in the workplace. No matter how many technical skills graduates have, if they have poor attitudes, they will have difficulty finding and keeping good jobs. The following activities will help students recognize the importance of a positive attitude and help them understand how their own attitude affects their day-to-day lives, and assist them in developing self-motivation and a positive attitude.

ACTIVITY 16-1
PHILOSOPHIES OF LIFE

What Students Will Learn

- To think about different life philosophies.

What You Will Need

- Cards made from Student Handout 16-1, Quotes.
- Whiteboard, chalkboard, or flip chart and appropriate writing utensil.

What To Do

1. Write a life-philosophy quote on the board on a regular basis (daily, weekly, etc.). You may use a quote from Student Handout 16-1, Quotes, or choose one of your own.

Student Handout **16-1**

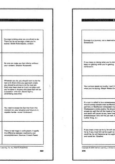

Student Handout **16-1**
(Continued)

Student Handout **16-1**
(Continued)

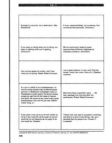

Student Handout **16-1**
(Continued)

Student Handout **16-1**
(Continued)

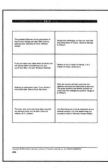

Student Handout **16-1**
(Continued)

2. Discuss the meaning of the quote with the students. Use this opportunity to help students understand positive attitudes and self-motivation.

3. Alternate activity: Cut apart the individual quotes on Student Handout 16-1 to make cards. Have each student randomly choose a card, read the quote out loud, and tell what he or she thinks it means.

Follow-up Discussion

1. What does each quote mean to you?

2. Do you think quotes might give you alternative views of life?

3. Why do people interpret quotes differently?

ACTIVITY 16-2
SELF-TALK

What Students Will Learn

- How negative and positive self-talk can affect what they do.

What You Will Need

- A copy of Student Handout 16-2, Self-Talk, for each student.
- Transparency 16-1, Self-Talk.

What To Do

1. Distribute Student Handout 16-2.

2. Ask students to change the negative self-talk to positive self-talk.

3. Use Transparency 16-1 to show examples of positive self-talk.

4. Ask students to share other negative self-talk and what they can use for positive self-talk.

Follow-up Discussion

1. How does self-talk affect your day-to-day life?

2. Do you think self-talk has an affect on your future success?

Transparency Master **16-1**

Transparency Master **16-1** *(Continued)*

Student Handout **16-2**

ACTIVITY 16-3
GIVE IT A POSITIVE SPIN

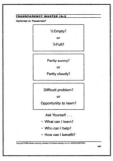

Transparency Master 16-2

Student Handout 16-3

What Students Will Learn

- To look for the positive in everyday problems and situations.

What You Will Need

- Transparency 16-2, Optimist or Pessimist?
- A copy of Student Handout 16-3, Make It Positive, for each student.
- A whiteboard, chalkboard, or flip chart and appropriate writing utensil.

What To Do

1. Using Transparency 16-2, discuss how difficult and disappointing situations can be handled either negatively or constructively—as either problems or as opportunities. For example, failing a test can serve as a wake-up call to learn better study habits, get needed help, or spend more time studying. A test is just that—a chance to see what we know before we are out working with patients.
2. Distribute Student Handout 16-3. The list of problems can be used in the following ways:
   - Divide the class into two teams. As you read off the problems, a member of each team goes to the board and writes as many ways the problem can be viewed positively he or she can think of in a designated period of time. The winner is the team with the most total positive views at the end of the game.
   - Divide the class into eight groups, one for each problem. Allow about 10 minutes for the groups to brainstorm positive views of their problem. The winning group is the one with the most positive views.
   - Pair off the students so they can give each other advice. One student says, "I have this problem . . . ." The other student offers advice and various ways to look at the problem. Students alternate until all situations have been used.

Follow-up Discussion

1. How many ideas did you generate working in groups (or pairs)?
2. What are some advantages of approaching difficult situations in this way?
3. Does getting angry or behaving negatively help improve difficult situations?

ACTIVITY 16-4
WHAT ARE MY STRENGTHS?

What Students Will Learn

- What others see in them that is good and positive.

What You Will Need

- Sheets of paper for each student.

What To Do

1. Have students list the names of the other students in the room on two sheets of paper, leaving a space between each name.
2. Instruct students to think of the nicest thing they can say about each of their classmates and write it down.

3. Collect the papers.
4. Type the name of each student on a separate piece of paper and list what everyone else said about that individual.
5. When complete, give each student his or her list.

Alternate activity: Have students use small pieces of paper, one for each classmate. This eliminates the need for typing lists.

Follow-up Discussion

1. Was it difficult to write something nice about each person?
2. Were some students more difficult than others? Why?
3. Did you find it easier to think of nice things about those you knew better, or did it not make any difference?
4. Are you surprised about what others have said about you?
5. Do you believe them?
6. Why do you think we have done this exercise? (Suggest that it gives each student something to use when he or she is feeling down or unmotivated.)

ACTIVITY 16-5
SUCCESS/FAILURE

What Students Will Learn

- To distinguish between succeeding and failing at something and being a success or failure as a person.

What You Will Need

- Whiteboard, chalkboard, or flip chart and appropriate writing utensil.

What To Do

1. Divide class into groups of four or five students.
2. Write the word "SUCCESS" on the board.
3. Allow 10 minutes for members of the group to share their ideas of what success means to them. Ask one member of each group to be a recorder and write down responses.
4. Have each recorder summarize his or her groups' definitions of success and write these on the board.
5. Next, write the word "FAILURE" on the board.
6. Allow 10 minutes for members of the group to discuss what failure means to them. Have the recorder takes notes and report as before.
7. Write the groups' definitions on the board.
8. Conduct a class discussion about the differences between success and failure and succeeding or failing as a person. Refer to the Follow-up Discussion questions.

Follow-up Discussion

1. Do you think succeeding or failing at something means that you have succeeded or failed as a person?
2. What does it mean to succeed or fail?

*A*CTIVITY 16-6
DREAM BOARD

What Students Will Learn

- To develop strategies for self-motivation.

What You Will Need

- Colored paper or cardstock.
- Magazines with lots of pictures.
- Scissors, glue, marking pens.

What To Do

1. Ask students to think about what is motivating them to pursue their education and become health care workers; for example, to provide a better life for their children, get a job that allows them to help people, buy a new car.
2. Ask them to bring something from home, such as a photograph of their children or a model car, or to look for appropriate pictures in magazines that illustrate their motivators. Explain that these will be used to make a display on a bulletin board or table entitled "Our Dream Board."
3. Allocate time during a class period for students to put together and set up their work.
4. Ask students to share their dreams with the class.

Follow-up Discussion

1. How do you think focusing on end results can help motivate you to study, and do what it takes to be a successful student?
2. What other ways do you think might help students motivate themselves to study and complete their education?

*A*CTIVITY 16-7
APPRECIATION

What Students Will Learn

- To develop a positive attitude by focusing on what's right about their lives.

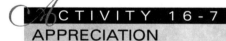

Student Handout **16-4**

What You Will Need

- A copy of Student Handout 16-4, Appreciation, for each student.

What To Do

1. Conduct a class discussion about how we sometimes see the world in terms of the negative instead of the positive. Ask students how often they think about all the things for which they can be grateful. Ask for examples of people who lack the life quality enjoyed by most Americans. Encourage them to think about places where the basics of life are difficult to find.
2. Distribute Student Handout 16-4.
3. Divide students into groups of three and ask them to discuss the questions on the handout.

Instructor's Note: If some of your students have particularly difficult living situations themselves, encourage them to think in terms of opportunities. You could also expand the exercise and have students think of ways they can help and support each other.

Follow-up Discussion

1. Were you able to list more opportunities and advantages than you expected?
2. What are some you would like to share with the class?
3. Do you believe that having opportunities brings with it the obligation to take advantage of them?
4. Can you think of examples of people who are successful in spite of difficulties, such as poverty and health problems?

ACTIVITY 16-8
HAPPINESS AND HEALTH

What Students Will Learn

- Results of recent research about the nature of happiness.
- How happiness is related to health and general well-being.

What You Will Need

- A copy of Student Handout 16-5, Happy Facts, for each student.

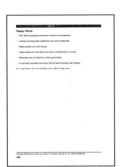

Student Handout **16-5**

What To Do

1. Conduct a short discussion about happiness and optimism (ask students to define), and how they have a positive impact on health and the immune system. (Research about the connection between happiness and health is starting to be accepted as a serious research topic.)
2. Distribute Student Handout 16-5. These statements were taken from a newspaper article reporting a study about happiness and optimism, which won a $250,000 award from the American Psychological Association.
3. The "Happy Facts" listed on the student handout can be used in the following ways:
   - Have students work in groups to make posters illustrating each "fact."
   - Conduct a class discussion and ask students whether they agree or disagree with the "facts" and to provide examples to support their opinions.

Follow-up Discussion

1. Conduct a class discussion to expand on the topic and include the role of humor and laughter in healing and recovery.

ACTIVITY 16-9
HAPPY SKITS

What Students Will Learn

- Proactive ways for people to increase their happiness.

What You Will Need

- A copy of Student Handout 16-6, Happiness-Building Strategies, for each student.

Student Handout **16-6**

What To Do

1. If you have not done Activity 16-5, conduct a short discussion about happiness and optimism (ask students to define) and how they have a positive impact on health and the immune system. If you have done Activity 16-5, proceed with this activity.
2. Distribute Handout 16-6. These statements were taken from a newspaper article reporting a study about happiness and optimism, which won a $250,000 award from the American Psychological Association.
3. Divide class into groups of two to five students.
4. Ask each group to choose a statement (or assign) and prepare a skit that presents and explains the idea.

Follow-up Discussion

1. Do you believe that people can choose to be happy?
2. What happens when people base their happiness on circumstances outside their control?

ACTIVITY 16-10
AFFIRMATIONS

What Students Will Learn

- To use affirmations to develop a positive self-image and achieve goals.

What You Will Need

- Transparency 16-3, Affirmations.

Transparency Master **16-3**

What To Do

1. Use Transparency 16-3 to introduce the concept of affirmations. Discuss the idea that people tend to become what they believe about themselves. Regarding self-fulfilling prophecies, a frequently used quotation from Henry Ford states something like this: "Whether you think you can or you can't, you're right." Discuss the concept of self-fulfilling prophecies.
2. Ask students to create two or three affirmations for themselves. These should be about things they hope for themselves or what they wish themselves to be. The statements do not have to be true. In fact, they should state something the student hopes for, but hasn't attained.
3. Ask students to conduct an experiment and say their affirmations aloud several times a day. Follow up in 2 or 3 weeks and ask students to report if they are feeling or acting any differently about what they've been affirming.

Follow-up Discussion

1. Conduct a discussion in which you invite students to share their experiences in trying affirmations.

Quotes

Cut along the dotted lines to make cards.

Life is about 10% how you make it . . . and 90% how you take it. (Unknown)	The more I want to get something done, the less I call it work. (Richard Bach)
Rings and jewels are not gifts, but apologies for gifts. The only true gift is a portion of thyself. (Ralph Waldo Emerson)	I've learned that going the extra mile puts you miles ahead of your competition. (*Live and Learn and Pass It On—Age 66*)
The greatest danger, that of losing one's own self, may pass off quietly as if it were nothing. Every other loss, that of an arm, a leg, five dollars, etc., is sure to be noticed. (Sören Kierkegaard)	It isn't evil that's running the earth, but mediocrity. The crime is not that Nero played while Rome burned, but that he played badly. (Ned Rorem)
Argue for your limitations, and sure enough, they're yours. (Richard Bach, *Illusions*)	You start growing up the day you have your first real laugh at yourself. (Unknown)
Diligence overcomes difficulties; sloth makes them. (Benjamin Franklin)	Wisdom is the reward you get for a lifetime of listening when you'd have preferred to talk. (Doug Larson)

You rise or fall, succeed or fail, by the image you hold in your own mind. (Unknown)	Only as high as I reach can I grow, Only as far as I seek can I go, Only as deep as I look can I see, Only as much as I dream can I be. (Karen Raun)
Test fast, fail fast, adjust fast. (Tom Peters, *In Pursuit of Excellence*)	The purpose of an organization is to make the strengths of people productive and their weaknesses irrelevant. (Peter Drucker)
What lies behind us and what lies before us are fine matters compared to what lies within us. (Ralph Waldo Emerson)	The difference between ordinary and extraordinary is that little extra. (Unknown)
Always bear in mind that your own resolution to succeed is more important than any other one thing. (Abraham Lincoln)	The future belongs to those who believe in the beauty of their dreams. (Eleanor Roosevelt)
Enthusiasm makes ordinary people extraordinary. (Unknown)	The reward of a thing well done is to have done it. (Ralph Waldo Emerson)

Destiny is not a matter of change, it is a matter of choice. (Unknown)

Courage is doing what you are afraid to do. There can be no courage unless you're scared. (Eddie Rickenbacker, aviator)

The price of greatness is responsibility. (Winston Churchill)

No one can make you feel inferior without your consent. (Eleanor Roosevelt)

The quality of a person's life is in direct proportion to their commitment to excellence, regardless of their chosen field of endeavor. (Vincent T. Lombardi)

Whatever you do, you should want to be the best at it. Every time you approach a task, you should be aiming to do the best job that's ever been done at it and not stop until you've done it. Anyone who does that will be successful—and rich. (David Ogilvy, advertising executive)

We are very short on people who know how to do anything. So please don't set out to make money. Set out to make something and hope you get rich in the process. (Andy Rooney)

You need to accept the fact that from this moment on, your situation and future is in capable hands—YOURS! (Unknown)

Be a yardstick of quality. Some people aren't used to an environment where excellence is expected. (Stephen Jobs, co-founder, Apple Computer Corp.)

There is real magic in enthusiasm. It spells the difference between mediocrity and accomplishment. (Norman Vincent Peale)

Success is a journey, not a destination. (Ben Sweetland)

It is our responsibilities, not ourselves, that we should take seriously. (Unknown)

If you keep on doing what you're doing, you keep on getting what you're getting. (Unknown)

We are continually faced by great opportunities brilliantly disguised as insoluble problems. (Unknown)

Your actions speak so loudly, I can't hear what you're saying. (Ralph Waldo Emerson)

I am a great believer in luck, and I find the harder I work, the more I have of it. (Stephen Leacock)

If a man is called to be a streetsweeper, he should sweep streets even as Michelangelo painted, or Beethoven composed music, or Shakespeare wrote poetry. He should sweep streets so well that all the hosts of heaven and earth will pause to say, here lived a great streetsweeper who did his job well. (Martin Luther King, Jr.)

Bad times have a scientific value . . . We learn geology the morning after the earthquake. (Ralph Waldo Emerson)

If you treat a man as he is, he will remain as he is; if you treat him as he ought to be and could be, he will become as he ought to be and could be. (Goethe)

There's only one way to succeed in anything, and that is to give it everything. I do, and I demand that my players do. (Vincent T. Lombardi)

The last of the human freedoms—to choose one's attitude in any given set of circumstances, to choose one's own way. (Viktor Frankl)

The words "I am . . . " are potent words; be careful what you hitch them to. The thing you're claiming has a way of reaching back and claiming you. (A. L. Kitselman)

I would prefer even to fail with honor than win by cheating. (Sophocles)

Only those who dare to fail greatly can ever achieve greatly. (Robert F. Kennedy)

Everything that irritates us about others can lead us to an understanding of ourselves. (Carl Jung)

The secret of joy in work is contained in one word—*Excellence.* To know how to do something well is to enjoy it. (Pearl Buck)

Learning is not attained by chance, it must be sought for with ardor and attended to with diligence. (Abigail Adams)

When facing a difficult task, act as though it is impossible to fail. If you're going after Moby Dick, take along the tartar sauce. (Unknown)

I think and think for months and years. Ninety-nine times, the conclusion is false. The hundredth time I am right. (Albert Einstein)

Take charge of your attitude. Don't let someone else choose it for you. (Unknown)

The greatest discovery of my generation is that human beings can alter their lives by altering their attitudes of mind. (William Jones)

Accept the challenges, so that you may feel the exhilaration of victory. (General George S. Patton)

If you can keep your head when all about you are losing theirs and blaming it on you . . . you'll be a Man, my son! (Rudyard Kipling)

Destiny is not a matter of chance, it is a matter of choice. (Unknown)

Nothing is particularly hard, if you divide it into small jobs. (Henry Ford, Ray Kroc)

Only the curious will learn and only the resolute overcome the obstacles to learning. The quest quotient has always excited me more than the intelligence quotient. (Eugene S. Wilson)

The man who wins may have been counted out several times, but he didn't hear the referee. (H. E. Jansen)

Any fact facing us is not as important as our attitude toward it, for that determines our success or failure. (Norman Vincent Peale)

Self-Talk

For each negative self-talk, write positive words you can use instead.

1. Negative: I'll never get this finished.

   Positive: _____

2. Negative: If I miss this, I've really blown it.

   Positive: _____

3. Negative: Why am I so anxious, I hate feeling like this.

   Positive: _____

4. Negative: I know (name) can do a better job than me.

   Positive: _____

5. Negative: I must get going, I must hurry.

   Positive: _____

6. Negative: I'll probably just fail anyway.

   Positive: _____

7. Negative: What will people think if I fall behind? No one will say anything, but I just know what they'll think!

   Positive: _____

8. Negative: What's the best way to proceed? A mistake may cost me too much time to get finished.

   Positive: _____

9. Negative: I hate myself.

   Positive: _____

10. Negative: I may as well stay home, I've already missed three days of class.

    Positive: _____

11. Negative: I'm never going to learn this stuff!

    Positive: _____

12. Negative: Everyone is so much younger than me. I'll never be able to get through this program.

    Positive: _____

13. Negative: It's been so long since I've been in school, I don't know if I remember how to study.

    Positive: _____

Make It Positive

Can You Give These a Positive Spin?

1. Your medical terminology class is more difficult than you expected.

2. The patient you've been assigned to work with is cranky and difficult.

3. The concert you were going to attend with friends has been cancelled.

4. You didn't get the job you applied for.

5. Your instructor has assigned you to work in a group with people you don't know.

6. Your best friend is moving to a town fifty miles away.

7. You failed your last test in pharmacology.

8. You didn't get the instructor you wanted for an important class that you must pass in order to graduate.

Appreciation

Develop an inventory of things the members of your group have to be thankful for. Expand on the ideas listed and add others.

- Good health

- Access to medical care

- Friends

- Family

- Opportunity to attend school

- Decent living conditions

- Sufficient food

- Mental ability to succeed in school

- Freedom to choose a lifestyle and occupation

Happy Facts

- Only 10% of happiness comes from individual circumstances.

- Actively pursuing goals is believed to be a key to happiness.

- Happy people have more energy.

- Happy people are more likely to be hired—and less likely to be fired.

- Happiness does not depend on winning the lottery.

- In one study, optimists were about half as likely to develop heart disease.

(From Susan Ferraro, New York Daily News article. 7/7/02 San Diego Union)

Happiness-Building Strategies

1. Do things. Be active.

2. Remember the big picture: where do you want to be in 5 years? 10? 20?

3. Don't compare yourself to others.

4. Don't regret decisions you've made. Instead, learn from them and move on.

5. Be kind to others.

6. Schedule time to appreciate what you have.

7. Stop obsessing about problems or negatives. Substitute positive thoughts.

(From Susan Ferraro. New York Daily News article. 7/7/02 San Diego Union)

Work with your group to make up a skit or other creative presentation that explains and demonstrates one of the strategies listed. The presentation can be funny or serious. Here are a few examples of what you can do:

- A conversation between friends

- A problem that people in the group handle in different ways

- A family situation showing how the individuals respond

- A poem

- A song

Self-Talk

1. Negative: I'll never get this finished.

   Positive: Just take it one step at a time.

2. Negative: If I miss this, I've really blown it.

   Positive: What can I do to make this up or get the information ahead of time?

3. Negative: Why am I so anxious? I hate feeling like this.

   Positive: I need to take a breath and only deal with that which I can take care of at this moment.

4. Negative: I know (name) can do a better job than me.

   Positive: We each have our own strengths. I will do the best I can. That is all that is important.

5. Negative: I must get going, I must hurry.

   Positive: I will do what I can reasonably do for today and not push to get more done.

6. Negative: I'll probably just fail anyway.

   Positive: I believe in myself and will do the best I can. If I fail, I'll get help and try again.

7. Negative: What will people think if I fall behind? No one will say anything, but I just know what they will think!

   Positive: No matter what I do I can't control what others think of me. I will do my best and feel good about what I have accomplished.

8. Negative: What's the best way to proceed? A mistake may cost me too much time to get finished.

   Positive: I know I can do this. Mistakes happen. Let the future take care of itself.

9. Negative: I hate myself.

   Positive: I did some great things today that I can be proud of. *Or,* I like myself.

10. Negative: I may as well stay home. I've already missed 3 days of class.

    Positive: I have set this education goal for myself and I'm not going to let anything get in my way.

11. Negative: I'm never going to learn this stuff!

    Positive: I will learn this in small, manageable pieces at a time

12. Negative: Everyone is so much younger than me. I'll never be able to get through this program.

    Positive: I have more life experiences than the others and can contribute a lot to the class.

13. Negative: It's been so long since I've been in school, I don't know if I remember how to study.

    Positive: I will take this one step at a time and use all the help the school and my classmates offer me.

Optimist or Pessimist?

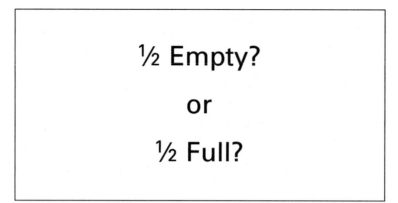

½ Empty?

or

½ Full?

Partly sunny?

or

Partly cloudy?

Difficult problem?

or

Opportunity to learn?

Ask Yourself . . .

- What can I learn?

- Who can I help?

- How can I benefit?

Affirmations

1. State them in the present tense.

2. Include your name.

3. Keep them positive.

4. Say them aloud several times a day.

Examples

I, Maria, am a capable student.

I, Jasmine, am a successful nursing assistant.

I, Hal, am a caring person.

CHAPTER 17

Time Management and Goal Setting

INTRODUCTION

Success in school, work, and our personal lives depends on the ability to set goals and manage our time effectively so we can meet those goals. If we go through life without knowing where we are going (without goals), we will be unable to make positive decisions for our families and ourselves. Goals help us stay focused so we can achieve things we might have thought were unachievable.

Good time management helps us to organize our busy lives so we can work on reaching our goals. It requires us to have an understanding of how we really spend our time each day and how we can utilize that time more effectively. The following activities will help students set realistic goals without becoming overwhelmed by the process. And they will aid students in evaluating and developing their own time management skills.

ACTIVITY 17-1
RUMBA

What Students Will Learn

- To write effective personal goals.*

What You Will Need

Student Handout **17-1**

- Transparencies 17-1, RUMBA: Characteristics of Effective Goals, and 17-2, Example of an Effective Goal.
- A copy of Student Handout 17-1, Goal Worksheet, for each student.

What To Do

1. Using Transparency 17-1, discuss the characteristics of effective goals.
2. Use Transparency 17-2 to show an example of an effective goal and its RUMBA analysis.
3. Distribute Student Handout 17-1.
4. Ask students to write goals, using the handout as a guide. (This may be done as homework.)

---

*Source: Adapted from B. Napier-Tibere & L. Haroun (2004). *Occupational therapy fieldwork survival guide: Strategies for success.* Philadelphia: F. A. Davis Company.

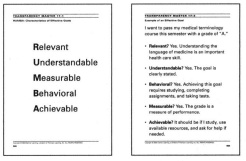

Transparency Master **17-1**   Transparency Master **17-2**

Follow-up Discussion

1. Conduct a general discussion about how written goals have been found to help people stay on track and be successful.
2. Ask students to share their experiences writing and achieving their goals.

ACTIVITY 17-2
SIMPLE GOAL SETTING

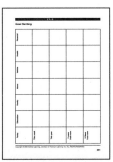

Student Handout **17-2**

What Students Will Learn

- To set short- and long-term goals.

What You Will Need

- A copy of Student Handout 17-2, Goal Setting, for each student.
- Transparency 17-3, Goal Setting.

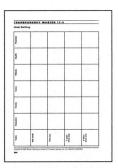

Transparency Master **17-3**

What To Do

1. Use Transparency 17-3 to demonstrate chart completion by writing sample goals in the squares.
2. Distribute Student Handout 17-2 and have students fill it in.
3. Have students share their goals and discuss in class.

Follow-up Discussion:

1. Are the goals specific enough?
2. Do they follow RUMBA?
3. Do they give a time frame?
4. Did students have trouble setting goals?
5. Which were harder, short- or long-term goals? Do any of the short-term goals help the student reach a long-term goal?

ACTIVITY 17-3
SHARE YOUR GOOD NEWS!

What Students Will Learn

- To clarify their 5-year goals.
- To set realistic goals.
- To be specific when goal setting.

What You Will Need

- No special materials are required for this activity.

What To Do

1. Discuss important goal-setting rules with students. These should include being realistic (but not being afraid to dream) and being specific.
2. Ask students to pretend it is 5 years in the future. They have graduated from school and have their dream job. Other areas of their lives are working just the way they want them to be.
3. Have students write a letter to a friend catching them up on what has been happening. Students should share news about their graduations, jobs, homes, relationships, cars, and the like.
4. Tell students to be as specific as possible. For instance, they should describe their car using make, model, year, color, and other specific details. Job information should include where they work, what they earn, what they do, and so on.
5. The letter should include all of the areas the student might want to have set goals for. Since it is 5 years in the future, the students should write as if they have achieved those goals.
6. Ask student volunteers to read their letters to the class.

Follow-up Discussion

1. Were the goals specific enough?
2. Did they tell what would happen or what would be different?
3. Did they tell how much or how many?
4. How can picturing your life in the future help you achieve that life?

ACTIVITY 17-4
ACTION PLANS

What Students Will Learn

- To create action plans to help them achieve their goals.

What You Will Need

- A copy of Student Handout 17-3, Action Plan Worksheet, for each student.

Student Handout **17-3**

What To Do

1. Discuss with students the need to determine the actions required to achieve their goal. These actions may include seeking information or asking for help. For the goal, pass medical terminology, the student might check out additional terminology books from the school library, make flash cards, listen to tapes, schedule regular study hours for this subject, seek help from the instructor, or join a study group. Action plans may consist of steps with target dates for completion. They are like stepping stones to goals.
2. Distribute Student Handout 17-3 and ask students to write action plans for the goals they wrote in Activity 17-1.
3. Designate a date in the future for students to be prepared to discuss their goals and action plans.

Follow-up Discussion

1. Were you able to follow through with your action plans?
2. If yes, how did you find them helpful?
3. If no, why do you think they did not work for you?
4. What are other methods you might utilize to achieve your goals?

ACTIVITY 17-5
HITCH YOUR GOALS TO THE STARS

What Students Will Learn

- To encourage themselves by displaying and sharing their goals with others.

Student Handout **17-4**

What You Will Need

- A copy of Student Handout 17-4, Star Pattern, for each student.
- Materials for making stars: Colored or plain cardstock, aluminum foil, plain paper for labels, tape or glue.
- Scissors for each student.

What To Do

1. Discuss with students the importance of believing that they can achieve their goals. Explain that it can be helpful to see the goals in written form and to share them with others.
2. Distribute Student Handout 17-4 and the supplies to make stars. Ask students to make one or two stars for goals they are willing to share with the class. The goals are written on the star or, if using aluminum to cover the card stock to make silver stars, on a label that is glued or taped to the star.
3. When students have completed their stars, ask them to share with the class, then put up the stars on a bulletin board or on the walls around the classroom.

Follow-up Discussion

1. Conduct a discussion about how seeing written goals can motivate us to put in the work necessary to achieve them.

ACTIVITY 17-6
THE UNIVERSE GOT IN MY WAY

What Students Will Learn

- Dealing with unexpected problems that interfere with reaching one's goals.

Student Handout **17-5**

What You Will Need

- Student Handout 17-5, Achieving Your Goals.

What To Do

1. Distribute Student Handout 17-5. Have each student choose a personal goal. If they have already done this in another activity, they may choose one of those goals. An alternative is for you to choose a goal such as graduating from school, completing your course, earning a certain grade in your course, and the like.

2. Have students write a short summary of the goal.
3. Next have students write three things that could keep them from achieving that goal (obstacles).
4. Have them write three ways to overcome these obstacles.
5. Ask students to share their obstacles and solutions.

Follow-up Discussion:

1. Can other students think of additional ways to overcome the problems?
2. How can friends, family, and a support group be included as part of the solution?

ACTIVITY 17-7
REACHING MY GOALS

What Students Will Learn

- Setting objectives that will help them reach their stated goals.*

What You Will Need

- Students: Their completed copies of Student Handout 17-2 from Activity 17-2.

What To Do

1. Explain to students that once goals are set, they will need a plan to reach those goals. For instance, if the goal is to become more physically fit, they will have to decide to set aside time several days each week to exercise. They will also have to decide what type of exercise to do and how much is needed to reach their goal. This analysis will help them to set objectives.
2. Have students write each of their goals (from Student Handout 17-2, if done) on a piece of paper. For each goal, have students write an objective that tells what will change or be different, how it will be different (by how many), and when it will be done. For example, if the goal is to complete school in 4 months, the student might write "Objective: Complete one class per month for four months."
3. For each goal, ask students to underline what will change, put a triangle around how it will be different, and a circle around when.
4. When completed, conduct a class discussion using the follow-up discussion questions.

Instructor's Note: Remind students that goals are not static. They can be changed as often as the students want.

Follow-up Discussion:

1. Was it hard to write objectives?
2. Were they able to include the three criteria in each objective?
3. Did this exercise help them to see their goals as more or less realistic?
4. Do they want to change any of the goals?

Source: Mindy Bingham (1987). *Mother daughter choices.* Santa Barbara, CA: Advocacy Press. Copyright © Girls Incorporated of Greater Santa Barbara. Reprinted with permission of Advocacy Press, P.O. Box 236, Santa Barbara, CA 93102. Not to be duplicated in any other form.

ACTIVITY 17-8
SHARING HELPFUL HINTS

What Students Will Learn

- Strategies for personal organization and time management.

What You Will Need

- At least one 3 × 5 card for each student.

What To Do

1. Give each student at least one 3 × 5 card.
2. Ask the students to write one organization or time management tip that works for them on the card(s). (Examples: do all gift shopping for each month or two months at one time; keep study flash cards in purse or pocket and review when waiting for bus, dentist, and so on.)
3. Collect the cards. Each class session, draw a card or two and share with the class. Ask the student who contributed the idea to expand.
4. Alternate version: Post the cards on a bulletin board. Give students a week to take a look at the cards and vote for the best idea. (You could number the cards to keep track of the votes.) Tally the votes and award a small prize to the creator of the winning entry.

Follow-up Discussion

1. Conduct a discussion about the importance of developing good personal organization habits for school and workplace success.

ACTIVITY 17-9
HOW DO I SPEND MY TIME?

What Students Will Learn

- To analyze their time management during one week.
- How time may be better spent.

What You Will Need

- A copy of Student Handout 17-6, Time Tracker, and 17-7, Time Tracker Questions, for each student.
- Transparency 17-4, Time Tracker.

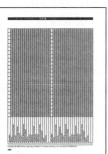

Student Handout **17-6**

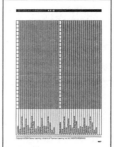

Student Handout **17-6**
(Continued)

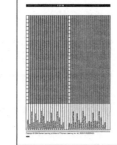

Student Handout **17-6**
(Continued)

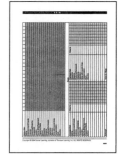

Student Handout **17-6**
(Continued)

Student Handout **17-6**
(Continued)

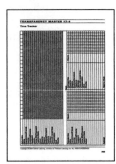

Transparency Master **17-4**

Student Handout **17-7**

What To Do

1. Explain to students that we each have 168 hours in each week. During the next week, students will track how they spend their time during those 168 hours.
2. Distribute Student Handout 17-6 and ask students to spend the next week recording how they spend their time.
3. You may want to use Transparency 17-4 to help students understand how to track their time.
4. Students may want to color code the chart for easier analysis. For example, use blue to mark hours spent sleeping, red for hours in class, green for meal preparation, yellow for entertainment, and so on.
5. Encourage students to be as specific as possible, indicating time spent on the telephone, in front of the TV, meeting with friends, studying, getting ready before going to school/work, with children, at worship, transportation, and the like.
6. At the end of the week, distribute Student Handout 17-7 and ask students to analyze their charts by answering the questions on the handout. You may have students answer these questions in writing or have a class discussion.

Follow-up Discussion

1. What kind of short-term goal can you set to improve your time management?

ACTIVITY 17-10
MANAGING YOUR PRECIOUS TIME

What Students Will Learn

- How effectively they manage their time.

What You Will Need

- A copy of Student Handout 17-8, Managing Your Precious Time, for each student.
- Transparency 17-5, Time Savers/Time Wasters.

What To Do

1. Distribute Student Handout 17-8 and have students complete it.
2. Display Transparency 17-5 and ask students to consider how the statements shown apply to the way they spend their time. During the discussion they should refer to their answers on the handout to see how they can apply this information.
3. Have students write down twenty jobs they are responsible for at home, at work, at school (such as paying bills, banking, writing papers, preparing meals, etc.)
4. Tell the students to underline the three jobs they enjoy doing most and to circle the three items that someone else could be paid for, assigned, or asked to do.
5. Remind students that asking for help is a great start to time management.

Follow-up Discussion:

1. Were you able to think of some time saving tips for yourself?
2. Was it easier to think of tips for yourself or for others?

Student Handout **17-8**

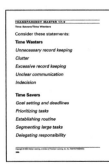

Transparency Master **17-5**

3. What is the most valuable tip you can think of?

4. What is your most difficult time waster to change?

ACTIVITY 17-11
PROCRASTINATION

What Students Will Learn

- Why people procrastinate.
- To break the procrastination habit.

What You Will Need

- Whiteboard, chalkboard, or flip chart and appropriate writing utensil.

What To Do

1. You may work with students as one large group.

2. Ask students to share with the class times when they procrastinate. Write their statements on one half of the board as they are offered. (Examples include putting tax information together, studying, large school reports or projects, cleaning house, exercising.)

3. Now ask students why they think people procrastinate and write these on the second half of the board. (Examples include too much to do, they are perfectionists and are sure they can't get it perfect, it's boring, it's hard, there are more fun things to do.)

4. Lead a discussion about strategies students have used or can use in the future to help them "kick the procrastination habit."

Follow-up Discussion:

1. How might your life change if you overcome your habit to procrastinate?

REFERENCES

Bingham, M., Stryker, S., & Edmondson, J. (1987). *Mother daughter choices*. Santa Barbara, CA: Advocacy Press.

Napier-Tibere, B., & Haroun, L. (2004). *Occupational therapy fieldwork survival guide: Strategies for success*. Philadelphia: F. A. Davis Company.

Goal Worksheet

Write a goal you would like to achieve by the end of the next 4 weeks. Then write a brief description of how it meets the criteria of RUMBA.

Goal _____

_____

_____

Targeted Completion Date _____

Relevant? _____

_____

_____

Understandable? _____

_____

_____

Measurable? _____

_____

_____

Behavioral? _____

_____

_____

Achievable? _____

_____

_____

Goal Setting

	Education	Family	Home	Vehicle	Health	Financial
Today						
This week						
This year						
2 years from now						
5 Years from now						

Action Plans Worksheet

Write an action plan for a goal.

Goal _____

_____

_____

Targeted Completion Date _____

Action Step #1

_____

Targeted Completion Date (if appropriate) _____

Resources or help needed _____

_____

_____

Action Step #2

_____

Targeted Completion Date (if appropriate) _____

Resources or help needed _____

_____

_____

Action Step #3

_____

Targeted Completion Date (if appropriate) _____

Resources or help needed _____

_____

_____

Star Pattern

Achieving Your Goals

Write a brief description of a goal that is important to you.

List Possible Obstacles	List Ways to Overcome Obstacles
1.	
2.	
3.	

Time Tracker

Use the attached time tracker to record your time use for 1 week.

1. Next to each day of the week, write the hours of the day beginning with the time you wake up. For example, if you wake at 6 A.M. on Monday, put a 6 in the larger box to the right of Monday. Track your activities by shading in the small boxes to represent 15-minute segments.

2. Your week has a total of 168 hours

3. At the end of the week, calculate how much total time you have spent on each activity and mark this information in the total columns at the bottom of the last page of the handout.

4. Tracking your time should help you see if you are spending too much time on time wasters such as watching television or chatting on the telephone.

Sunday
Eating
Entertainment/Friends
Exercise
Grooming/Dressing
Housework
Laundry
Paying Bills/Paperwork
Preparing Meals
School
Shopping
Sleeping
Studying/Homework
Telephone
Television
Time with Loved Ones
Transportation
Work
Worship

Monday
Eating
Entertainment/Friends
Exercise
Grooming/Dressing
Housework
Laundry
Paying Bills/Paperwork
Preparing Meals
School
Shopping
Sleeping
Studying/Homework
Telephone
Television
Time with Loved Ones
Transportation
Work
Worship

Tuesday

Eating
Entertainment/Friends
Exercise
Grooming/Dressing
Housework
Laundry
Paying Bills/Paperwork
Preparing Meals
School
Shopping
Sleeping
Studying/Homework
Telephone
Television
Time with Loved Ones
Transportation
Work
Worship

Wednesday

Eating
Entertainment/Friends
Exercise
Grooming/Dressing
Housework
Laundry
Paying Bills/Paperwork
Preparing Meals
School
Shopping
Sleeping
Studying/Homework
Telephone
Television
Time with Loved Ones
Transportation
Work
Worship

Thursday
Eating
Entertainment/Friends
Exercise
Grooming/Dressing
Housework
Laundry
Paying Bills/Paperwork
Preparing Meals
School
Shopping
Sleeping
Studying/Homework
Telephone
Television
Time with Loved Ones
Transportation
Work
Worship

Friday
Eating
Entertainment/Friends
Exercise
Grooming/Dressing
Housework
Laundry
Paying Bills/Paperwork
Preparing Meals
School
Shopping
Sleeping
Studying/Homework
Telephone
Television
Time with Loved Ones
Transportation
Work
Worship

Saturday

Eating
Entertainment/Friends
Exercise
Grooming/Dressing
Housework
Laundry
Paying Bills/Paperwork
Preparing Meals
School
Shopping
Sleeping
Studying/Homework
Telephone
Television
Time with Loved Ones
Transportation
Work
Worship

Categories	Hours
Eating	
Entertainment/Friends	
Exercise	
Grooming/Dressing	
Housework	
Laundry	
Paying Bills/Paperwork	
Preparing Meals	
School	
Subtotal	

Totals

Categories	Hours
Shopping	
Sleeping	
Studying/Homework	
Telephone	
Television	
Time with Loved Ones	
Transportation	
Work	
Worship	
Total for Week	

Time Tracker Questions

Review the Time Tracker chart you kept for one week, and answer the following questions.

1. How hard was it to keep the chart?

2. Were you surprised by what you learned? How?

3. Are there places you tend to waste time?

4. How much time did you spend on relaxation or fun?

5. Are you happy with the way your time is spent? Why or why not?

6. What items are you spending too much time on?

7. What are you doing that does not need to be done at all?

8. What are you spending too little time on?

9. What are you doing that could be done better (more economically, more effectively) by others?

10. Where can you make your most important time savings?

11. How can you avoid overusing the time of others?

Managing Your Precious Time

Survey of Time-Management and Organizational Habits

There are three steps to time management:

1. Establish your goals.
2. Analyze your present time usage.
3. Establish procedures to allow you to achieve your goals.

Write the number in the blank that best reflects your habits.

4 = almost always   3 = often   2 = sometimes   1 = seldom   0 = never

_____ 1. Do you have a regular written schedule you attempt to follow?

_____ 2. Do you know how much time you average each week for various responsibilities you have?

_____ 3. Do you assign specific periods of time for each activity during the week?

_____ 4. Do you find that you are well-prepared for special events?

_____ 5. Do you use small amounts of time productively?

_____ 6. Do you plan ahead so that it is not necessary to rush around at the last minute to meet deadlines?

_____ 7. Do you allow time in your schedule for regular relaxation and recreation?

_____ 8. Do you watch fewer than 2 hours of TV per day on the average?

_____ 9. Do you feel that you have a good balance between home and work responsibilities?

_____ 10. Do you know what you plan to accomplish and generally how you plan to do it before you start on a given task?

_____ 11. Do you feel that you work to your fullest potential?

_____ 12. Do you adjust your priorities and complete required work so that you don't worry about your job while you are on vacation?

_____ 13. Is your work area organized and functional?

_____ 14. Do you know what you have done at the end of each day?

_____ 15. Do you control or direct distractions and interruptions so that you can complete your work?

_____ 16. Do you know what to do next?

_____ 17. Do you emphasize major ideas and goals rather than minor, insignificant details?

_____ 18. Can you find any items you have at home or at work in 5 minutes or less?

_____ 19. Do you clear your desk, notebook, or work area at least once each week?

_____ 20. Can you adjust your schedule when unexpected events arise and then return to complete you work?

_____ Total (maximum total is 80)

Scoring

75–80 points— Excellent, congratulations! You manage your time well.
60–74 points—Good. A little more effort needed.
45–59 points—Fair. You need to analyze your time usage and take control of your time.
30–44 points—Poor. Your life could be easier if you learn some time management.

RUMBA: Characteristics of Effective Goals

Relevant

Understandable

Measurable

Behavioral

Achievable

I want to pass my medical terminology course this semester with a grade of "A."

- **Relevant?** Yes. Understanding the language of medicine is an important health care skill.

- **Understandable?** Yes. The goal is clearly stated.

- **Behavioral?** Yes. Achieving this goal requires studying, completing assignments, and taking tests.

- **Measurable?** Yes. The grade is a measure of performance.

- **Achievable?** It should be if I study, use available resources, and ask for help if needed.

Goal Setting

	Financial	Health	Vehicle	Home	Family	Education
Today						
This week						
This year						
2 years from now						
5 Years from now						

Time Tracker

Saturday

Categories	Hours
Eating	
Entertainment/Friends	
Exercise	
Grooming/Dressing	
Housework	
Laundry	
Paying Bills/Paperwork	
Preparing Meals	
School	
Shopping	
Sleeping	
Studying/Homework	
Telephone	
Television	
Time with Loved Ones	
Transportation	
Work	
Worship	

Totals

Categories	Hours	Categories	Hours
Eating		Shopping	
Entertainment/Friends		Sleeping	
Exercise		Studying/Homework	
Grooming/Dressing		Telephone	
Housework		Television	
Laundry		Time with Loved Ones	
Paying Bills/Paperwork		Transportation	
Preparing Meals		Work	
School		Worship	
Subtotal		Total for Week	

Consider these statements:

Time Wasters

Unnecessary record keeping

Clutter

Excessive record keeping

Unclear communication

Indecision

Time Savers

Goal setting and deadlines

Prioritizing tasks

Establishing routine

Segmenting large tasks

Delegating responsibility

CHAPTER 18

Work Habits, Ethics, and Confidentiality

INTRODUCTION

Medical ethics and confidentiality are two concepts that can be confusing for some students. One's ethnic or cultural background or upbringing may influence one's view of what is ethical and what information should be kept confidential. But in a medical office, there are specific guidelines and laws that must be followed closely. The activities included here will help students understand their own views of ethics and confidentiality as well as what is appropriate in the typical health care facility.

ACTIVITY 18-1
IF I WERE THE BOSS

What Students Will Learn

- Employee behaviors that are important to employers.
- The impact employee behavior can have on others in the workplace.

What You Will Need

- A copy of Student Handout 18-1, If I Were the Boss, for each student.

What To Do

1. Distribute Student Handout 18-1.
2. Divide class into groups of three to five students.
3. Give groups about 15 minutes to discuss the questions on the handout.

Student Handout **18-1**

Follow-up Discussion

1. Did this exercise help you understand the employer's point of view when dealing with employee behaviors? Explain your answer.
2. What effect can an individual employee's actions have on others in the workplace?
3. Why is it important for employers to encourage positive behaviors and work habits?

ACTIVITY 18-2
IF I WERE THE PATIENT

What Students Will Learn

- To consider health care employee behaviors from the patient's perspective.
- To understand the impact of employee behavior on patients.

What You Will Need

- A copy of Student Handout 18-2, If I Were the Patient, for each student.

Student Handout 18-2

What To Do

1. Distribute Student Handout 18-2.
2. Divide class into groups of three to five students.
3. Give groups about 15 minutes to discuss the questions on the handout.

Follow-up Discussion

1. Did this exercise help you understand the patient's point of view when dealing with employee behaviors? Explain your answer.
2. What effect can an individual employee's actions have on patients?
3. Do you believe that patient health and recovery can be influenced by the attitudes of health care workers? Explain your answer.
4. What are some characteristics of health care workers that are important when working with all patients?

ACTIVITY 18-3
OUTSTANDING EMPLOYEES

What Students Will Learn

- The behaviors exhibited by outstanding employees.

What You Will Need

- No special materials are required for this activity.

What To Do

1. Conduct a brainstorming session with the class to create a list of the 10 most important characteristics of a health care employee. Encourage the class to suggest as many as possible. (If students are unfamiliar with brainstorming, refer to Activity 11-8.)
2. Work as a group to choose the final 10, asking students to explain and defend their choices.
3. Post the final list on the wall.

Follow-up Discussion

1. How do you plan to develop the skills and attitudes you have identified for outstanding employees?
2. What can you do now while you are in school to practice these workplace behaviors?

ACTIVITY 18-4
IT'S THE LAW

What Students Will Learn

- Facts about a variety of federal employment laws.

What You Will Need

- A copy of Student Handout 18-3, Oral Presentation Guidelines, for each student.

Student Handout **18-3**

What To Do

1. Divide class into five groups (one for each law).
2. Assign one of the following laws to each group:
   - Americans with Disabilities Act
   - Civil Rights Act of 1964
   - Equal Pay Act of 1963
   - Family Medical Leave Act
   - Occupational Safety and Health Act
3. Tell students they are to work in their groups to prepare an oral presentation for the class about their assigned law.
4. Distribute Student Handout 18-3 to each student for use in their groups as a guide in preparing their reports.

Follow-up Discussion

1. Why is it important for employees to understand the basics of major employment laws?
2. Who do you think you should talk with first if you have a problem at work?

ACTIVITY 18-5
SEXUAL HARASSMENT QUESTIONNAIRE

What Students Will Learn

- Facts about the nature of sexual harassment.

What You Will Need

- A copy of Student Handouts 18-4, Sexual Harassment Questionnaire, and 18-5, Facts About Sexual Harassment, for each student.
- Transparency 18-1, Facts About Sexual Harassment.

Student Handout **18-4**   Student Handout **18-5**   Transparency Master **18-1**

What To Do

1. Distribute Handout 18-4 and ask students to answer the questions.
2. When they have completed the questionnaire, discuss the nature of sexual harassment using Transparency 18-1.
3. Distribute Student Handout 18-5 for future reference.

Follow-up Discussion

1. What might be the consequences of sexual harassment in the health care workplace?
2. What can you do to discourage sexual harassment?
3. What can you do to avoid being accused of sexual harassment?

Instructor's Note: More information about sexual harassment is available at http://www.eeoc.gov/facts/fs-sex.html.

ACTIVITY 18-6
RUMORS

What Students Will Learn

- How information can become distorted as it is passed from one person to the next.

What You Will Need

- No special materials are required for this activity.

What To Do

1. Explain that students will be playing a version of the telephone game, which many of them will already know, in which one student starts by whispering something to the next student. The message is passed around the room until it reaches the last person who says aloud what he or she hears.
2. Start by asking students to each think of a medically related message to pass on. It might be instructions for taking a medication, facts about a patient, or the like. Allow as many students to start their "rumor" as time permits to play the game.

Follow-up Discussion

1. How does this game demonstrate the importance of clear communication when interacting with patients and co-workers?
2. How does it demonstrate the danger of sharing unnecessary or confidential information about others, especially patients?
3. How can rumors damage interpersonal relationships in the workplace?
4. Why is it important to speak directly to people if you are having problems with them instead of complaining to others?

ACTIVITY 18-7
ETHICAL PRINCIPLES

What Students Will Learn

- Eight guiding principles of health care ethics.

What You Will Need

- A copy of Student Handout 18-6, Eight Guiding Principles of Health Care Ethics, for each student.
- Transparency Master 18-2, Eight Guiding Principles of Health Care Ethics.
- Instructor Sheet 18-1, Application of Ethics by Health Care Workers.

What To Do

1. Distribute Student Handout 18-6.
2. Divide class into eight groups, one for each of the ethical principles.
3. Assign one principle to each group.
4. Ask students to discuss their principle, what they think it means, and how it applies to health care work. Encourage them to think of examples to show how health care workers might apply them on the job. Allow approximately 15 minutes for this portion of the activity.
5. When groups have finished their discussions, use Transparency 18-2 to conduct a discussion of the principles. As part of the discussion, ask a representative from each group to share their conclusions and examples. Instructor sheet 18-1 contains examples of health care worker responsibilities.
6. Suggest that students make notes on their handouts.

Follow-up Discussion

1. How important do you believe it is to practice these ethical principles?
2. How might patient care be affected if health care workers did not follow ethical principles?
3. What are some examples of student behaviors that are related to the principles? (For example, cheating on a test.)

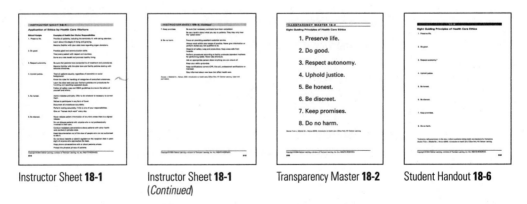

Instructor Sheet **18-1**

Instructor Sheet **18-1** (*Continued*)

Transparency Master **18-2**

Student Handout **18-6**

ACTIVITY 18-8
WHAT DO YOU THINK?

What Students Will Learn

- Many ethical and legal issues are complex and do not have easy answers.

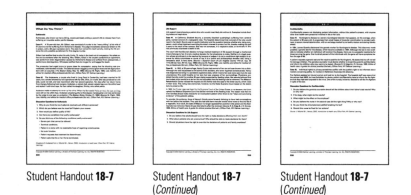

Student Handout **18-7**

Student Handout **18-7**
(*Continued*)

Student Handout **18-7**
(*Continued*)

What You Will Need

- A copy of Student Handout 18-7, What Do You Think? for each student.
- Dictionaries available for student use (some of the words in cases might be unfamiliar to students).

What To Do

1. Distribute Student Handout 18-7.
2. Allow time for students to read the cases in class or assign as homework.
3. Conduct a class discussion using the questions on the handout.

Follow-up Discussion

1. A general discussion of medical ethics that includes other current topics would be appropriate.

ACTIVITY 18-9

IT'S CONFIDENTIAL!

What Students Will Learn

- Ways to protect patient confidentiality.

What You Will Need

- Instructor Sheet 18-2, Suggested Methods for Maintaining Patient Confidentiality.

Instructor Sheet **18-2**

What To Do

1. Divide class into three groups.
2. Assign each group one of the following: computer, written, spoken.
3. Each group is to list as many ways as possible to protect confidentiality in their assigned method of communication. Allow approximately 15 minutes for this portion of the activity.
4. Ask each group to share its list with the class.
5. Ask students for additional ideas.
6. Use Instructor Sheet 18-2 for additional suggestions.
7. Collect the ideas and put together a student handout. Or, have a student in each group type on the computer, then combine into one document for copying.

Follow-up Discussion

1. Why is it critical to maintain patient confidentiality?
2. What are some possible results of breaking patient confidentiality?

ACTIVITY 18-10
WHERE DO I STAND?

What Students Will Learn

- A better understanding of where they stand on ethical issues.

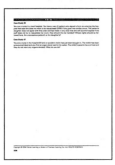

What You Will Need

- Instructor Sheet 18-3, Ethics Case Studies.

What To Do

1. Read each case study to the class.
2. Ask the students to write down what they think they would do.
3. Discuss student answers using the discussion questions following the scenarios.

Instructor Sheet **18-3**

Follow-up Discussion

1. Conduct a class discussion using the questions scenario on Instructor Sheet 18-3.

ACTIVITY 18-11
SHOW YOUR ETHICS

What Students Will Learn

- To deal with ethical situations that may arise in the medical office.

What You Will Need

- A copy of Student Handout 18-8, Skit Case Studies, for each student.

What To Do

1. Distribute Student Handout 18-8.
2. Divide class into groups of three to five students.
3. Assign a different case study from the handout to each group.
4. Have groups create skits of their assigned case study that will show how they might handle the ethical situation.

Student Handout **18-8**

Alternative activity: Use case studies for discussion instead of skits.

Follow-up Discussion

1. After each skit, discuss the situation and solution with the entire class.

Student Handout **18-8**
(*Continued*)

REFERENCES

Edge, R., & Groves, J. (1999). *Ethics of health care: A guide for clinical practice.* Clifton Park, NY: Delmar Learning.

Flight, Myrtle. (1998). *Law, liability, and ethics for medical office professionals* (3rd ed.). Clifton Park, NY: Delmar Learning.

Mitchell, J., & Haroun, L. (2002). *Introduction to health care.* Clifton Park, NY: Delmar Learning.

Application of Ethics by Health Care Workers

Ethical Principle	Examples of Health Care Worker Responsibilities
1. Preserve life.	Provide all patients, including the terminally ill, with caring attention.
	Learn about the stages of dying and grieving.
	Become familiar with your state laws regarding organ donations.
2. Do good.	Practice good oral communication skills.
	Treat every patient with respect and courtesy.
	Serve as a role model and promote healthy living.
3. Respect autonomy.	Be sure that patients have consented to all treatment and procedures.
	Become familiar with the state laws and facility policies dealing with advance directives.
4. Uphold justice.	Treat all patients equally, regardless of economic or social background.
	Know the rules for handling all categories of controlled substances.
	Learn the state laws and your facility's policies and procedures for handling and reporting suspected abuse.
	Follow all safety rules and OSHA guidelines to ensure the safety of yourself and others.
5. Be honest.	Admit mistakes promptly. Offer to do whatever is necessary to correct them.
	Refuse to participate in any form of fraud.
	Document all procedures accurately.
	Perform coding accurately, if this is one of your responsibilities.
	Give an "honest day's work" every day.
6. Be discreet.	Never release patient information of any kind unless there is a signed release.
	Do not discuss patients with *anyone* who is not professionally involved in their care.
	Conduct necessary conversations about patients with other health care workers in private areas.
	Keep documentation out of the view of people who are not authorized to see it.
	Do not leave records or patient registers on the reception desk in plain sight of anyone who approaches the desk.
	Keep phone conversations with or about patients private.
	Protect the physical privacy of patients.

7. Keep promises.

Be sure that necessary contracts have been completed.

Be very careful about what you say to patients. They may only hear the "good news."

8. Do no harm.

Focus on providing excellent customer service.

Always work within your scope of practice. Never give information or perform duties you not qualified to do.

Observe all safety rules and precautions. Keep areas safe from hazards.

Perform procedures according to facility protocols (standard methods for performing tasks). Never take shortcuts.

Ask an appropriate person about anything you are unsure of.

Keep your skills up-to-date.

Keep certifications current (CPR, first aid, professional certifications or licenses).

Stay informed about new laws that affect health care.

Source: J. Mitchell & L. Haroun, 2002, *Introduction to health care,* Clifton Park, NY: Delmar Learning. Used with permission.

Suggested Methods for Maintaining Patient Confidentiality

Computer

- Allow only authorized personnel access to computers containing patient records.
- Allow only authorized personal to enter confidential patient information.
- Do not use obvious passwords that someone else might guess.
- Clear monitor screens before leaving the work area.
- Close programs containing patient information when not in use.
- Do not allow patients or other unauthorized persons to enter the area where data entry is taking place.
- Shred discarded printouts before throwing them in the trash.
- Take care when working on a laptop in a public area to prevent others from reading the data on the screen.
- Do not leave laptops where they can be accessed by others.

Source: Adapted from J. Mitchell, & L. Haroun (2002). *Introduction to health care.* Clifton Park, NY: Delmar Learning.

Written

- Shred any documents containing patient information before throwing them in the trash.
- Do not leave patient sign-in sheets out on the reception desk where patients and others can see them.
- Do not leave medical records or charts unattended in areas such as examining rooms where other patients might see them.
- Take care with materials that seem harmless, such as appointment reminder letters with the patients' names on them.
- Secure areas, such as physician's office, when they are unoccupied.

Spoken

- Do not discuss patients in public areas where you might be overheard.
- Do not discuss patient issues with your friends and family members.
- Be discrete when speaking on the telephone so that the patient's name is not overheard.
- Take care when giving highly confidential information, such as test results, over the telephone.
- Provide patient privacy as appropriate by closing examination room doors, pulling curtains between beds, or providing a private place to hold a conversation.

Ethics Case Studies

#1. You and your best friend have returned to school. You are both single parents and have promised to support each other through the 9-month Medical Assisting program that you are taking. Your instructor has given a small assignment that must be done, but that will not have a huge impact on your grade. Your friend's baby has been sick and your friend has not had time to complete the assignment, so she asks you to copy yours. What do you do?

#2. You and your best friend have returned to school. You are both single parents and have promised to support each other through the 9-month Medical Assisting program that you are taking. Your instructor has given an assignment that must be done because it will count as 25% of your grade. Your friend's baby has been sick and your friend has not had time to complete the assignment, so she asks you to copy yours. What do you do?

#3. You and your best friend have returned to school. You are both single parents and have promised to support each other through the 9-month Medical Assisting program that you are taking. Your instructor has given a small assignment that must be done, but that will not have a huge impact on your grade. Your friend has a new boyfriend and partied so much that she has a hangover and cannot complete the assignment, so she asks you to copy yours. What do you do?

#4. Your instructor believes it is very important for you to learn about diabetes, a major health concern in the United States. He has given a research assignment to help students gain a full understanding of this disease process. Your friend put off completing the assignment until the last minute, and now has been called into work and will not have the time to do the research. He has asked you if you will share what you have found so he can write his paper during his lunch hour. Do you give him the material?

#5. Your instructor believes it is very important for you to learn about diabetes, a major health concern in the United States. She has given a research assignment to help students gain a full understanding of this disease process. Someone in the class that you are just beginning to get to know has had a very sick child and has not had time to do the necessary research for the project. He asks you if you will share your material. What do you do?

Discussion Questions

1. Did you find that the type of assignment affected your decision?

2. Did you find that the circumstances affected your decision? (Were you more likely to let your friend use your material because of the sick baby or work assignment, than if the friend couldn't do the assignment because she or he was partying?)

3. Are there circumstances when it is okay to let someone copy your work?

4. Are there circumstances when it is very wrong to let someone copy your work?

5. Could you have done anything in any of these scenarios to prevent being put in these difficult situations? (For example, help the friend take care of the sick baby so the friend can complete the assignment without copying.)

If I Were the Boss

1. Angela is friendly and helpful with patients, but does not always follow safety rules.

2. Brian's uniform is often spotted and his shoes could use a good cleaning.

3. Cassandra is a few minutes late for work at least once a week.

4. Keshia is a very efficient medical coder, but her co-workers are tired of her negative attitude.

5. Juan works efficiently when he is in the clinic, but he often returns late from lunch.

6. Jossy is unwilling to do any extra work that is not in her job description, even when it is at her skill level.

7. Sanjay is so shy he does not always communicate effectively.

8. Jason does not always put equipment back where it belongs, so his co-workers spend time looking around for things when they need them.

Group Discussion Questions

- How would you handle each of these employees?

- How might their actions affect their co-workers?

- How might their actions affect their patients?

- What would you tell them?

- How might you help them improve?

If I Were the Patient

1. You are elderly and hard of hearing. You do not understand what part of your treatment expenses will be covered by Medicare.

2. You are 11 years old and broke your arm while riding your new scooter.

3. You are a 52-year-old career woman and have just been told you have breast cancer.

4. You are a mother whose child has a painful earache. You are trying to make an appointment to see the pediatrician as soon as possible.

5. You are a young woman expecting your first child. You speak very little English and are having trouble explaining that you think you are in labor.

6. You are 4 years old and are having your teeth cleaned by a hygienist for the first time.

7. You have been sent to the lab to have your blood drawn. You are both terrified of the procedure and embarrassed because you think you are too old to have such fears.

8. You are in the emergency room of the hospital closest to your home because you cut your finger badly. You have no health insurance and did not know where else to go.

Group Discussion Questions

• How might you feel if you were the patient in these situations?

• How would you want to be treated by health care workers?

• What do you think are the most important characteristics of health care workers from the patient's point of view?

Oral Presentation Guidelines

As a group, prepare a presentation for the class that includes the following:

- The purpose of the law.

- Who the law protects.

- Which organizations are affected by the law.

- Which government agency oversees enforcement of the law.

- Examples of how the law is applied.

- Where to get more information.

Sexual Harassment Questionnaire

Sexual harassment is a problem in many workplaces. Test your knowledge of the facts about harassing behaviors by answering the following questions.

1. Studies have shown that between _____ and _____ % of women have experienced sexual harassment in the workplace.

	Agree	Disagree
2. Only young and attractive women are harassed.	☐	☐
3. Men are the only ones who do the harassing.	☐	☐
4. Bosses are the only ones who have the power to sexually harass.	☐	☐
5. The way a woman dresses influences whether or not she is harassed.	☐	☐
6. Sexual harassment is only a problem between two individuals.	☐	☐
7. We have laws to protect people against sexual harassment.	☐	☐
8. Ignoring sexual comments and advances is the best way to handle them.	☐	☐

Source: Adapted from M. Flight (1998). *Law, liability, and ethics for medical office professionals* (3rd ed.). Clifton Park, NY: Delmar Learning.

Facts About Sexual Harassment

- Between 40 and 70% of women and between 10 and 20% of men report being sexually harassed in the workplace.

- The harasser's conduct must be unwelcome.

- The victim as well as the harasser may be a woman or a man. Victims are not necessarily young, attractive, or even female.

- The harasser can be the victim's supervisor, someone who represents the employer, a supervisor in another area, a co-worker, or a nonemployee.

- The victim does not have to be the person harassed but could be anyone affected by the offensive conduct.

- Sexual harassment is a form of sex discrimination that violates Title VII of the Civil Rights Act of 1964.

- It is helpful for the victim to directly inform the harasser that the conduct is unwelcome and must stop.

- If the behavior does not stop, the victim should use the employer's complaint process or grievance system.

Eight Guiding Principles of Health Care Ethics

1. Preserve life.

2. Do good.

3. Respect autonomy.*

4. Uphold justice.

5. Be honest.

6. Be discreet.

7. Keep promises.

8. Do no harm.

*Autonomy: self-government; in this case, it refers to patients making health care decisions for themselves.
Source: From J. Mitchell & L. Haroun (2002). *Introduction to health care.* Clifton Park, NY: Delmar Learning.

What Do You Think?

Euthanasia

Euthanasia, also known as mercy killing, means painlessly ending a person's life to release them from suffering an incurable and/or painful disease.

Case #1.   A 75-year-old man, Mr. Gilbert, was convicted of murder in the "mercy killing" of his wife of 51 years to end her suffering from Alzheimer's disease. The judge immediately sentenced Gilbert to life in prison, with a 25 year mandatory term. The state had waived the death penalty, making the life sentence the only possible punishment for first-degree murder.

Gilbert had testified that he shot his wife, Emily, 73, twice in the head out of compassion. He called police and surrendered after the shooting. Mrs. Gilbert, killed in the couple's condominium apartment, was senile from brain degeneration caused by Alzheimer's disease and suffered from osteoporosis, a painful bone disintegration. Witnesses testified that she longed for and begged for death.

The prosecutor had urged jurors to ignore pleas for compassion, saying that the shooting was premeditated, cold-blooded murder. The defense lawyer begged jurors to ignore laws and set legal precedent with an acquittal. [*The Boston Globe*, May 10, 1985] (*Source:* M. Flight, 1998, *Law, liability, and ethics for medical office professionals* (3rd ed.), Clifton Park, NY: Delmar Learning.)

Case #2.   The Andersons, a couple who lived in Long Pond in Centerville, had been married for 52 years, but a stroke followed by two operations left the wife, Olive, an invalid. She was paralyzed on one side, could not talk, and was incontinent after her second operation. Ten days after her return home from therapy following brain surgery, Anderson, a retired chef, placed a plastic bag over his wife's head and sealed it with duct tape. He then called his daughter, Shirley, who called police.

Anderson made no attempt to cover up his crime. When the Barnstable Police arrived, the tape and bag were still on his wife's face. Anderson pleaded guilty to first-degree manslaughter and was sentenced by the judge to one year on probation. [*The Boston Globe*, October 31, 1985] (*Source:* M. Flight, 1998, *Law, liability, and ethics for medical office professionals* (3rd ed.), Clifton Park, NY: Delmar Learning.)

Discussion Questions for Euthanasia

1. Why do you think the two husbands received such different sentences?

2. Which do you believe was the most fair? Explain your answer.

3. How would you define quality of life?

4. Are there any conditions that justify euthanasia?

5. Do you think any of the following conditions justify euthanasia?

   • Severe pain that cannot be relieved.

   • Terminal conditions.

   • Patient in a coma with no reasonable hope of regaining consciousness.

   • No brain function.

   • Patient requests that treatment be discontinued.

   • Patient asks that his or her life be terminated.

(Questions 2–5 adapted from J. Mitchell & L. Haroun, 2002, *Introduction to health care.* Clifton Park, NY: Delmar Learning.)

Life Support

Life support means keeping a patient alive who would most likely die without it. Examples include feeding tubes and respirators.

Case #1. In California, Elizabeth Bouvia, a severely disabled quadriplegic suffering from cerebral palsy, wanted removal of a nasogastric tube. The hospital determined that removal of the tube would result in her death. Bouvia was in a public institution and the question became whether she, being competent, could refuse treatment overriding the state's interest to protect her life, thereby making the staff a party to the result of her conduct. She was not comatose, in a vegetative state, or terminally ill. She had previously expressed a desire to die.

The court held that Bouvia's decision to forgo medical treatment of life support through a mechanical means belongs to her. It is not a medical decision for her physicians to make. Neither is it a legal question whose soundness is to be resolved by lawyers or judges. It is not a conditional right subject to approval by ethics committees or courts of law. It is a moral and philosophical decision that, being a competent adult, is hers alone. [*Bouvia v. Superior Court of Los Angeles County* 179 Cal. App. 3d 1172,225 Cal. Rptr. 297 (Ct. App. 1986)] (*Source:* M. Flight, 1998, *Law, liability, and ethics for medical office professionals* (3rd ed.), Clifton Park, NY: Delmar Learning.)

Case #2. In 1983, at 25 years of age, Nancy Cruzan lost control of her car and was thrown into a ditch. Although she was resuscitated at the scene of the accident, she never regained consciousness. Nancy was diagnosed as being in a persistent vegetative state, which means her eyes were open but she was unconscious. She could breathe on her own but was unaware of her surroundings. Physicians predicted that she could live another 30 years being supported by feeding tubes. Her parents believed that the kindest action would be to let her die and requested that the feeding tube be removed. The Missouri Rehabilitation Center refused the request and the family took the case to the lower courts, which ruled in their favor. This ruling was overturned, however, by the State Supreme Court based on the state's duty to preserve life.

In 1989, the Cruzan case was heard by the Supreme Court of the United States. In its decision, the Court upheld the Missouri Supreme Court that denied removal of the feeding tube. The reason was that not even families should make choices for an incompetent patient when there is not "clear and convincing evidence" of the patient's wishes.

To provide this evidence, three of Nancy's friends came forward claiming to have had conversations with her before the accident. They said she had told them that she would never want to live the life of a vegetable. As a result, the state of Missouri no longer opposed her parents in this action and the feeding tube was removed. Nancy Cruzan died shortly after the removal. (*Source:* R. S. Edge & J. R. Groves, 1999, *Ethics of health care: A guide for clinical practice* (2nd ed.), Clifton Park, NY: Delmar Learning.)

Discussion Questions for Life Support

1. Do you believe that adults should have the right to make decisions affecting their own death?

2. What about patients who are unconscious? Who should be able to make decisions for them?

3. Should physicians have the right to override the decisions of patients and family members?

Confidentiality

Confidentiality means not disclosing patient information, without the patient's consent, with anyone other than health care personnel involved in his or her care.

Case #1.   Huntington's disease is a severe neurological disorder that appears, on the average, when the patient is 36 years old. It progresses from small losses of muscular coordination to constant jerkiness, to severe mental deterioration, with an end stage marked by no bodily motion and staring blankly ahead.

In 1984, James Gusella discovered the genetic marker for Huntington's disease. This discovery made possible a genetic test for the disease, which became available in 1994. Although the test is now available to indicate whether an individual will contract the disease, there are no successful treatments for those carrying the gene. One hundred percent of the individuals with the gene will have symptoms before the age of 65.

A patient requests a genetic test and the result is positive for Huntington's. He states that he will not tell his teenage children. The genetics counselor must decide whether to break the parent's confidentiality and inform the children who may want to be tested. (*Source:* R. S. Edge & J. R. Groves, 1999, *Ethics of health care: A guide for clinical practice* (2nd ed.), Clifton Park, NY: Delmar Learning.)

Case #2.   Individual rights to privacy sometimes conflict with the public's right to be informed about matters concerning safety. An incident in Baltimore illustrates this dilemma.

Fire fighters assisted an injured woman and took her to the hospital. The hospital staff was aware that the woman had AIDS, but was forbidden by doctor–patient confidentiality laws to inform the fire fighters that they had been exposed to the virus. One of the nurses, however, decided to tell the fire fighters in spite of the law.

Discussion Questions for Confidentiality

1. Do you believe the genetics counselor should tell the children about their father's test results? Why or why not?

2. If he does, what might be the results?

3. What might be the effect on his employer?

4. Do you believe the nurse in the second case did the right thing? Why or why not?

5. Do you think the circumstances justified breaking the law?

6. Should this nurse be fired for her actions?

Source: J. Mitchell & L. Haroun, 2002, *Introduction to health care,* Clifton Park, NY: Delmar Learning.

Skit Case Studies

Case Study #1

You work for an ophthalmologist who has just completed a second cataract surgery on a 28-year-old Asian woman. This woman came to the office with cataracts in both eyes. It is unusual for a 28-year-old to have cataracts in both eyes, so during the initial history, the physician questioned the woman thoroughly regarding what type of work she did in her native country, genetic background, exposure to chemicals, and any other indication for bilateral cataracts. No significant history was found. The woman had surgery on her right eye and had a minor post-op complication of scleral hemorrhage. One week after surgery on her left eye, the woman again presented with the minor complication of scleral hemorrhage. Since this is so unusual, the doctor began to question the woman and she tearfully admitted that her husband is physically abusive and banged her head against a wall. At the time of the exam, her husband and three small children are sitting in the waiting room. How should the medical staff handle this situation?

Case Study #2

You work for a family practice physician. The Smith family has had the same physician for many years and the doctor and staff know all of the family members very well. Tamara Smith, the family's 15-year-old daughter has come to the doctor for contraceptives because she has a new boyfriend and wants to become sexually active. You are good friends with Tamara's mom and feel as if Tamara is your own daughter. Tamara's mom finds an appointment card on her daughter's dresser and, because she is worried, calls the office to verify the appointment. How do you handle the call?

Case Study #3

Mrs. Wolinski has been brought to the office by her daughter, who waits in the waiting room while Mrs. Wolinski is being seen for her history of heart disease. While taking her history and chief complaint, Mrs. Wolinski, who seems a little confused, complains that her family is mean to her. You notice that Mrs. Wolinski has a bruise on her upper arm as if someone has grabbed her and left a fingerprint. What do you do?

Case Study #4

You work for a family practice physician. The Smith family has had the same physician for many years and the doctor and staff know all of the family members very well. Tamara Smith, the family's 15-year-old daughter has come to the doctor for a pregnancy test, which is positive. Tamara would like to have an abortion and does not want either of her parents to know. You are good friends with Tamara's mom and feel as if Tamara is your own daughter. You don't really believe in abortion, though the doctor you work for does refer patients to the local Ob-Gyn for termination of pregnancy if the patient requests it. Do you try to talk Tamara out of the abortion? Do you talk to Tamara's mom?

Case Study #5

The office you work for has a 54-year-old patient who has a degenerative disease that is slowly shutting down his body. He can no longer use his arms or legs, cannot speak, has difficulty swallowing, and has lost bladder and bowel control. The patient is not expected to live more than a year. He has been having difficulty breathing, and, because he can't speak, has difficulty communicating. He does manage to get across to you and the doctor that he would like to have a prescription for enough pills to commit suicide. How should this be handled? Do you think some physicians quietly help their terminally ill patients die? Do patients have a right to make this decision for themselves?

Case Study #6

You are a nurse in a local hospital. You have a very ill patient who signed a form on entering the hospital that says she does not want to be resuscitated (DNR) if she goes into cardiac arrest. The patient's daughter does not agree with this order and has made it very clear that she will sue the hospital if the staff does not try to resuscitate her mom. How should this be handled? Whose rights should be followed here, the unconscious patient's or the daughter's?

Case Study #7

You are a nurse in the hospital ER and an accident victim has just been brought in. The victim has been pronounced dead and you find an organ donor card in his wallet. The victim's parents have arrived and they do not want any organs donated. What do you do?

Facts About Sexual Harassment

1. *Studies have shown that between 40 and 70% of women report being sexually harassed in the workplace. (And between 10 and 20% of men.)*

2. Only young and attractive women are harassed.
   False. Victims are not necessarily young, attractive, or even female.

3. Men are the only ones who do the harassing.
   False. Although few in numbers, females also engage in sexual harassment.

4. Bosses are the only ones who have the power to sexually harass.
   False. Harassers can be supervisors, but they also can be anyone who represents the employer, a co-worker, or a nonemployee.

5. The way a woman dresses influences whether or not she is harassed.
   False. The victim should never be blamed.

6. Sexual harassment is only a problem between two individuals.
   False. Improper behavior, such as telling off-color jokes, may be considered harassment of more than one individual.

7. We have laws to protect people against sexual harassment.
   True. Sexual harassment is a form of sex discrimination that violates Title VII of the Civil Rights Act of 1964.

8. Ignoring sexual comments and advances is the best way to handle them.
   False. The victim should directly tell the harasser that the comments and/or advances are unwelcome and that they should stop immediately.

Source: Adapted from M. Flight (1998). *Law, liability, and ethics for medical office professionals* (3rd ed.) Clifton Park, NY: Delmar Learning.

Eight Guiding Principles of Health Care Ethics

1. Preserve life.

2. Do good.

3. Respect autonomy.

4. Uphold justice.

5. Be honest.

6. Be discreet.

7. Keep promises.

8. Do no harm.

Source: From J. Mitchell & L. Haroun (2002). *Introduction to health care.* Clifton Park, NY: Delmar Learning.